INSIGHTS INTO INFERTILITY MANAGEMENT

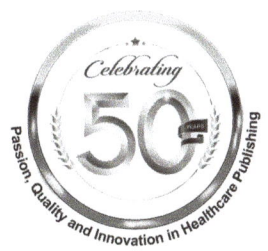

INSIGHTS INTO INFERTILITY MANAGEMENT

Editor

K Jayakrishnan DGO MD DNB
Managing Director
Chief Consultant in Reproductive Medicine
KJK Hospital, Fertility Research and Gynecology Center
Nalanchira
KJK Fertility and Well Woman Center, Vazhuthacud
Thiruvananthapuram, Kerala, India

Foreword

M Subhadra Nair

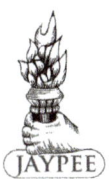

JAYPEE BROTHERS MEDICAL PUBLISHERS
The Health Sciences Publisher
New Delhi | London | Panama

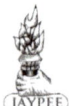 **Jaypee Brothers Medical Publishers (P) Ltd**

Headquarters
Jaypee Brothers Medical Publishers (P) Ltd
4838/24, Ansari Road, Daryaganj
New Delhi 110 002, India
Phone: +91-11-43574357
Fax: +91-11-43574314
Email: jaypee@jaypeebrothers.com

Overseas Offices

J.P. Medical Ltd
83 Victoria Street, London
SW1H 0HW (UK)
Phone: +44 20 3170 8910
Fax: +44 (0)20 3008 6180
Email: info@jpmedpub.com

Jaypee-Highlights Medical Publishers Inc
City of Knowledge, Bld. 235, 2nd Floor
Clayton, Panama City, Panama
Phone: +1 507-301-0496
Fax: +1 507-301-0499
Email: cservice@jphmedical.com

Jaypee Brothers Medical Publishers (P) Ltd
Bhotahity, Kathmandu, Nepal
Phone: +977-9741283608
Email: kathmandu@jaypeebrothers.com

Website: www.jaypeebrothers.com
Website: www.jaypeedigital.com

© 2019, Jaypee Brothers Medical Publishers

The views and opinions expressed in this book are solely those of the original contributor(s)/author(s) and do not necessarily represent those of editor(s) of the book.

All rights reserved. No part of this publication may be reproduced, stored or transmitted in any form or by any means, electronic, mechanical, photocopying, recording or otherwise, without the prior permission in writing of the publishers.

All brand names and product names used in this book are trade names, service marks, trademarks or registered trademarks of their respective owners. The publisher is not associated with any product or vendor mentioned in this book.

Medical knowledge and practice change constantly. This book is designed to provide accurate, authoritative information about the subject matter in question. However, readers are advised to check the most current information available on procedures included and check information from the manufacturer of each product to be administered, to verify the recommended dose, formula, method and duration of administration, adverse effects and contraindications. It is the responsibility of the practitioner to take all appropriate safety precautions. Neither the publisher nor the author(s)/editor(s) assume any liability for any injury and/or damage to persons or property arising from or related to use of material in this book.

This book is sold on the understanding that the publisher is not engaged in providing professional medical services. If such advice or services are required, the services of a competent medical professional should be sought.

Every effort has been made where necessary to contact holders of copyright to obtain permission to reproduce copyright material. If any have been inadvertently overlooked, the publisher will be pleased to make the necessary arrangements at the first opportunity. The **CD/DVD-ROM** (if any) provided in the sealed envelope with this book is complimentary and free of cost. **Not meant for sale.**

Inquiries for bulk sales may be solicited at: jaypee@jaypeebrothers.com

Insights into Infertility Management

First Edition: 2012

Second Edition: **2019**

ISBN: 978-93-5270-597-9

Dedicated to
Dr Thomas Chandy who inspired me to take this specialty
Dr Subhadra Nair who motivated me to choose this subspecialty
Dr K Radhakumari who moulded me into a Reproductive Medicine Specialist
Radha K Pillai, my mother whose determination, strength and
passion gave me the courage to pursue my dreams
and
Lekha, Niranjana and Ashwin for making this journey worthwhile.

Contributors

Abhimanyu Sinde

Aby K Koshy
Consultant in Reproductive Medicine and Gynecology
Sunrise Hospital
Kochi, Kerala, India

Alexander Quaas

Ameet Patki
Medical Director ReGenesis
Reliance Life Sciences
Mumbai, Maharashtra, India

Arati Gupte-Shah
Consultant
Pulse Women's Hospital, Ahmedabad and Gupte Hospital and Center for Research in Reproduction
Pune, Maharashtra, India

Ava Desai
Cancer Institute
Ahmedabad, Gujarat, India

Christian De Geyter
Women's Hospital
University of Basel, Switzerland

Gabriella Garruti
Assistant Professor
Department at Endocrinology
University of Bari, Italy

HJA Carp
Professor
Department of Obstetrics and Gynecology
Sheba Medical Center
Tel Hashomer and University of Tel Aviv
Israel

Judith Menezes
Fertilitetscentrum Stockholm
Sweden

Katharina Rüther-Wolf

K Jayakrishnan
Managing Director
Chief Consultant in Reproductive Medicine
KJK Hospital, Fertility Research and Gynecology Center, Nalanchira
KJK Fertility and Well Woman Center
Vazhuthacud
Thiruvananthapuram, Kerala, India

Madhupriya
Associate Consultant
Apollo Hospitals Chennai, Tamil Nadu, India

Madhuri Patil
Consultant
Dr Patil's Fertility and Endoscopy Clinic
Bengaluru, Karnataka, India

Majumdar Abha
Director
Center of IVF and Human Reproduction
Department of Obstetrics and Gynecology
Sir Ganga Ram Hospital
New Delhi, India

Manish Banker
Director
Pulse Women's Hospital and Melbourne IVF
Ahmedabad, Gujarat, India

Maria De Geyter
Women's Hospital
University of Basel, Switzerland

Mridhubashini Govindarajan
Director and Consultant
Womens Clinic, Coimbatore, Tamil Nadu, India

Niranjana Jayakrishnan
Consultant in Reproductive Medicine
KJK Hospital, Fertility Research
and Gynocology Center
Thiruvananthapuram, Kerala, India

Padmini Raviraj
Clinical Director
Department of Obstetrics and Gynecology
Liverpool Hospital
Sydney South West Area Health Service, Australia

Pankaj Desai
Associate Professor
Department of Obstetrics and Gynecology
Medical College
SSG Hospital and
Baroda, Gujarat, India

Partha Guha Roy
Senior Consultant
Fertility Clinic and IVF Center
Mumbai, Maharashtra, India

Peter Sjoblom
Nurture Fertility
University of Nottingham
Nottingham, United Kingdom

Pratap Kumar
Professor and Head
Department of Obstetrics and Gynecology
Kasturba Medical College and Hospital
Manipal, Karnataka, India

Praveena Pai

Pravin Patel
Director
Pulse Women's Hospital and Melbourne IVF
Ahmedabad, Gujarat, India

Raffaella Depalo
Unit of Pathophysiology of Human Reproduction and Gametes Cryopreservation
Department of Gynecology, Obstetrics and Neonatology
University of Bari "Aldo Moro", Italy

Rajat Gyaneshwar
Clinical Director
Department of Obstetrics and Gynecology
Liverpool Hospital
Sydney South West Area
Health Service, Australia

Ramya Jayaram

Ranjana Mangoli
Laboratory Director
Fertility Clinic and IVF Center
Mumbai, Maharashtra, India

Rohit V Bhatt
Chief, Department of Obstetrics and Gynecology
Bhailal Amin General Hospital
Baroda, Gujarat, India

Sadhana Desai
Director, Fertility Clinic and IVF Center
Mumbai
Emeritus Professor
Department of Obstetrics and Gynecology
Bombay Hospital Institute of Medical Sciences
Mumbai, Maharashtra, India

Sameer Dixit
Hon. Sonologist
Nowrosjee Wadia Maternity Hospital
Mumbai, Maharashtra, India

Sarat Battina
Senior Consultant and Head
Department of Obstetrics, Gynecology and Reproductive Medicine
Apollo Hospitals
Chennai, Tamil Nadu, India

Silvia de Stefani

Simone Palini

Singh Tejshree A
Consultant Infertility Unit
Department of Obstetrics and Gynecology
Kolmet Hospital and Research Center
New Delhi, India

Sonia Golani

Suresh Kattera
IVF Scientific Consultant
Singapore

Vijay Mangoli
Laboratory Director
Fertility Clinic and IVF Center
Mumbai, Maharashtra, India

Foreword

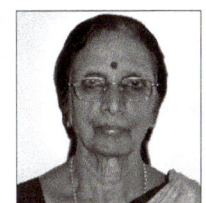

I am delighted to write the foreword for the second edition of *Insights into Infertility Management*. The first edition of the book was well received. Now six years later, Dr Jayakrishnan and his able editorial staff have carefully updated this book, with the same multidisciplinary approach that has been the hallmark of success of the first edition.

Newer concepts, innovations and technology have practically revolutionized the decision-making and management of various gynecological problems relating to infertility. With the explosion of information flooding the field, it became easier for an average clinician to keep pace with the advances and changes that are needed from time to time; since modern health care demands clinicians a practice of evidence-based medicine.

The consumers are also better informed and demand the latest information on the diagnosis of their problem. Moreover, rapid progress in Assisted Reproduction Technology (ART) has identified treatable causes of infertility; thus, more people have been able to achieve a successful pregnancy. Pregnancy wastage is also reduced by preimplantation genetic diagnosis that enables the birth of a genetically normal baby.

For a busy clinician, the access to clinically relevant information should be useful and readily accessible. This is exactly where the book *Insights into infertility Management* by Dr Jayakrishnan steps in.

Starting from the role of semen analysis in the investigation for infertility, it goes on to anovulation and induction of ovulation, to polycystic ovarian disease, to hyperprolactinemia in infertility, and to unexplained infertility. It goes on to setting up of an ART clinic, intrauterine insemination (IUI), methods of enhancing the IUI success rates. It explores the laboratory set-up for *in vitro* fertilization (IVF) and intracytoplasmic sperm injection (ICSI) and embryo culture, discusses the current scenario of IVF and ICSI, selection of human oocytes, and finally, it ends up by telling us when to stop infertility treatment with a few facts about the ART bill and its implications, which all of us have to be aware of.

I congratulate Dr Jayakrishnan and all the contributors who have generously contributed to the book *Insights into Infertility Management* which will be of immense benefit to all gynecologists and postgraduate students of gynecology.

I thank Dr Jayakrishnan for the privilege he has given me, by asking me to be the one to write the foreword for his marvellous work. I wish the second edition of this book, all success.

M Subhadra Nair
Senior Consultant, Obstetrician and Gynecologist
Cosmopolitan Hospital, Thiruvananthapuram
Formerly, Director and Professor
Obstetrics and Gynecology Medical College
Thiruvananthapuram, Kerala, India

Preface

Reproductive medicine is an evolving specialty with new advances made every day. When I set out to write this book, my aim was to give a comprehensive coverage of all aspects of infertility that was relevant in day-to-day practice. Most books I felt were either too concise or too elaborative; so, it was necessary to strike a balance between the two. Thus was born the idea of writing what I felt, was most relevant.

The first edition of *Insights into Infertility Management* was extremely successful and well received. In the second edition, my editorial staff and I, have kept the same concise format in order to remain a practical quick reference guide. Yet we have also added new content and features based on the valuable feedback from readers. All chapters have been revised and include the latest studies and techniques. Newer chapters have also been included.

We have again strived to maintain a balance of including the most important information for practitioners, while also limiting the size of the book so that it did not become a full-fledged textbook.

It is important that even as we practice, we follow evidence-based medicine, and I for one have been a firm believer in it. Most chapters in this book are based on the latest evidence and concepts. Each chapter has been written in a way that is lucid and at the same time tells all that we need to know while dealing with our patients. For every practitioner who wishes to practice reproductive medicine, this book serves as a primer. For the established practitioner, it acts as a refresher and a quick reference. For the postgraduate with interest in infertility, it simplifies things and answers all queries.

We are grateful to all the contributing authors, including multiple new ones, for their hard work and dedication. I believe that *Insights into Infertility Management*, will continue to be an invaluable resource for students, residents, fellows and other practitioners of Infertility and Reproductive Medicine.

K Jayakrishnan

Acknowledgments

First and Foremost, I would like to thank the God. In the process of putting this book together I realized how true this gift of writing is for me. You have given me the power to believe in my passion and pursue my dreams. I could have never done this without the faith I have in you, the Almighty.

To my mother, Radha K Pillai, who is no longer with me. Thank you for your unconditional love, support and wisdom.

I would like to express my gratitude to many people who saw me through the second edition of this book. To all those who provided support, talked things over, read, wrote, offered comments, assisted in the editing, proof reading and design.

This book is a culmination of my desire to demystify reproductive medicine, making it simple and understandable for both the generalists and the specialists.

I would not have been able to achieve this dream, without my colleagues, who have contributed to various segments of this book. I am deeply indebted to them for their useful inputs and kind contributions, despite their busy work schedule.

I am thankful to, Dr M Subhadra Nair, my teacher, for having been kind enough to write the foreword to the second edition of the book. Having been the one who initiated me into this specialty, this foreword holds a special place in my heart.

My gratitude to Mr PV Nair, Manager and Mr Sanal Kumar, Laboratory-in-Charge, KJK Hospital, Nalanchira, Thiruvananthapuram, Kerala, India, for overseeing the smooth functioning of the hospital; so that I could devote my time towards this book.

Above all, I want to thank my wife, Lekha and the rest of my family, who supported me and encouraged me in spite of all the time it took me away from them. It was a long and difficult journey for them.

Last but not least, I beg forgiveness of all those who have been with me over the course of the years and whose names I have failed to mention.

Contents

Chapter 1 Is the Prevalence of Infertility Increasing? 1
Rajat Gyaneshwar, Padmini Raviraj

• How Common is Infertility? 2 • Is Infertility Becoming more Common? 2 • Infertility and Sexually Transmitted Infections 4 • Infertility and Aging 4 • Infertility and Stress 5

Chapter 2 Female Reproductive Endocrinology: An Insight 7
Aby K Koshy

• Embryology and Development 7 • Functional Components 9 • Hormones 9 • Hypothalamic-pituitary-ovarian Axis 11 • Two-cell, Two-gonadotropin Hypotheses 12 • Menstrual Cycle 12 • Follicular (Proliferative) Phase 13 • Ovulation 13 • Luteal (Secretory) Phase 14 • Other Changes 14 • Menopause 15

Chapter 3 Male Infertility: Evaluation and Management 17
K Jayakrishnan, Aby K Koshy

• Physiology 17 • Semen and its Analysis 18 • Sperm Function Tests 19 • History-taking and Examination 19 • Treatment 21 • Medical Management 21 • Surgical Management 22 • Intrauterine Insemination 22 • Donor Insemination 23 • Assisted Reproductive Technologies 23 • Azoospermia 24 • Level of Evidence 25 • Information Resources 25

Chapter 4 Recurrent Pregnancy Losses in Assisted Reproduction 28
HJA Carp

• Causes of Recurrent Pregnancy Loss and Infertility 28 • Abnormal Embryo 28 • Antiphospholipid Syndrome 29 • Alloimmune Factors 30 • Prognosis 31 • Investigation Protocol 31 • Treatment 32 • Progesterone Supplementation 32 • hCG Supplementation 32 • Aspirin 33 • Heparin 33 • Immunoglobulin 34 • Assisted Reproductive Technology as Treatment of Recurrent Pregnancy Loss 34 • Pregestational Screening 34 • Gamete Donation 35 • Surrogacy 35

Chapter 5 Evaluation of Fertilizing Ability and DNA Damage in Spermatozoa ... 37
Suresh Kattera

• Functional Tests 38 • Hamster Penetration Test 38 • Assessment of Acrosome Reaction 38 • Sperm Morphology Assessment using Kruger's Strict Criteria 38 • Assessment of Motility and Sperm Survival Test 39 • Computer Assisted Semen Analyzer 39 • Newer Sperm Function Tests 39 • Recent Technological Advances 40

Chapter 6 The Role of Semen Analysis in the Investigation of Infertility 43
Peter Sjoblom

• Semen Analysis 44 • Semen Analysis Variables and their Physiological Significance 44 • Semen Volume 44 • Sperm Count 45 • Sperm Motility 46 • Morphology 46 • Antisperm Antibodies 47 • Postwash Motile Sperm Count 47 • Inflammatory Cells 47 • Sperm DNA Integrity Tests 47 • Diagnostic Use of Semen Analysis: Threshold Values 48

Chapter 7	Optimizing Ovulation Induction: Back to Basics................... 51

Niranjana Jayakrishnan, K Jayakrishnan

- Excess Body Weight   52   • Clomiphene Citrate   52
- Dosage   52   • Complications   54
- Metformin   54   • Dosage   55   • Thiazolidinediones   56   • Aromatase Inhibitors   56   • Letrozole   57   • AI and Unexplained Infertility   58   • AI and Endometriosis   58   • Safety of Aromatase Inhibitors   59   • Gonadotropins   59

Chapter 8	Polycystic Ovarian Syndrome: Diagnosis, Management and Recent Advances... 63

Praveena Pai, Pratap Kumar

- Pathophysiology   63   • Clinical Features and Diagnosis   64   • Diagnosis of PCOS in Adolescence   66   • Management   66   • Menstrual Irregularity   66   • Hyperandrogenism   66   • Metabolic Syndrome   67   • Subfertility   67

Chapter 9	Ovarian Hyperstimulation Syndrome: Newer Concepts 71

Ameet Patki, Abhimanyu Shinde

- Early and Late Forms of OHSS   71   • Classification of OHSS   71   • Risk Factors Associated with OHSS   72   • Pathophysiology   72   • Management of OHSS   72   • Prevention   74   • Primary Prevention   74   • Secondary Prevention   75   • OHSS and Pregnancy   76

Chapter 10	GnRH Agonist Versus GnRH Antagonist in *In Vitro* Fertilization and Embryo Transfer.................................. 78

Raffaella Depalo, Gabriella Garruti

- Gonadotropin-releasing Hormone Analogs   78   • Treatment Regimens with GnRH Agonist   79   • GnRH Agonist: Long versus Short and Ultrashort Protocol   80   • GnRh Agonists: Low and Long Acting Doses   81   • Treatment Regimens with GnRH Antagonist   81   • Single versus Multiple Dose GnRH Antagonist Protocol   81   • Fixed versus Flexible Antagonist Administration   81   • Dose of Exogenous FSH in GnRH Antagonist Cotreatment Cycles   82   • LH Supplementation in GnRH Antagonist Cotreatment Cycles   82   • Oral Contraceptive Pill Pretreatment in Ovarian Stimulation with GnRH Antagonists   83   • GnRH Antagonist in IUI Cycles   83   • Long Acting Gonadotropins   83   • GnRH Agonist versus GnRH Antagonist Regimens   84   • GnRH Antagonist versus GnRH Agonist in Poor Ovarian Responders   85   • GnRH Agonist Trigger for Final Oocyte Maturation   85

Chapter 11	Hyperprolactinemia and Infertility............................. 91

Mirudhubashini Govindarajan, Ramya Jayaram

- Prolactin Gene and Structure   92   • Prolactin Variants   92   • Lactotrophs   92   • Extrapituitary Prolactin   92   • Prolactin Receptor   92   • Regulation of Prolactin Secretion   93   • Functions of Prolactin   93   • Mammary Gland Development and Lactation   93   • Other Reproductive Functions   93   • Nonreproductive Functions   94   • Prolactin Secretion and Assays   94   • Hyperprolactinemia   95   • Macroprolactinemia (Big-Big Prolactin)   96   • Prolactin-Secreting Adenomas   97   • Treatment of Hyperprolactinemia   97   • Prolactin-secreting Adenoma   97   • Clinical Features   98   • Galactorrhea   98   • Hypogonadism and Menstrual Cycle Dysfunction   98   • Treatment Strategies   99   • Observation   99   • Oral Contraceptives for Hypogonadism   99   • Medical Therapy   99   • Time Course of Clinical Response   101   • Definition of Dopamine Agonist Resistance   101   • Dopamine Agonist Withdrawal   101   • Surgery   102   • Radiotherapy   102   • Management of Prolactinomas in Pregnant Women   103   • Microprolactinoma Treatment in Pregnancy   103   • Macroprolactinoma in Pregnancy   104   • Hyperprolactinemia in Men   104   • Prolactinomas in Multiple Endocrine Neoplasia   106   • Giant Prolactinomas   106   • Malignant Prolactinomas   106

Contents **xvii**

Chapter 12 **Poor Responder in Ovulation Induction: Management Options** 108
Sadhana Desai, Partha Guha Roy

• Cause of Decrease Ovarian Reserve 108 • Poor Responders: Definition 108 • Prediction of Ovarian Response 109 • Various Protocols 110 • Precycle Adjuvants 110 • Adjuvants at the Initiation of the Cycle 112 • Gonadotropins 114 • Corifollitropin Alpha 116 • Other Approach 116

Chapter 13 **Laparoscopic Treatment of Endometriosis Focusing on Fertility Outcomes** 122
K Jayakrishnan

• Diagnosis of Endometriosis 123 • Newer Classifications for Endometriosis 123 • Treatment 124 • Preoperative and Postoperative Ovarian Suppression 124 • Surgery 124 • Deep Infiltrating Endometriosis 126 • Ovarian Endometrioma and Assisted Reproduction Technique 127 • General Principles of Management of Endometriosis 129

Chapter 14 **Congenital Malformations of Uterus and Reproduction** 131
Pankaj Desai, Sameer Dixit

• Embryology of the Female Genital Tract 132 • Genetics of Müllerian Abnormalities 132 • Techniques to Assess the Female Genital Tract 133 • History 133 • Clinical Examination 133 • Hysterosalpingography 133 • Standard Sonography 133 • Saline Infusion Sonography 134 • Three Dimensional Sonography 134 • Laparoscopy 135 • Congenital Malformations of the Uterus 139 • Class I: Agenesis or Hypoplasia—Segmental or Complete 139 • Class II: Unicornuate Uterus with or without Rudimentary Horn 139 • Class III: Didelphys Uterus 140 • Class IV:-Bicornuate Uterus—Complete or Partial 141 • Class V: Septate Uterus—Complete or Partial 140 • Class VI: Arcuate Uterus 141 • Class VII: DES Related Abnormalities 141 • Defects not Classified by the AFS 141 • Management 142 • Müllerian Aplasia 142 • Creation of Neovagina 142 • Fertility Treatment 143 • Unicornuate Uterus 143 • Uterus Didelphys 143 • Bicornuate Uterus 143 • Septate Uterus 143

Chapter 15 **Medical Management of Fibroids** 146
K. Jayakrishnan, Niranjana Jayakrishnan

• Oral Contraceptive Pills 146 • Tranexamic Acid 148 • Medical Management 149 • Progesterone Receptor Agonists and Modulators 149 • Ulipristal Acetate 150 • Telapristone 150 • Progestogen-releasing Intrauterine System 150 • Gonadotropin-releasing Hormone Agonist 151 • Practice Guidelines: Ulipristal versus GnRHa 151 • Gonadotropin-releasing Hormone Antagonist 152 • Promising GnRH Antagonist (Elagolix) 152 • Somatostatin Analogs 152 • Aromatase Inhibitors 153 • Selective Estrogen Receptor Modulator 153 • Raloxifene and Tamoxifen 154 • Potential of Novel Therapies Enabled by Smart Nanocarriers 154 • Halofuginone 155

Chapter 16 **Current Treatment Options and Emerging Strategies for Fibroid Management** 158
K Jayakrishnan

• Pharmacologic Treatment Options 158 • Hysterectomy 159 • Myomectomy 159 • Myolysis and Cryomyolysis 160 • MRI-guided Focused Ultrasound Surgery 161 • Fibroid Treatment via Uterine Artery Occlusion or Embolization 162 • Uterine Artery Embolization 162 • Laparoscopic Uterine Artery Occlusion 163 • Doppler-guided Uterine Artery Occlusion 164 • Proposed Mechanism of Action of Uterine Artery Occlusion and Embolization 165

Chapter 17   Unexplained Infertility 170
Madhuri Patil

• Definition 170 • Incidence 171 • Prevalence 171 • Standard Basic Investigations 171 • RCOG Guidelines (1998) and National Guideline Clearinghouse (2000) 171 • American Society of Reproductive Medicine 172 • Medical History 172 • Physical Examination 173 • Basic Semen Analysis 173 • Supplementary (Advanced) Investigations 176 • Laparoscopy 176 • Hysteroscopy 177 • Ultrasound 177 • Endometrial Biopsy 178 • Evaluation of Cervical Score and Postcoital Test 180 • Assessment of Ovarian Reserve 180 • Specialized Clinical Tests on Semen and Sperm 181 • Zona-free Hamster Oocyte Test 181 • Hypo-osmotic Swelling Test 182 • *In Vitro* Sperm Nuclear Chromatin Decondensation Test 182 • Sperm Mitochondrial Activity Index 182 • Hemizona Binding Assay 182 • Sperm DNA Fragmentation 183 • ESHRE Task Force on Unexplained Infertility 184 • Possible Causes (Identified/Unidentified) 186 • Diagnosis 187 • Treatment 187 • Selection of Treatment Option 187 • Treatment Modalities 188 • Antibiotic Therapy 188 • Expectant Management and Lifestyle Changes 188 • Clomiphene Citrate 189 • Letrozole 190 • Gonadotropins 191 • Artificial Insemination 192 • Controlled Ovarian Hyperstimulation and Artificial Insemination 192 • Assisted Reproductive Technology 193 • Oil Soluble HSG 194 • Comparison of Different Treatments for Unexplained Infertility 194 • NICE Guidelines: Unexplained Infertility 194

Chapter 18   Intrauterine Insemination: At a Glance 202
Sarat Battina, Madhupriya

• Pre-intrauterine Insemination Workup 202 • Various Insemination Techniques 203 • Intravaginal Insemination 203 • Intracervical Insemination 204 • Intrafallopian Insemination 204 • Intraperitoneal Insemination 204 • Intrauterine Insemination Procedure 204 • Patient Selection for IUI 204 • Center Selection for IUI 204 • Steps Involved in Artificial Insemination (AI) Techniques 205 • Different Methods for Extraction of Sperm from Seminal Plasma 206 • Success Rates of IUI 207 • Complications of IUI 208 • RCOG Guidelines on OHSS 208 • Artificial Insemination of Donor 209 • Indications for Use of Donor Semen for IUI 209 • Instructions to Prospective Sperm Donor 209 • Semen Cryopreservation 209 • Technique of Cryopreservation of Human Sperm 209 • Technique of Human Sperm Thawing 209 • IUI Procedure Steps at a Glance 210 • Single versus Dual IUI Treatment Cycles 210 • IUI–One of the Fertility Options for HIV Patients/HIV Discordant Couple 211

Chapter 19   Enhancing IUI Success Rates 213
Madhuri Patil

• Progress in IUI 214 • Literature Search on Use of IUI for Different Etiologies 214 • Unexplained Infertility 214 • Male Factor Infertility (WHO) 214 • Success of IUI 216 • Success Rates are Contingent Upon Procedure being Performed 216 • Factors Affecting Success of IUI 216 • Trials which Revolutionized IUI 218

Chapter 20   IVF and ICSI: Current State of the Art 220
Christian De Geyter, Alexander Quaas, Maria De Geyter, Katharina Rüther-Wolf

• Infrastructure and Organization Needed for IVF and ICSI including Quality Assurance 221 • Outline of the Diagnostic Workup Prior to ART 222 • Controlled Ovarian Hyperstimulation 225 • Ovulation Induction 226 • Semen Preparation 227 • IVF or ICSI? 227 • Embryo Transfer 227 • Luteal Phase Support 230 • The Major Complications of ART 230 • Ovarian Hyperstimulation Syndrome 230 • Monitoring the Outcome of Assisted Reproduction 231 • Quality Assurance through Data Reporting 231

Chapter 21	Embryo Culture Systems 234

Judith Menezes

- Physiology and Metabolism of the Preimplantation Embryo   235
- pH Control   236   • Temperature and Osmolarity   237   • Oxygen Concentration   239   • Oil   239   • Culture Media   240

Chapter 22	Laboratory Set-up for IVF-ICSI................................ 246

Vijay Mangoli, Ranjana Mangoli

- Location of the Laboratory   247   • Structural Requirements   247   • Layout   248   • Reception Area   248   • Nurse's Work Area   248   • Changing Room   248   • Semen Collection Room   248   • General Laboratory   249   • Sterilization Area   249   • Scrubbing Area   249   • Operation Theater   249   • Culture Room   249   • Administration Office   249   • Embryologist and Staff Rest Room and Discussion Room   250   • Storage Space   250   • Gas Cylinders and Liquid Nitrogen Tanks   250   • Electricity Control Room   250   • Instruments   250   • Instruments for Operation Theater   250   • Instruments and Materials for Laboratory   251   • Instruments and Materials for Culture Room   252   • Laboratory Personnel   255   • Record Keeping   256   • Quality Control   256

Chapter 23	Noninvasive Strategies for Selection of Human Oocytes and Embryos 258

Simone Palini, Silvia de Stefani, Raffaella Depalo

- Noninvasive Strategies for Selection of Human Oocytes and Embryos   258   • Oocytes   259   • Oocytes Investigations: New Approaches   260   • Embryos   262   • Embryos Investigation: New Approaches   265

Chapter 24	Fertility Preservation in Women with Gynecologic Cancer 270

Ava Desai

- Fertility and Ovarian Cancer   270   • Fertility Preservation in Invasive Epithelial Ovarian Cancer   270   • Fertility Preservation in Borderline Epithelial Ovarian Cancer   273   • Pregnancy and Epithelial Ovarian Cancer   274   • Fertility Preservation in Germ Cell Ovarian Tumors   275   • Pregnancy and Germ Cell Tumors   277   • Fertility Preservation in Granulosa Cell Tumors   277   • Fertility and Cervical Cancer   277   • Cone Biopsy in Stage IA1 Microinvasive Disease   277   • Stage IA2 Microinvasive Disease   278   • Ovarian Transposition   280   • Pregnancy and Cervical Cancer   280   • Fertility and Endometrial Cancer   280   • Ovarian Preservation in Endometrial Cancer   282   • Fertility and Gestational Trophoblastic Disease   283   • Preservation of Ovarian Function in Cancer Patients   283   • Cryopreservation of Embryos/Oocytes or Ovarian Tissue   283

Chapter 25	Ectopic Pregnancy: Current Management 287

Majumdar Abha, Singh Tejshree A

- Incidence   287   • Risk Factors   287   • Cilia Damage and Tubal Occlusion   288   • Altered Tubal Motility   288   • Idiopathic   288   • Previous History of Ectopic Pregnancy   288   • Infertility Treatment   288   • Other Risk Factors   288   • Clinical Presentation   288   • Diagnosis   289   • Tubal Ectopic Pregnancy   289   • Ovarian Ectopic Pregnancy   291   • Cervical Ectopic Pregnancy   291   • Abdominal Pregnancy   291   • Cesarean Scar Ectopic   292   • Heterotopic Pregnancy   292   • Treatment   292   • Expectant Management   292   • Nonsurgical Management   292   • Surgical Management   296   • Current Evidence on Surgery, Systemic Methotrexate and Expectant Management in the Treatment of Tubal Ectopic Pregnancy   298   • Ectopic Pregnancies in Unusual Locations   299   • Interstitial (Cornual) Pregnancy   299   • Cervical Ectopic Pregnancy   299   • Ovarian Pregnancy   300   • Abdominal Pregnancy   300   • Cesarean Scar Ectopic   301   • Heterotopic Pregnancy   301   • Chance of Future Pregnancy   302

Chapter 26   Gonadotropins: The Future 305
Madhuri Patil

• Structure of Corifollitropin Alfa (Org 36286)   306   • Method of Administration   306   • Pharmacokinetics   307   • Efficacy   308   • Follicular Growth   308   • Hormone Levels   309   • Results with Corifollitropin Alfa   309   • Disadvantages of Corifollitropin Alfa   310   • Safety   311   • Cost Effectiveness of Corifollitropin Alfa   311   • Conclusion on Corifollitropin Alfa   311   • Recombinant LH-Lutropin Alfa for Injection (Luveris)   312   • Follitropin Alfa and Lutropin Alfa (2:1 Ratio) (Pergoveris)   (r-hFSH 150 IU and r-hLH 75 IU)   312   • Follitropin Delta   313   • Dosing and Administration of Follitropin Delta   313   • For Subsequent Treatment Cycles   313   • In Research   314   • In Humans   314

Chapter 27   Infertility Treatment: When to give up? 319
Rohit V Bhatt, Sonia Golani

• When to Stop Infertility Treatment?   319   • Material and Methods   320   • When should Friends and Relatives Give Up?   321   • When should Religious Leaders, Soothsayers and Astrologers Give Up?   322   • When should Quacks Give Up?   323   • When should Family Physician Give Up?   323   • When should Obstetric and Gynecologic Specialist and ART Expert Give Up?   324   • How many Attempts at Induction of Ovulation before Giving Up?   324   • When to Give Up after Intrauterine Insemination?   325   • When to Give Up after Donor Insemination?   325   • When to Give Up after Microtubal Surgery?   325   • When to Give Up ART Procedures?   325   • Reactions of Infertile Couple Who Discontinued Further Treatment   326   • When to Give Up for Medical Reasons?   327   • Embryo Donation, Surrogacy and Adoption   327   • Future Hopes for Infertile Couples   328

Chapter 28   The ART Bill: Its Implications 329
Manish Banker, Pravin Patel, Arati Gupte-Shah

• Setting Up an ART Clinic   329   • Primary (Level 1) Infertility Care Units   329   • Secondary (Level 2) Infertility Care Units   331   • Tertiary (Level 3) Infertility Care Units   331   • Requirements of an ART Clinic   331   • Space   331   • The Nonsterile Area   331   • The Sterile Area   331   • Staff   332   • Registration and Accreditation   333   • Which Clinics should be Registered?   333   • Grant of Registration   334   • Information and Counseling of Patients   334   • Confidentiality and Consent   334   • Penalties   335

Index 337

CHAPTER 1

Is the Prevalence of Infertility Increasing?

Rajat Gyaneshwar, Padmini Raviraj

Chapter outline

- How Common is Infertility?
  - Is Infertility Becoming more Common?
  - Infertility and Sexually Transmitted Infections
- Infertility and Aging
- Infertility and Stress

INTRODUCTION

The right to reproduce is a basic human right. This right was first formally recognized by representatives from 179 countries at the International Conference on Population and Development (ICPD) held in Cairo in the early 1990s. The conference reaffirmed the 1948 declaration of human rights.[1] The ICPD declaration maintains that couples should have a choice about their fertility. This implies that reproductive health care should include a range of services directed to assisting couples when they are ready to have a child, space pregnancies, so that they have as many children as they desire and stop having babies when they have completed their family. Those couples who cannot conceive need to be managed as well.

The World Health Organization (WHO) has listed infertility as a global public health issue. Dr Mahmoud Fathalla in his opening remarks at a WHO international meeting argued that a major millennium development challenge will be to make management of infertility more accessible to the estimated 80 million couples in the world who are unable to conceive.[2]

Human beings are remarkably fertile. Most females are capable of conceiving within 2 years of trying. However, infertility has been reported since ancient times. The book of Samuel in the Bible recounts Hannah's story. She was childless for many years and was taunted by her more fertile cowife Peninnah. After much anguish and praying she conceived and bore a son Samuel. Yet another heart-rending tale is that of Jacob and Rachael who were unable to have a child. Rachael said to her husband "Here take my maid Bilhah. Consort with her, that she may bear on my knees and that through her I too may have children". Abraham and Sarah were without issue. Sarah finally conceived when she was ninety! The early Indian writings such as the *Ayurveda* gave details on the physiology of fertility and recognized that the causes of infertility were multifactorial.[3] In the Ramayana, King Dashrath had no issues although he had three wives. Much prayer led to a boon and all three wives conceived.

Rama, the son of the first wife has impacted on Hindu society for many millennia. Aristotle, Plato's pupil and Alexander the Great's teacher wrote a treatise on the 'generation of animals—infertility and semen'. Not unreasonably his understanding of the semen was somewhat different to ours, but his basic notions on fertility were not very different to what was written in the *Ayurveda*.[4] Human kind has recognized fertility as a natural consequence of couples coming together and childbearing and rearing an important responsibility.

Infertility has been recognized for many a millennia. It leads to social ostracism, which in many situations is condoned, by deep-seated religious beliefs. In the Koran, it states "He makes whom he pleases barren; verily he is knowing, powerful." The Hindu belief that infertility is due to karma is shared by almost all religions and hence there is a sense that the inability to conceive is some form of punishment.

In the 21st century due to better understanding of reproductive physiology, factors contributing to infertility are better understood. Social ostracism is less of an issue. Couples who cannot conceive are more open in seeking help and society generally is more sympathetic to their plight.

HOW COMMON IS INFERTILITY?

Infertility is a common human burden, but there are few hard data regarding its incidence. The lack of a standardized definition, and inaccuracies in interpreting them in surveys makes the task more difficult. The definition of infertility has varied from couples trying to conceive unsuccessfully for 12 months or 24 months.[5] Most studies are anecdotal or biased by examining skewed populations. In some populations, where there is a high incidence of pelvic inflammatory disease, the incidence of tubal factor infertility is high. In a study from the United States, the infertility rates amongst blacks is 18% compared to the whites whose rate is 9%. This may be indicative of the epidemiology of pelvic inflammatory disease.[6] In Sweden, Hogberg et al. asserted that as many as 1 in 13 couples were infertile.[7] Hull et al. reported that 1 in 6 couples required professional help to conceive.[8] Trussell and Wilson included data from 1550 to 1850 when effective contraception was not available. They reported that 8% of females who married remained sterile and that the likelihood of remaining childless rose sharply with age. This study might suggest that the rates of infertility have tended to remain somewhat stable over the years.[9] It is difficult to find any good data on the trends in infertility rated over the last century.

The Journal of Human Reproduction under the title 'New Debate' published an interesting article entitled 'International estimates of infertility prevalence and treatment seeking potential need and demand for infertility medical care'.[6] The authors looked at 14 studies, which provided estimates of infertility prevalence in 10 more developed countries based on surveys of over 50,000 women. A further study looked at data from 5 European countries involving 1600 infertile women. They reported that the prevalence of current infertility ranges from 3.5% to 16.7%. The median was 9% for 12-month delay amongst women aged 20–44, in married and consensual unions. The authors also reported that lifetime infertility rates ranged from 5% to 25.7%. Interestingly enough there does not seem to be an overall difference in rates between the developed and developing countries.[10] *The 1995 National Survey of Family Growth performed by the national health statistics in United States found the infertility rate to be 10.2%, which in comparison with earlier survey in 1965 has not significantly changed.*[10]

Is Infertility Becoming more Common?

As stated earlier, no reliable information regarding global infertility trends is available.

Hence, it is difficult to do any more than speculate. However, the perception in recent years is that the rate of infertility is increasing. This perception does not seem unreasonable as more and more couples seek treatment. In addition, almost all the factors contributing to subfertility appear to have become more prevalent. These include both male and female factors including increasing rates of ovulatory failure, tubal blockage, and conditions such as endometriosis. Delaying pregnancy to an older age when the couple are less fecund is an additional significant factor.

Throughout the developed world fertility rates have decreased dramatically.[11] This has occurred because of the availability of more reliable contraception and a deliberate policy to slow the global population growth. So more and more individuals and couples are deliberately trying to postpone first pregnancies, have fewer children and use permanent contraception once their family is complete. The world average total fertility rate in the five years to 2005, was 2.7 babies per woman, which when compared to the fertility rates of 4.5 babies per woman in 1970s is a marked decline. In most countries, the age of marriage has been legislatively increased.[11] Women are better-educated and seeking career opportunities. All this has led to a decline in the overall fertility rates. Governments have targeted family planning and reduced fertility rates as an essential strategy for socioeconomic development. A key strategy to achieving Millennium Development Goals 4 and 5 is to reduce the incidence of unwanted, unplanned pregnancies.

A medical survey conducted in various cities in India revealed a shocking truth that rate of infertility is increasing in urban India. This is more among the IT professionals. According to the survey about 15 out of 100 couples from this sector faces infertility and 40% of such cases are related to male infertility.

According to the expert, the main culprit is the competitive working atmosphere. IT sector faces a tough competition that makes people to work for extra hours and even in odd hours. This really is taking toll on the family relations. Absence of proper and regular sexual relations, stress and tensions in the work place, etc. are the major causes of infertility in this sector. Secondly, the amphibian lifestyle followed by the IT professionals also plays an important role. Irregular food habits, more consumption of junk foods, etc. are classified under this lifestyle.

The decrease in fertility rates is a measure of socioeconomic development. As couples are better educated they are more empowered to seek treatment for infertility. It has been estimated that 10–15% of couples are unable to fall pregnant without any assistance. This figure has probably been fairly stable, but with the advent of reproductive technology, there is an increasing demand the world over for couples seeking treatment. This may give an impression that the prevalence of the condition is increasing. Anecdotes of reports from skewed populations, a growing interest in infertility management and less stigma attached to infertility may all be contributing to the perception that infertility rates are rising. Adding to this perception is a rapid rise in the number of specialists providing infertility management services. There is a risk that this might lead to an over reporting of the incidence. More physicians trained in the area of infertility services reflects demand for their services. Availability of more trained specialists helps improve access to care. The rapid progress in assisted reproductive technology has identified treatable causes of infertility thus more couples are able to achieve a successful pregnancy. This is a positive development as a consequence of better fertility control has been a decline in the number of babies available for adoption.

Infertility and Sexually Transmitted Infections

The increasing prevalence of sexually transmitted infections (STIs) may also be contributing to an increase in infertility rates. With change in social mores, greater population mobility, addressing gaps in economic opportunities due to gender, in the last few decades, young people have become sexually more active and at an earlier age. Lack of safe sex practices increases the risk of STIs. It has been estimated that about 3 million adolescent girls contract STIs annually.[12] Untreated they can result in pelvic inflammatory disease (PID), which has negative impact on fertility.

In industrialized countries, the annual incidence of PID in women aged 15–39 is reported to be 10–13/1000 women with a peak incidence of 20 per 1000 in 20–24 age group. The PID rate has almost doubled since 1960. Tubal infertility occurs in 8% of women after one episode of PID, 20% after two episodes of PID and 40% after three episodes of PID.[13] The fraction of women rendered infertile as a consequence of PID is thought to have risen by a factor of 1.6 since 1960. More recently, there are reports that the incidence of PID is decreasing. This may be related to the advent of acquired immunodeficiency syndrome (AIDS) and the promotion of safe sex. Availability of more sexually transmitted disease (STD) clinics provide counseling services, identify at risk population and encourage them to get treated also contribute to the reversal of trends in STDs.[13]

The STDs also equally affect men by causing deoxyribonucleic acid (DNA) damage in their sperm.[13]

Infertility and Aging

After one year of trying to conceive 75% of women aged 30 or below will conceive and deliver. However, at 35 only 66% will and at 40 only 44% will.[14] Primary infertility was observed in 7% of the women aged 45+, while 20% were considered subfertile in one of the studies.[15]

Postponement of pregnancy to a later age means that couples may be missing their peak age of fecundity for starting a family. It is well known that advancing maternal age is associated with decline in fertility rates in women. The pregnancy rate is inversely proportional to the female woman's age. There may be many explanations for this including decreased coital frequency, decreased overall time to try for a pregnancy and diminished ovarian reserve.

Fertility rates are at its peak between the ages of 25 and 30 and begin to decline at the age of 30 and steeper decline begins at 35 years. About 75% of women trying to conceive at the age of 30 will achieve a pregnancy within 1 year and 91% will do so within 4 years. At age 40 only 44% will conceive within one year and 64% within 4 years. The estimated infertility rate for women aged 19–26 is 8%, 27–34 years is 13–14% and 18% for women aged 35–39 years.[10]

In a computer-simulated model of reproduction combining monthly probability of conceiving, risk of miscarriage and probability of becoming permanently sterile due to age Leridon et al. calculated that assisted reproductive technology as it exists today cannot compensate for births lost by natural decline in fertility after the age of 35.[16]

Biologically women without contraceptive intervention were either pregnant or were breastfeeding. Life expectancy was much shorter. Thus, women were amenorrheic for much of their life. The current tendency to menstruate for much of her ovulatory life may well be responsible for many of the modern conditions associated with infertility. Experimentally, baboons who are regularly menstruating are more likely to have endometriosis than those who are predominantly amenorrheic due to pregnancy and lactation.[17]

Another disturbing observation is that the quality of mammalian sperm has declined steadily over the last ten decades or so. This has been attributed to chemical pollutants in the atmosphere, which mimic hormones. The human male has not escaped this. In addition to reduced sperm counts aging adversely affects the quality of sperm.[18]

With advancing age, medical comorbidities such as hypertension, diabetes become more prevalent as does obesity. Obesity is becoming a major threat to most of the countries and in fact obesity rates have doubled in the last two decades. By causing hormonal imbalance that contribute to anovulatory cycles and by reduction in sexual drive it increases infertility rates. Obese women are 2.7 times more likely to be infertile compared to normal women.

It equally affects men by causing erectile dysfunction and reduces libido. In addition as people grow older they are more likely to be on medications, more likely to have been exposed to harmful radiation and other deleterious influences of their reproductive potential.

Infertility and Stress

Busy daily routines and other modern lifestyle imperatives have an adverse effect on couples being able to conceive. Shift work, work-related travel, the need for both couples to work can mean that there is no time to make babies so to speak. So young couples tend to postpone infertility management till an age when help is less likely to be possible.

Psychological stress leads to problems with relationships, reduced frequency of coitus and other sexual problems.

CONCLUSION

Fertility rates are likely to continue to decline globally. This will occur as a deliberate policy on the part of national governments and also due to empowerment of women through education and socioeconomic development.

The rates of infertility may increase primarily due to childbearing being postponed to older age when both men and women are less fecund. Less fecund couples requiring assisted reproductive technology assistance to conceive may pass on their problem to the next generation.

However, preimplantation genetic diagnosis will increase the chance of a genetically normal pregnancy, which may reduce pregnancy wastage.

REFERENCES

1. International Conference of Population and Development; 1994.
2. Vayena E, Rowe PJ, Griffin PD. Medical, ethical and social aspects of assisted reproduction. Current practices and controversies in assisted reproduction: report of a WHO meeting, Geneva, Switzerland; 2001.
3. Babu G, Babu A, Bhuyan GC, et al. Vandhyatva—a medico-historical study. Bull Inst Hist of Med Hyderabad. 2006;36(1): 83-6.
4. Trompoukis C, Kalaitzis C, Giannakopoulos S, et al. Semen and the diagnosis of infertility in Aristotle. Andrologia 2007;39(1):33-7.
5. Dunson DB, Baird DD, Colombo B. Increased infertility with age in men and women. Obstet Gynecol. 2004;103:51-6.
6. Boivin J, Bunting L, Collins JA, et al. International estimates of infertility prevalence and treatment seeking: potential need and demand for infertility medical care. Hum Reprod: 2007;22(6):1506-12.
7. Hogberg U. Reproductive patterns among Swedish women born 1936-1960 Acta Obstetricia et Gynecologica Scandinavica 1992;171:207-14.
8. Hull MG, Glazener CM, Kelly NJ, et al. Population study of causes, treatment and outcome of infertility. BMJ. 1985;291:1693-7.

9. Trussel J, Wilson C. Sterility in a population with natural fertility. Popul Stud. 1985;39(2):269-86.
10. Sonya Norris. Royal Commission on New Reproductive Technologies Canada, 1990.
11. International Fertility Comparison—Australian Bureau of Statistics; 2007.
12. National Institute of Allergy and Infectious Diseases. (2018). Sexually Transmitted Diseases. [online] Available from https://www.niaid.nih.gov/diseases-conditions/sexually-transmitted-diseases [Accessed Sept., 2018].
13. Westrom L. Incidence, prevalence and trends in acute PID and its consequence in industrialised countries. AMJOG. 1980;138:880-92.
14. Menken J, Trussell J, larsen LL. Age and infertility. Science. 1986;233:1389-94.
15. Omar MM, Högberg U, Bergström B. Fertility infertility and child survival of Somali women. Scand J Soc Med. 1944;22(3):194-200.
16. Leridon H. Can assisted reproductive technology compensate for the natural decline in fertility with age? A model assessment. Hum Reprod. 2004;19:1548-53.
17. Carlsen E, Giwircman A, Keiding N, et al. Evidence for decreasing quality of semen during past 50 years. BMJ 1992;305:609-13.
18. Hastings JM, Fazleabas AT. A baboon model for endometriosis: implications for fertility. Reproductive Biology and Endocrinology. 2006;4(suppl 1):57.

CHAPTER 2

Female Reproductive Endocrinology: An Insight

Aby K Koshy

Chapter outline

- Embryology and Development
- Functional Components
  - Hormones
  - Hypothalamic-pituitary-ovarian Axis
  - Two-cell, Two-gonadotropin Hypotheses
- Menstrual Cycle
  - Follicular (Proliferative) Phase
  - Ovulation
  - Luteal (Secretory) Phase
- Other Changes
- Menopause

INTRODUCTION

Knowledge is a process of piling-up facts; wisdom lies in their simplification.
–Martin Fisher

For a clinician, a good understanding of the working of the male and female reproductive system is essential for the evaluation and the treatment of infertility. Reproductive endocrinology forms the basis of this understanding. Though a vast subject, this chapter does not endeavor to extensively cover it, but aims to give the reader a brief and concise outline of the working of female endocrine system with respect to reproductive medicine.

EMBRYOLOGY AND DEVELOPMENT

The *in utero* differentiation of the primitive gonads is genetically determined. In contrast, the development of genitalia is dependent on the presence or absence of a functional testis.

Primordial germ cells originate in the endoderm of the yolk sac and migrate to the genital ridge to form the indifferent gonad. The genital ridge is a condensation of tissue near the adrenal gland. Around the sixth week of development, this genital ridge gives rise to the primitive gonad, which then develops a cortex and medulla. During the seventh and eighth week, further development of the gonads occurs—in males, the testes develop from the medulla and in females the ovaries from the cortex.

In the female fetus, primordial ova differentiate from the germinal epithelium and migrate into the substance of the ovarian cortex. Around each primordial ovum there collects a layer of cells from the ovarian stroma—the granulosa cells. These cells are initially spindle shaped, but later take on epithelioid characteristics. The ovum surrounded by a single layer of granulosa cells is called a primordial follicle.

The external and internal genitalia arise from the primordial genital ducts. In the seventh week of gestation, the embryo has both male and female primordial genital ducts. Absence of functioning testicular tissue results in development of female genitalia. In the female fetus, the Müllerian duct system develops into fallopian tubes and the uterus. The Wolffian duct disappears, though its remnants persist into adult life.

In males, the Y chromosome is necessary for the differentiation and development of the testes.[1] The sex-determining region of the Y chromosome (SRY), located near the tip of the short arm of the Y chromosome initiates transcription of a cascade of genes necessary for testicular differentiation.[2] Testosterone begins to be elaborated by the male fetal testes at about the seventh week of embryonic life (by the Leydig cells). Under the influence of testosterone, epididymis and vas deferens develop from the Wolffian duct. The Müllerian inhibiting substance (MIS) or anti-Müllerian hormone (AMH) secreted by the Sertoli cells of the testis causes regression of the Müllerian ducts by apoptosis.

The external genitalia are bipotential until the eighth week. Thereafter, testosterone, secreted first by the genital ridges and later by the fetal testes leads to the development of a penis and a scrotum. Dihydrotestosterone, a metabolite of testosterone plays an important role in the formation of male external genitalia and later of the male secondary sex characteristics. In the absence of testosterone, the urogenital slit remains open and female genitalia form.

A female is born with a finite number of germ cells. During fetal development, the ovaries contain over 7 million primordial follicles. Many of these undergo atresia before birth and at the time of birth, they number around 2 million.[3] As nearly half of these are atretic, around 1 million ova undergo the first part of the first meiotic division and get arrested in prophase. Atresia continues during development, and the number of ova in both of the ovaries at the time of puberty is less than 300,000. The number further decreases as the process of recruitment of primordial follicles for folliculogenesis continues at a relatively constant rate during the first three decades of a woman's life. Between about 13 years and 46 years of age, 400–500 of the primordial follicles develop enough to expel their ova one each month. In addition, the rate of loss of nongrowing follicles to atresia is continuously accelerating. As a result, the ovarian reserve is reduced leading to decreased fecundity by age 30 and a marked decrease by age 35.[4] In older mothers, the long time that surviving oocytes spend arrested in meiotic prophase may account for the increased incidence of genetically abnormal pregnancies.

Circulating luteinizing hormone (LH) and follicle-stimulating hormone (FSH) levels are elevated at birth, but fall to low levels within a few months and remain low until puberty. The ovaries remain quiescent until gonadotropins from the anterior pituitary bring about the changes related to puberty and adolescence. The period of final maturation activated by gonadotropins from the pituitary to bring about the final maturation of the reproductive system is known as 'adolescence'. 'Puberty' is the period when the endocrine and gametogenic functions of the gonads have first developed to the point where reproduction is possible. Physical changes of puberty occur sequentially during adolescence. In girls, the first event is thelarche, the development of breasts, followed by pubarche, the development of axillary and pubic hair, and then by menarche, the first menstrual period. Menarche usually occurs about 2 years after breast budding. The initial periods are generally anovulatory, and regular ovulation appears about a year later. During this period there is a change in the body habitus—the pelvis and hips widen and body fat increases and accumulates in the hips and thighs.

The exact endocrinal changes during puberty are still far from clear. Central influences may inhibit release of gonadotropin-releasing hormone (GnRH) during childhood, and then initiate its release to induce puberty in early adolescence. An increase in pulsatile GnRH secretion, the cause of which remains unknown promotes LH and FSH secretion. This stimulates production of sex hormones, primarily estrogen, which in turn stimulates development of secondary sexual characteristics. Pubic and axillary hair growth may be stimulated by the adrenal androgens.

Over the last 150 years, the age at which puberty begins has been decreasing, primarily because of improved health and nutrition, but this trend has stabilized. In the United States in recent years, puberty generally occurs between the ages of 10 and 13 in girls, with the median age being 12.43 years.[5] Data from a large Indian survey shows the mean age at menarche among Indian women was 13.76 years.[6] It occurs earlier in girls with more than normal body mass index (BMI), those living in urban areas, in the blind and those whose mother had early puberty. Girls with less than normal BMI tend to have a delayed puberty.

FUNCTIONAL COMPONENTS

Though the hypothalamus, the pituitary and the gonads form the principal component of the reproductive axis, it receives many input and influences from other organ systems. The important organs of the human female reproductive tract include the ovaries, fallopian tubes, uterus, and vagina.

Hormones

Gonadotropin-releasing hormone is a peptide containing 10 amino acids (Glu-His-Trp-Ser-Tyr-Gly-Leu-Arg-Pro-Gly-NH2). It is secreted by neurons whose cell bodies are located mostly in the arcuate nuclei of the hypothalamus. The endings of these neurons terminate mainly in the median eminence of the hypothalamus, where they release GnRH. It is transmitted by hypothalamic-hypophysial portal vascular system to stimulate the gonadotropes of the anterior pituitary. GnRH is secreted intermittently in pulses lasting 5–25 minutes at a time once every 1–3 hours. GnRH stimulates the synthesis and secretion of the gonadotropins, FSH and LH. Secretion depends on size and frequency of GnRH pulses. When GnRH is infused continuously, its ability to cause the release of LH and FSH by the anterior pituitary gland is lost. This forms the basis of the therapeutic action of GnRH agonists.

Both FSH and LH are small glycoproteins having molecular weights of about 30,000 secreted by the anterior pituitary. The secretion of LH is also cyclical and follows the pulsatile release of GnRH. In contrast, FSH secretion increases and decreases only slightly with each fluctuation of GnRH secretion. Instead, it changes more slowly over a period of many hours in response to longer-term changes in GnRH.

The FSH is responsible for the maturation of germ cells. In males, FSH stimulates Sertoli cells and thus maintains spermatogenesis. It is also essential in the conversion of the spermatids to sperm (spermiogenesis). In females, FSH is responsible for the early growth of ovarian follicles.[7]

In males, LH acts on the interstitial cells (Leydig cells) of the testes stimulating them to synthesize and secrete testosterone. In males, it is thus also called the interstitial cell stimulating hormone (ICSH). In females, LH stimulates the follicle to secrete estrogen in the first half of the menstrual cycle; a surge of LH triggers the completion of meiosis I of the oocyte and ovulation. In the secretory phase of the menstrual cycle, it stimulates the now-empty follicle to develop into the corpus luteum, which secretes progesterone.

Prolactin (PRL) is a polypeptide secreted by lactotrope cells of the anterior pituitary. During pregnancy, it helps in the preparation of the breasts for future milk production.

After birth, prolactin promotes the synthesis of milk. Prolactin also inhibits the effects of gonadotropins, possibly by an action at the level of the ovary. Prolactin thus prevents ovulation in lactating mothers. Prolactin secretion is stimulated by thyrotropin-releasing hormone (TRH) and repressed by estrogens and dopamine.

Androgens and estrogens, which are the steroid sex hormones, are normally secreted in both sexes. They can be synthesized either from cholesterol or directly from acetyl coenzyme A. Androgens include testosterone, dihydrotestosterone and androstenedione. Though testosterone is much more abundant than the other androgens, most of it is eventually converted into the more active hormone dihydrotestosterone in the target tissues. The testes secrete large amounts of androgens, principally testosterone, but they also secrete small amounts of estrogens. The Leydig cells of the testis secrete testosterone, and the Sertoli cells secrete Müllerian inhibiting substance (MIS/AMH). The ovaries secrete large amounts of estrogens and small amounts of androgens. Androgens are secreted from the adrenal cortex in both sexes, and some of the androgens are converted to estrogens in fat and other extragonadal and extra-adrenal tissues. The ovaries also secrete progesterone, a steroid that has special functions in preparing the uterus for pregnancy. Androgen, estrogen and progesterone circulate in the bloodstream almost entirely bound to plasma proteins. Only unbound hormones appear to be biologically active.

The naturally occurring estrogens are 17β-estradiol, estrone, and estriol (C18 steroids). Though secreted primarily by the granulosa cells of the ovarian follicles, it is also secreted by the corpus luteum and the placenta. The principal estrogen secreted by the ovaries is β-estradiol. Small amounts of estrone are also secreted; mostly in the peripheral tissues from ovarian and adrenal androgens. Estriol is produced mainly in the liver as an oxidative product derived from both estradiol and estrone. Both estrone and estriol are weak estrogens; the estrogenic potency of β-estradiol is 12 times that of estrone and 80 times that of estriol. Estrogens are responsible for the feminizing changes in the breasts, the reproductive organs and other parts of the body at the time of puberty. Changes in estrogen levels during different phases of the menstrual cycle are responsible for the changes in the uterus, endometrium, fallopian tubes, cervix, vagina and the blood flow to these organs. In addition, estrogens have an important role in other body systems. These include stimulation of bone growth and prevention of osteoporosis. Estrogens also have multiple actions on the central nervous system (CNS).

Progesterone, a C21 steroid is secreted by the corpus luteum and during pregnancy by the placenta. Though also secreted during the follicular phase of the menstrual cycle, the major production occurs after ovulation during the luteal (secretory) phase. Progesterone is responsible for the changes in the endometrium and the cyclic changes in the cervix and vagina. It stimulates the development of lobules and alveoli in the breast. It induces differentiation of estrogen-prepared ductal tissue and supports the secretory function of the breast during lactation.

Other hormones secreted by the ovary include the polypeptide hormone relaxin which during pregnancy loosens the ligaments of the pubic symphysis and softens the cervix, thus facilitating labor and delivery.

Inhibin is a polypeptide that down regulates FSH synthesis and inhibits FSH secretion. It is secreted by the granulosa cells in females and in the Sertoli cells in males.

Activin is produced in the gonads, pituitary gland and the placenta. It enhances FSH biosynthesis and secretion, and participates in the regulation of the menstrual cycle. It increases FSH binding and FSH-induced aromatization in the ovarian follicle. In the male, activin enhances spermatogenesis.

Hypothalamic-pituitary-ovarian Axis

The changes during puberty and establishment of menstrual cycles result from a unique harmonious interaction between the hypothalamus, the pituitary and the ovaries (Fig. 2.1).

The hypothalamus secretes GnRH into the portal hypophysial vessels, which stimulates the secretion of FSH as well as LH. Estrogen in small amounts has a strong effect to inhibit the production of both LH and FSH (negative feedback). At the time of ovulation, high estrogen levels cause the LH surge (positive feedback).

Progesterone decreases the number of estrogen receptors in the endometrium and increases the rate of conversion of 17β-estradiol to less active estrogens.

The feedback effects of progesterone are complex and are exerted at both the hypothalamic and pituitary levels. Large doses of progesterone inhibit LH secretion and potentiate the inhibitory effect of estrogens, preventing ovulation. This feedback operates mainly on the anterior pituitary gland directly, but they also operate to a lesser extent on the hypothalamus.

Inhibin B, which is secreted by the granulosa cells of the ovarian corpus luteum, has a negative feedback, inhibiting the secretion of FSH and, to a lesser extent, LH by the anterior pituitary gland. It is believed that inhibin might be especially important in causing the decrease in secretion of FSH and LH at the end of the menstrual cycle.

In the early follicular phase of the menstrual cycle, inhibin B levels are low, FSH levels gradually increase leading to follicular growth. Levels of estrogen, particularly estradiol, increase exponentially (Fig. 2.2).

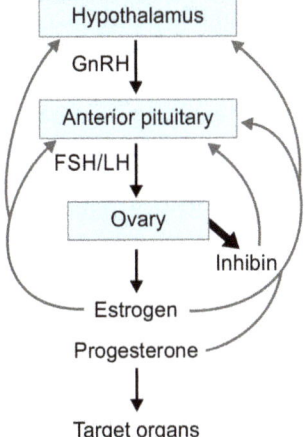

Fig. 2.1: Hypothalamic-pituitary-ovarian axis.

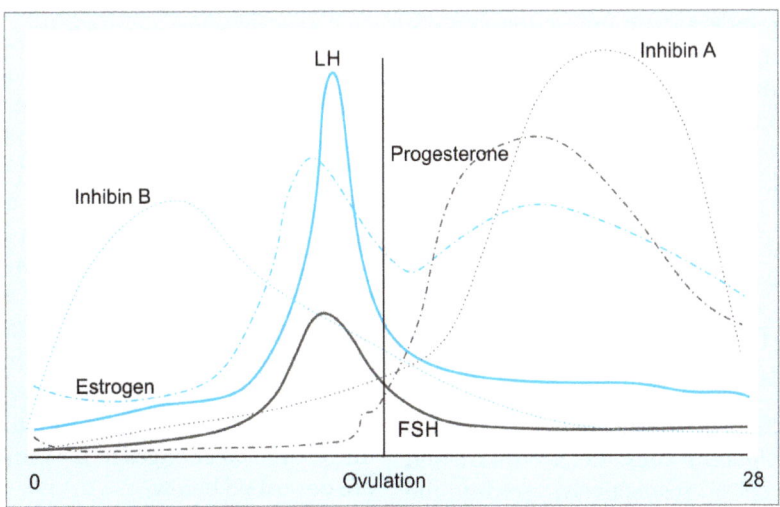

Fig. 2.2: Hormonal changes during the menstrual cycle.

The levels of LH also increase moderately though not as much as FSH. The rising estrogen levels keep LH secretion under check. When a follicle reaches an optimum size, the estrogen level reaches a peak and the negative feedback on LH secretion changes to a positive one and causes the LH surge. It is postulated that a sustained level of estrogen over an unknown period of time is essential to cause the LH surge. For the positive feedback effect of LH release to occur, estradiol levels must be greater than 200 pg/mL for approximately 50 hours duration. The rise in estrogen also augments the responsiveness of the pituitary to GnRH and triggers a burst of LH secretion. Ovulation follows after 36–48 hours after the initiation of the LH surge (and 9 hours after the LH peak). There is a smaller FSH surge similar to the LH surge. Estradiol levels fall dramatically immediately prior to the LH peak.

Following ovulation, secretion of estrogen, progesterone and inhibin occurs. This keeps the FSH and LH low during the luteal phase of the cycle. Inhibin secreted by the lutein cells also inhibits secretion by the anterior pituitary. Progesterone stimulates development of the secretory endometrium, which is necessary for embryonic implantation. Because progesterone is thermogenic, basal body temperature increases by 0.5°C for the duration of this phase.

In the absence of pregnancy, regression of the corpus luteum occurs. PGF 2α and ET-1 appears to be responsible for luteolysis.[8] Following this, the estrogen and progesterone levels fall and menstruation occurs. The secretion of FSH and LH increases and the next cycle begins.

Two-cell, Two-gonadotropin Hypotheses

The production of androgens and estrogens from two different cells, i.e. by theca and granulosa cells, respectively, under the influence of two different gonadotropins LH and FSH is termed as "two-cell two-gonadotropin hypothesis". LH principally stimulates androstenedione production, and to a lesser degree testosterone production through the adenylyl cyclase pathway in the theca cells. The androstenedione synthesized in the theca cells freely diffuses to the granulosa cells. FSH activates the aromatase enzyme in granulosa cells. Androstenedione is aromatized to estrone and finally converted to estradiol by 17-β-hydroxysteroid dehydrogenase type I.[9] The estradiol then diffuses into the blood vessels (Fig. 2.3).

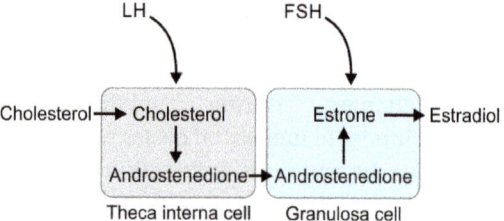

Fig. 2.3: Two-cell two-gonadotropin hypotheses.

MENSTRUAL CYCLE

The menstrual cycle reflects the periodic preparations for fertilization and pregnancy. The length of a menstrual cycle is the number of days between the first day of menstrual bleeding of one cycle to the onset of menses of the next cycle. The median duration of a menstrual cycle is 28 days with most cycle lengths between 25 days and 36 days, although abnormal cycle length is frequently associated with decreased fertility.[10,11] The average duration of menses is 5 (± 2) days and is usually greatest on the 2nd day. The menstrual cycle can be divided into follicular (proliferative or preovulatory), ovulatory, and luteal (secretory or postovulatory) phases. These cyclical changes in the different organs are described below.

Follicular (Proliferative) Phase

This phase of the menstrual cycle varies more compared to the other ones. The primary event is the process of folliculogenesis. This occurs within the cortex of the ovary, which contains the primordial follicles. Recruitment of a number of primordial follicles occurs several days before actual folliculogenesis. Follicle recruitment and the initial stages of follicle growth are independent of gonadotropins. In addition to follicular growth, there occurs accumulation of increased numbers of granulosa cells that form multiple layers around the oocyte. The arrangement of the granulosa cells changes from a simple cuboidal epithelium to a stratified or pseudostratified columnar epithelium. Spindle cells derived from the ovary interstitium collect in several layers outside the granulosa cells, giving rise to a second mass of cells called the theca. The inner layer—the theca interna, consists of cells which take on epithelioid characteristics similar to those of the granulosa cells. These cells secrete additional steroid sex hormones. The outer layer, the theca externa, develops into a highly vascular connective tissue capsule that becomes the capsule of the developing follicle. The acquisition of a second layer of granulosa cells and development of the theca leads to transition from a primary follicle to a secondary follicle.

As these follicles enlarge, follicular fluid rich in estrogen is secreted from the granulosa cells. Accumulation of this fluid causes an antrum to appear within the mass of granulosa cells (antral follicle). The total number of antral follicles present in a woman's ovaries early in the menstrual cycle is the antral follicular count (AFC). This along with AMH is presently considered the best indicator for assessing a woman's ovarian reserve.

Though many follicles start growing, one of them, the dominant follicle starts growing rapidly around the sixth day, whereas the others undergo atresia. The reason why a particular follicle becomes dominant is still not clear. Selection of the dominant follicle possibly occurs depending on the number of FSH receptors, concentration of follicular fluid FSH and the amount of estrogen secreted by the follicle. The 'FSH window' theory is an attempt to explain this. In response to negative feedback from rising estradiol and inhibin levels, FSH levels fall in the late follicular phase. The dominant follicle has increased sensitivity to the falling FSH levels and continues growing. Follicles that initiate the latter stages of development after FSH levels begin to fall undergo atresia. The duration of this FSH window during which FSH levels are above the threshold required to stimulate ongoing development determines the number of follicles that can develop to the preovulatory stage. Recognition of this concept has resulted in use of exogenous FSH to recruit more follicles during treatment for *in vitro* fertilization.[12]

Atresia of the nondominant follicles follows activation of apoptosis in the oocyte and granulosa cells. This process of atresia allows only one follicle to grow large enough to ovulate and thus prevent multiple pregnancies.

During the latter part of the proliferative stage, rapid growth of the follicles occurs transforming the antral follicles into vesicular follicles. Increased secretion of estrogens from the granulosa cells causes an increase in the FSH receptors and appearance of LH receptors. This in turn causes accelerated growth of the follicles. The granulosa and theca cells proliferate extensively with the antrum becoming filled with follicular fluid.

Ovulation

At around the 14th day (in a 28-day cycle), ovulation—rupture of the distended dominant follicle occurs. To produce the critical concentration of estradiol needed to initiate the positive feedback, the dominant follicle is almost always greater than 15 mm in diameter on ultrasound. The LH surge stimulates enzymes that initiate breakdown of the follicle wall and release of the now mature ovum. This ovum, which is released into the peritoneal cavity is picked up by the fimbrial ends of the fallopian tube and gets transported medially. Fertilization may occur if spermatozoa are present during this time. In the absence of fertilization, the ovum is shed from the uterine cavity through the vagina.

Simultaneous changes occur at the cellular level during ovulation. The oocyte, which was arrested in diplotene stage of prophase of the first meiotic division, resumes meiosis and completes the first meiotic division. This is an unequal division and one of the daughter cells, the secondary oocyte, receives most of the cytoplasm. The other daughter cell, the first polar body, fragments and disappears. The secondary oocyte immediately begins the second meiotic division, but this division stops at metaphase and is completed only when a sperm penetrates the oocyte. If fertilization occurs, the second polar body is cast off.

Luteal (Secretory) Phase

Following ovulation, the follicle fills with blood (corpus hemorrhagicum). Many women perceive ovulation as a fleeting lower abdominal pain ("mittelschmerz") which results from peritoneal irritation due to minor bleeding from the follicle into the abdominal cavity. Proliferation of the granulosa and theca cells occurs and the corpus hemorrhagicum is rapidly replaced with yellowish, lipid-rich luteal cells, forming the corpus luteum. These luteal cells secrete estrogens and progesterone.[13] If pregnancy does not occur, the corpus luteum begins to degenerate. These changes of the corpus luteum become apparent histologically 8 days after ovulation. The corpus luteum is eventually replaced by scar tissue, forming a corpus albicans. If implantation occurs, the corpus luteum persists till the placenta takes over the function of maintaining the pregnancy. In this situation, the corpus luteum is supported by human chorionic gonadotropin (hCG) that is produced by the developing embryo.

OTHER CHANGES

When these changes are happening in the ovary, the uterus prepares for the implantation of the embryo. The endometrium, which consists of glands and stroma, has a basal layer, an intermediate spongiosa layer, and a layer of compact epithelial cells that line the uterine cavity. The functionalis—the spongiosa and epithelial layers taken together is sloughed during menstruation. After menstruation, the endometrium is typically <2 mm thick with dense stroma and narrow, straight, tubular glands lined with low columnar epithelium. There is proliferation of endometrium under the influence of estrogen secreted by the ovarian follicles (proliferative phase). The mucosa thickens and the glands lengthen and coil. The secretory or luteal phase begins after ovulation. The length of this phase is the most constant, averaging 14 days, after which the corpus luteum degenerates. The endometrium, under the influence of estrogen and progesterone from the corpus luteum becomes more highly vascularized and slightly edematous. The glands become coiled and tortuous. All these changes facilitate successful implantation of the embryo.[14] The late follicular endometrium characteristically has a trilaminar pattern on transvaginal sonography, with hyperechoic basal and luminal layers and an intervening hypoechoic layer. After ovulation, the endometrium appears homogeneously echogenic.

In the absence of pregnancy, regression of the corpus luteum causes a fall in the levels of estrogen and progesterone. Progesterone withdrawal results in increased coiling and constriction of the spiral arterioles. Vasospasm leading to prostaglandin secretion along with appearance of areas of necrosis, this causes bleeding and sloughing of endometrium—menstruation. Menstrual blood contains both arterial and venous blood, with the former contributing nearly three quarters of all blood. It also contains tissue debris, desquamated endometrial tissue, inflammatory exudates, proteolytic enzymes and large quantities of fibrinolysin which prevents blood from clotting. Menstrual flow averages between four to six days, but the normal range in women can be from two to eight days. The average amount of menstrual blood loss is 30 mL and volumes greater than 80 mL is considered abnormal.

During the menstrual cycle, the quality and quantity of the mucus changes in the cervix. Immediately after menstruation, the cervical mucus is scant and viscous. During the proliferative phase of the cycle, under the influence of rising estradiol levels, there is an increase in cervical vascularity and edema. As a result, the cervical mucus becomes clear, copious and elastic. These changes promote the survival and transport of sperms. If spread on a slide, it dries in a palm-leaf arborizing, fern like pattern. This indicates increased sodium chloride in cervical mucus. At the time of ovulation, a drop of mucus can be stretched into a long, thin thread that may be 8–12 cm or more in length (spinnbarkeit). During the luteal phase, increasing progesterone levels make the cervical mucus thicker, less elastic and cellular. The fern pattern is now minimal or absent.

Early in the follicular phase, when estradiol levels are low, the vaginal epithelium is thin and pale. During the proliferative phase, the vaginal epithelium becomes cornified under the influence of estrogens. These cornified epithelial cells can be identified in the vaginal smear as they have vesicular nuclei and are basophilic. After ovulation, the epithelium proliferates and becomes infiltrated with leukocytes under the influence of progesterone. These vaginal cells have pyknotic nuclei and are acidophilic.

In the fallopian tubes, estrogens cause the proliferation of the glandular tissues and an increase in the number of ciliated epithelial cells. These cilia beat toward the uterus and thus helps propel the fertilized ovum in that direction. This action is enhanced by the presence of estrogens. Progesterone promotes increased secretion by the mucosal lining of the fallopian tubes. These secretions are necessary for nutrition of the fertilized, dividing ovum as it traverses the fallopian tube before implantation.

Cyclical changes occur in the breast due to the influence of hormones. Estrogens cause proliferation of mammary ducts, whereas progesterone causes growth of lobules and alveoli. Many women experience breast swelling, tenderness, and pain during the days preceding menstruation. This is probably due to distention of the ducts, hyperemia, and edema of the interstitial tissue of the breast. These physiological changes regress during menstruation.

MENOPAUSE

Menopause is the period of permanent cessation of menstruation, usually occurring between the ages of 45 and 55. The average age at onset of the menopause has been increasing since the end of the 19th century and is currently around 51 years. In India, the average age of menopause is 46 years.[15,16] It is usually defined as absence of menstrual periods for about one year. Prior to menopause, the menstrual cycle usually becomes irregular, and ovulation often fails to occur. After a few months to a few years, the cycle ceases altogether.

Menopause occurs as a result of exhaustion in the number of follicles in the ovaries. During a woman's life, about 400 of the primordial follicles grow into mature follicles and ovulate, and hundreds of thousands of ova degenerate. At the time of menopause, the ovaries no longer secrete progesterone and 17β-estradiol in appreciable quantities, and estrogen is formed only in small amounts by aromatization of androstenedione in peripheral tissues. When estrogen production falls below a critical value, the estrogens can no longer inhibit the production of the gonadotropins FSH and LH and they (mainly FSH) are produced after menopause in large and continuous quantities.

The loss of estrogens often causes marked physiological changes of which the most disturbing are the "hot flushes (hot flashes)" characterized by extreme flushing of the skin. Other symptoms include irritability, fatigue and anxiety. There is decreased strength and calcification of bones predisposing the woman to osteoporosis. Many of these symptoms can be ameliorated by estrogen supplementation.

REFERENCES

1. Gustafson ML, Donahoe PK. Male sex determination: current concepts of male sexual differentiation. Annu Rev Med. 1994;45:505-24.
2. Fiddler M, Abdel-Rahman B, Rappolee DA, et al. Expression of SRY transcripts in preimplantation human embryos. Am J Med Genet. 1995;55(1):80-4.
3. Baker TG. A quantitative and cytological study of germ cells in human ovaries. Proc R Soc Lond B Biol Sci. 1963;158:417-33.
4. Faddy MJ, Gosden RG, Gougeon A, et al. Accelerated disappearance of ovarian follicles in mid-life: implications for forecasting menopause. Hum Reprod. 1992;7(10):1342-6.
5. Chumlea WC, Schubert CM, Roche AF, et al. Age at Menarche and racial comparisons in US Girls. Pediatrics. 2003;111(1):110-3.
6. Pathak PK, Tripathi N, Subramanian SV. Secular trends in mencharcheal age in India-evidence from the Indian human development survey. PLoS One. 2014;9(11):e111027.
7. Hillier SG. Gonadotropic control of ovarian follicular growth and development. Mol Cell Endocrinol. 2001;179(1-2):39-46.
8. Wentz AC, Jones GS. Transient luteolytic effect of prostaglandin F2 alpha in the human. Obstet Gynecol. 1973;42(2):172-81.
9. Short RV. Steroids in the follicular fluid and the corpus luteum of the mare. A 'two-cell type' theory of ovarian steroid synthesis. J Endocrinol. 1962;24:59-63.
10. Haman JO. The length of the menstrual cycle. Am J Obstet Gynecol. 1942;43:870.
11. Chiazze L Jr, Brayer FT, Macisco JJ Jr, et al. The length and variability of the human menstrual cycle. JAMA 1968;203(6):377-80.
12. Macklon NS, Fauser BC. Follicle-stimulating hormone and advanced follicle development in the human. Arch Med Res. 2001;32(6):595-600.
13. Browning HC. The evolutionary history of the corpus luteum. Biol Reprod. 1973;8(2):128-57.
14. Markee JE. Menstruation in intraocular endometrial transplants in the rhesus monkey. Contr Embryol Carneg Instn. 1940;28:219-308.
15. Singh M. Early age of natural menopause in India, a biological marker for early preventive health programs. Climacteric. 2012;15(6):581-6.
16. Ahuja M. Age of menopause and determinants of menopause age: A PAN India survey by IMS. J Midlife Health. 2016;7(3):126-31.

CHAPTER 3

Male Infertility: Evaluation and Management

K Jayakrishnan, Aby K Koshy

Chapter outline

- Physiology
- Semen and its Analysis
- Sperm Function Tests
- History-taking and Examination
- Treatment
  - Medical Management
  - Surgical Management
- Intrauterine Insemination
- Donor Insemination
- Assisted Reproductive Technologies
- Azoospermia
- Level of Evidence
- Information Resources

INTRODUCTION

A gynecologist is often the first person to evaluate an infertile couple and is often expected to assess the male partner too. An understanding of the male reproductive function, its assessment and treatment modalities is expected of every practicing gynecologist.

The male partner may contribute to 30–40% cases of infertility and he may be solely responsible in 20% of cases.[1] Introduction of micromanipulation techniques in the last decade has revolutionized the way male infertility is treated.[2]

This chapter aims to brush up the readers understanding of the anatomy and physiology of the male reproductive system and the methods of evaluating it. This will be followed by a discussion on the treatment modalities.

PHYSIOLOGY

The male reproductive organs are influenced by hormones secreted in the hypothalamus and the pituitary. Gonadotropin releasing hormone (GnRH) is released from the medial basal hypothalamus in a pulsatile pattern approximately every 70-90 minutes. The half-life of GnRH is 2-5 minutes. GnRH release is inhibited by testosterone and inhibin. Its secretion is also decreased by corticotropin-releasing hormone (CRH) and opiates. This is clinically evident at times of illness and stress, when there is a decreased production of gonadotropins.

Follicle stimulating hormone (FSH) and luteinizing hormone (LH) are glycopeptides secreted by the gonadotrophs in the anterior pituitary in response to GnRH secretion. LH acts on the interstitial cells of Leydig to increase steroidogenesis (synthesis and secretion of testosterone and other androgens). LH release is controlled by the feedback of steroids from the testicle. FSH participates in protein synthesis and the initiation of spermatogenesis at the level of the seminiferous tubules in conjunction with testosterone. It stimulates the Sertoli cells to secrete inhibin. FSH release is controlled by the feedback of inhibin from the testicle. Androgens at physiological levels do not suppress FSH secretion. LH and FSH also control their own release by negative feedback to the hypothalamus. FSH binds to Leydig cells and increases the number of LH receptors on the cells.

Spermatogenesis occurs in the testes at the seminiferous tubules, which form most of the testis. Sertoli cells, which rest on the basement membrane of the seminiferous tubules, serve mainly to support, nourish and protect the developing germ cells. Spermatogonia undergo mitotic division to form the primary spermatocytes. They undergo meiotic division to form secondary spermatocytes. These secondary spermatocytes mature to become spermatids and undergo spermiogenesis to become spermatozoa. This involves casting excess cytoplasm away as a residual body, the formation of the acrosome and flagella, and the migration of cytoplasmic organelles to their final cellular location. These sperms travel to the epididymis before appearing in the ejaculate. Here they mature and acquire the capacity to fertilize. Sperms take around two to three weeks to traverse the epididymis. Sperms are stored near the tail portion and in the vas deferens until they are ejaculated. The whole process takes around 72–74 days. Semen is composed of secretions from the prostate, the vas deferens, the seminal vesicles, bulbourethral glands and the periurethral glands. The seminal vesicles contribute prostaglandins and fructose and are responsible for two-thirds of the volume of the ejaculate. The prostate contributes acid phosphatase, zinc and citric acid. Qualitative fructose is useful for verifying the presence of the vas deferens.

SEMEN AND ITS ANALYSIS

Semen is collected by masturbation after a period of abstinence of 2–3 days. A longer period of abstinence may show a lower sperm count. Semen should be collected in a wide mouthed, dry and clean container and should be brought to the laboratory within one hour of collection. Till then it should be kept at a temperature close to the body temperature. For those uncomfortable with collecting semen by masturbation, it should be collected in a nontoxic sheath. Condoms should not be used. The WHO reference values for semen analysis are described in Table 3.1.[3]

Semen consists of spermatozoa and seminal plasma from the accessory glands. Before being able to fertilize the ovum, liquefaction of semen, capacitation of sperm and the acrosome reaction must occur. Semen normally liquefies in 20–30 minutes. Semen might be abnormally viscid and may take a longer time for liquefaction. Analysis may be performed after repeatedly pushing the semen through a No. 19 needle. If the postcoital test is negative, such abnormal semen might be implicated as a cause for infertility and intrauterine insemination might be helpful.

Before going into the further parameters of a semen analysis, it must be understood that the World Health Organization (WHO) criteria are described as 'reference' values rather than 'normal' values. Variations in

Table 3.1: Semen analysis: Normal reference values (WHO, 2010).

Volume	1.5 mL
pH	>7.2
Sperm concentration	15 million/mL
Total sperm number	39 million/ejaculate
Percent motility (PR+NP %)	40% or PR:32%
Normal morphology	4%
Vitality	58% live spermatozoa
White blood cells	1 million/mL

PR: rapid progressive motility; NP: non-progressive motility
Grade B: Slow or sluggish progressive motility 30%; or 15% if based on strict morphological criteria

reports might be seen between samples from the same person, in the same sample when analyzed by two different persons and even when analyzed by the same person at two different occasions. Automated methods have not been able to correct this problem. Though computer-aided semen analysis (CASA) produces good qualitative data, it is a labor-intensive procedure that includes a high initial cost and is plagued with inaccuracies when sperm concentrations are very high or very low. Hence, it is important to understand that a better picture might be obtained only by repeated testing. Semen analysis is usually performed after an interval of two to four weeks, even though the optimal time for checking a second sample is at least three months after the initial study [III]. Another important aspect is that a person who has semen parameters below the 'normal' values might not be infertile and fertile men do occasionally have values in the 'abnormal' range. Individual tests evaluate only one aspect of a quality necessary for fertility and do not imply the ability or inability to achieve conception. Table 3.2 summarizes causes of abnormal semen parameters.

Assessment of sperm morphology may vary from one laboratory to another. Most andrology laboratories follow the 'strict' or the Tygerberg criteria[4] and that has been mentioned in the latest WHO recommendations.[3] Though it classifies even minor abnormalities as 'abnormal sperms,' it has a better correlation with fertilization and pregnancy rates at *in vitro* fertilization (IVF) and other assisted reproductive technology (ART) procedures.[4] Results were more reproducible when the strict criteria were adopted. When the routine criteria are followed, 30% or more sperms should be of normal morphology.

SPERM FUNCTION TESTS

Many tests have been used to study sperm function as a semen analysis gives an idea about the sperm quality only. Most tests try to assess a particular function of the sperm. These tests are more of academic interest and are not commonly performed even at specialized infertility centers; as most of them are cumbersome, do not provide a clear prognosis, may not be standardized and sometimes not very specific [IV]. The more important sperm function tests are elaborated in Table 3.3.

Intrauterine insemination is currently used for the treatment of infertility in unexplained as well as those due to immunological causes. Empirical treatment with corticosteroids is therefore not recommended now. Considering the above facts, testing for immunological causes of infertility itself is controversial.

HISTORY-TAKING AND EXAMINATION

A careful history might be useful in pointing out the cause for infertility. The duration of infertility and details regarding prior workup and treatment should be asked for. Enquiries regarding previous medical and surgical problems, chemotherapy, radiation, use of therapeutic and recreational drugs, smoking and alcohol intake should be made. Ask for any history of trauma or surgery to the testes and testicular involvement during mumps. It is also important to enquire about the sexual habits of the couple. The frequency of sexual intercourse and problems related to erection and ejaculation should be specifically asked or they are likely to be missed.

Following a general and systemic examination, local examination of the genitals should be performed. Look for anatomical abnormalities of the penis; presence, size, and consistency of the testicles and palpate the epididymis, vas deferens and the spermatic cord. To check for the presence of a varicocele, the patient should perform a Valsalva maneuver in the sitting and standing

Table 3.2: Abnormalities in semen parameters.

Parameter	Causes	Comments
Reduced semen volume	• Short period of abstinence • Spillage of sample • Retrograde ejaculation • Absence of the vas deferens or seminal vesicles • Ductal obstruction • Hypogonadotropism	• Postejaculation urine microscopy Transrectal USG • Hormonal evaluation
Increased semen volume	• Prolonged abstinence • Accessory gland inflammation • Contamination with urine	• Semen culture • Antibiotics
Semen that does not coagulate	• Ejaculatory duct obstruction • Absence of seminal vesicles	Transrectal USG Semen fructose
Reduced sperm concentration (oligospermia)	• Idiopathic (most common) • Accessory gland infection • Chemotherapy • Cryptorchidism	• Physical examination for varicocele • Antisperm antibody evaluation Hormonal analysis • Transrectal USG
Decreased motility (asthenospermia)	• Drugs • Endocrine • Environmental toxins • Epididymal causes	Toxins include pesticides, lead, carbon disulfide
Increased morphologically abnormal sperms (teratospermia)	• Increased scrotal temperature • Occupational • Radiation • Smoking • Systemic illnesses • Varicocele	Drugs which may affect semen parameters include spironolactone, cyproterone, ketoconazole, cimetidine, tetracycline, nitrofurantoin, sulfasalazine, colchicine, methadone, methotrexate, phenytoin, thioridazine and calcium channel blockers
Azoospermia	Obstructive azoospermia • Congenital bilateral absence of vas deferens (CBAVD) • Vasectomy • Infective causes Nonobstructive azoospermia • Klinefelter's syndrome • Young syndrome • Cryptorchidism • Chemotherapy • Radiation	• Examination • Serum FSH levels • Semen fructose • Karyotyping • Sperm centrifuged to verify azoospermia • Postejaculation urine (retrograde ejaculation) • Hormonal evaluation • Testicular biopsy (testicular failure) • Transrectal USG (ejaculatory duct obstruction) • CBAVD – evaluate for cystic fibrosis mutations and renal tract abnormality
Increased in WBCs	• Prostatitis • May be mistaken for immature sperm cells	Increased round cells may reflect poor prognosis of fertilization

(USU: ultrasonography; FSH; follicle stimulating hormone)

Table 3.3: Sperm function tests.

Sperm penetration assay (SPA) or zona free hamster oocyte test	Tests the ability of sperm to penetrate the egg. Patients with a poor SPA should proceed directly to ICSI
Human zona binding assay	Tests zona penetrating or zona binding ability of human sperm
Hypo-osmotic swelling test	Assessment of functional disturbance of the tail membrane to differentiate between viable but immotile sperm and dead sperm. Used clinically to select viable (but nonmotile) sperm for ICSI
Capacitation assay	To evaluate the ability of sperm to undergo capacitation, sperm that do not undergo capacitation portend a poor response to IVF, and ICSI should be considered
Acrosome reaction	Tests the ability of the sperm to undergo the acrosome reaction when exposed to inducing substances. Results correlate with IVF success; abnormal test require ICSI
Postcoital test	Effect of cervical mucus on sperm viability and function
Test for sperm antibodies	Immunobead test Mixed agglutination test (SpermMar)

(ICSI: intracytoplasmic sperm injection; IVF: *in vitro* fertilization)

positions in a warm room. Grade 1 varicocele is defined as one palpable only with Valsalva, while grade 2 is palpable at standing, and grade 3 is visible at rest.

TREATMENT

Encourage patients to stop smoking cigarettes [IIb] and to limit environmental exposures to harmful substances and/or conditions. Stress relief therapy and consultation of other appropriate psychological and social professionals may be advised. Broad management protocols are outlined first, management of specific conditions are elaborated latter.

Medical Management

Treatment of disorders diagnosed during evaluation should be undertaken. This would include correction of endocrine disorders like hyperprolactinemia, thyroid disorders, etc. Infections should be treated with antibiotics [Ib]. Counseling and medications like sildenafil may be required for patients with erectile dysfunction [Ia]. Retrograde ejaculation may be treated with imipramine or alfa-sympathomimetics, such as pseudoephedrine. If medical treatment of retrograde ejaculation fails, the use of penile electrovibration stimulation and sperm recovery from the urine can be considered.

A variety of empirical treatments has been used in an attempt to improve semen characteristics and fertility. The use of such medications for improving semen parameters is controversial. Clomiphene citrate which increases serum levels of FSH, LH and testosterone may improve the total sperm count, but has not yet been proven to increase pregnancy rates when compared with those who receive no treatment[5] [Ia]. The use of androgens like mesterolone and testosterone undecanoate has no difference when compared to placebo in the treatment of patients with oligoasthenospermia[6,7] [Ia]. Human chorionic gonadotropin has been used in a dose of 2500 IU twice weekly for 6–8 weeks in men with hypogonadism[8] [II] and those with isolated Leydig cell dysfunction.[9] Its use in normogonadotropic oligozoospermia though is not effective[10] [Ib]. Antioxidants like vitamins C and E, selenium and glutathione have shown some promise in improving semen parameters but further studies are required[11-13] [Ib]. Other commonly prescribed drugs like L carnitine, coenzyme Q derivatives, N acetyl cysteine and arginine may have shown improvement in semen parameters in some studies but good evidence regarding improvement in pregnancy rates is lacking.

Surgical Management

Surgical correction of penile deformities is sometimes required. The most common surgical procedure though is that for correcting a varicocele. A varicocele is an abnormal tortuosity and dilatation of the veins of the pampiniform plexus within the spermatic cord. It is more commonly seen in the left side, because of the insertion of the vein into the renal vein in contrast to the right side where it drains into the inferior vena cava. Varicoceles are seen in 20-40% of infertile males and in 10-15% of fertile men! Rise in testicular temperature, reflux of toxic metabolites from the renal vein and germ cell hypoxia have been attributed to varicoceles as a cause of infertility. Surgical correction by open or laparoscopic routes is possible. Whether surgery results in higher fertility is controversial. Studies showing improvement in fertility[14,15] and no differences abound.[16-21] Though evidence-based on clinical trials lacks support for varicocelectomy [Ia], most clinicians will recommend surgical correction, if varicoceles are diagnosed by examination.[22] Those diagnosed purely by scrotal ultrasound probably will not benefit by surgical correction.

Men who desire to have children after a vasectomy may be offered a microsurgical vasovasostomy or vasoepididymostomy. Success rates for couples with female partner aged 40 or older was lower than for those with the female partner aged 39 or younger (14% vs 56%).[23] Patients with a known or suspected obstruction of the ejaculatory ducts may be eligible for a transurethral resection of the ejaculatory ducts (TURED) [III]. Recovery and cryopreservation of spermatozoa for use in assisted reproduction should be considered during surgical reconstruction to avoid a second surgical procedure at a later date.

Intrauterine Insemination

This involves placement of processed semen into the uterine cavity. Intrauterine insemination (IUI) allows the sperm to be placed past the inhospitable cervical mucus and increases the chance of natural fertilization. IUI involves placement of 0.3-0.5 mL of semen which is processed by various techniques using a very thin flexible catheter via the transcervical route into the uterine cavity. IUI is indicated in male factor infertility, in those with antisperm antibodies, infertility due to cervical factors and in cases of unexplained infertility. Placement of unprocessed semen into the uterine cavity is not practiced as prostaglandins and proteins in semen can cause uterine cramping and occasionally allergic reactions.

Processing of semen aims to obtain a sperm population of uniform morphology and good motility, devoid of dead sperm, miscellaneous cellular elements and seminal plasma which is resuspended in a medium. The commonly used methods are described. In conventional washing, semen is washed and centrifuged in commercial media, the supernatant discarded and the pellet overlaid with media again. This process may be repeated 2-3 times. After the final wash, the pellet is resuspended in media and used for IUI. Such a technique is used with near normal samples. Alternatively in the swim-up technique, following sperm preparation by the conventional method, the tube is incubated and sperms 'swim-up' from the pellet to the overlaying media, which is then used for insemination. Such inseminates have lesser levels of contamination from dead sperms and cellular debris. The gradient method involves centrifugation through a dense liquid phase (density gradient). Commercially available gradient media are overlaid with semen and subjected to centrifugation. Motile sperm cells migrate to the bottom of the tube, which are used for IUI after further washing. The swim up and gradient density techniques have better results than the conventional method, the gradient density technique being used when the sperm concentration is lower and the number of dead and abnormal cells are high.

The IUI is usually combined with superovulation in the female partner [Ib]. Follicular monitoring with transvaginal sonography is followed by an ovulation trigger with human choronic gonadotropin (hCG). Some centers time IUI after a natural LH surge demonstrated on a urinary LH kit.

Protocols regarding timing and number of IUIs performed vary. When a single IUI is performed, it may be performed after 36 hours after the administration of hCG. Those centers which advocate two IUIs usually spaced at least 12 hours apart between 24 hours and 48 hours after the hCG. Both protocols have their advocates, with studies showing either no difference in pregnancy rates[24,25] or a significant increase.[26] The Cochrane review states that double IUI showed no significant benefit over single intrauterine insemination in the treatment of subfertile couples with husband semen [Ia].[27]

Success rates per cycle in various studies vary from 8% to 30%. Variables which determine success rates depend on semen parameters (total number of sperms per inseminate and morphology), method of preparation, age and presence of uterine, tubal or ovarian pathology in the female partner and the use of medications for superovulation.[28-30] IUI is more successful in unexplained infertility than in pure male factor infertility. A couple may be offered 3-6 cycles of superovulation with IUI before moving to ARTs. Generally, IUIs are performed, if the total inseminate contains more than one million sperms. If this is not achieved, an early recourse to intracytoplasmic sperm injection (ICSI) should be made.

Donor Insemination

Therapeutic donor insemination (TDI) is useful in patients with azoospermia or severe oligospermia, when ICSI is not possible or desired. This may be in cases of nonobstructive azoospermia; when there is a possibility of a disease being transmitted from the male partner (inherited, sexually transmitted) or due to financial reasons.

Donor semen available from sperm banks should be collected from healthy young donors after screening by history and appropriate laboratory test for transmittable diseases (HIV, hepatitis B, hepatitis C, syphilis, gonorrhea, chlamydia, and cytomegalovirus) [IV]. Semen thus obtained is cryopreserved. Tests which may become positive after an incubation period should be repeated and only then semen should be made available for TDI (e.g. HIV, which should be tested after 6 months). A freeze and thaw cycle results in sperms which are of an inferior quality compared to a fresh sample [Ib]. Success rates up to 30% per cycle have been reported. TDI may be performed for 6-12 months [III]. If conception does not occur, the female partner should be assessed.

Assisted Reproductive Technologies

Assisted reproductive technologies (ARTs) involves fertilization of the human oocyte by human sperm *in vivo*. In IVF, oocytes are obtained following controlled ovarian hyperstimulation followed by ultrasound-guided transvaginal aspiration. Semen is washed in a way similar to that before an IUI and 50,000 to 100,000 capacitated sperms are placed in culture with a single oocyte. Fertilization is assessed after 16–20 hours and embryos are transferred into the uterine cavity between days 2 and 5.

In vitro fertilization (IVF) was very useful in cases of male factor infertility, but what really revolutionized treatment in severe male factor infertility was ICSI. This involves micromanipulation techniques to inject a viable sperm into the ooplasm of the egg. After cumulus and corona cell removal (denudation), oocytes are used for microinjection. ICSI is carried out on metaphase II oocytes. Motile sperms are selected and immobilized under an inverted microscope equipped with micromanipulators and microinjectors. The microinjectors are used to either fix or release the oocyte with the holding pipette, or to aspirate and inject a spermatozoon with the injection pipette. The oocyte is held in position by means of minimal suction by the holding pipette. The oocyte is manipulated so that the polar body is located at the six o'clock position, which avoids damage to the spindle. The oolemma is ruptured using the injection needle and the sperm is released into the oocyte (Fig. 3.1). ICSI is also useful in azoospermia when sperm can be retrieved from the testes or the epididymis. Sperms can be collected from the epididymis by microsurgical epididymal sperm aspiration (MESA) or percutaneous epididymal sperm aspiration (PESA). The latter might be a less invasive procedure, but the number of sperms obtained is less and pregnancy rates slightly lower [III]. Testicular sperm is obtained by open microsurgical testicular sperm extraction (TESE) or testicular sperm aspiration (TESA). Both open procedures might provide for more quantity of sperms which can be cryopreserved for future use. Fresh and frozen-thawed spermatozoa appear to have comparable fertilization and ongoing pregnancy rates when used for ICSI. Fertilization and pregnancy rates in pure male factor infertility depends on the etiology. The rates are lower in patients with testicular when compared to post-testicular causes.

An area of concern has been about the possibility of congenital malformation in children conceived following ART. Current evidence confirms the higher risk of major malformations in IVF and ICSI children in comparison to spontaneously conceived children, but there was no significant difference in the risk when IVF and ICSI were compared.

Azoospermia

Absence of sperm in the ejaculate is seen in 1% of all men.[31] Azoospermia has been traditionally classified into 'obstructive' and 'nonobstructive'. Because of overlapping and confusion with respect to certain etiologies, azoospermia is currently divided into causes due to deficient hormonal stimulation of the testis, testicular dysfunction, and seminal ducts obstruction or dysfunction— pretesticular, testicular, and post-testicular causes respectively (Table 3.4).[32]

Management of azoospermia depends on the cause. In pretesticular azoospermia, low levels of gonadotropins (LH and FSH) and testosterone are seen. Treatment involves

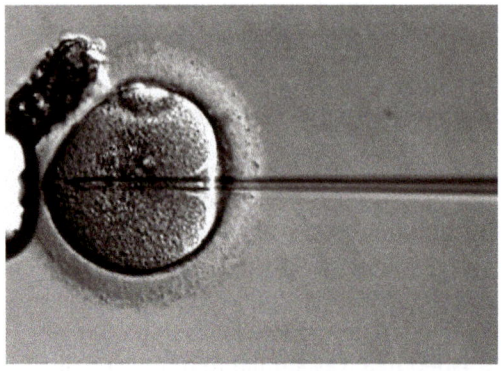

Fig. 3.1: Intracytoplasmic sperm injection.

Table 3.4: Causes of azoospermia.

Types	Causes
Pretesticular	• Hypogonadotropic hypogonadism • Congenital (Kallmann's syndrome, Noonan syndrome) • Acquired (trauma, tumor) • Idiopathic
Testicular	• Congenital (Klinefelter's syndrome, Y-deletion) • Acquired (radiotherapy, chemotherapy, torsion, mumps, orchitis) • Developmental (testicular maldescent)
Post-testicular	• Ductal obstruction • Dysfunction (retrograde ejaculation)

pulsatile GnRH therapy or sequential therapy with hCG (1,000-2,500 IU twice a week) followed by human menopausal gonadotropin (hMG) (150 IU three times weekly) after serum testosterone and estradiol levels are back in the normal range. In testicular azoospermia, LH and FSH levels are elevated and serum levels of testosterone are low. Testicular biopsy and karyotyping is indicated. Testicular azoospermia can be treated, if spermatozoa are obtained from the testes for ICSI. ICSI is also indicated in post-testicular azoospermia. Exceptions include patients who have undergone vasectomy who can initially opt for a reversal surgical procedure; and in retrograde ejaculation, where sperms obtained from urine can be used for IUI or ART depending on the yield. Truly azoospermic patients should be evaluated for ejaculatory duct obstruction by transrectal ultrasound (TRUS). A TRUS is indicated in patients with azoospermia or severe oligospermia to rule out a complete or partial ejaculatory duct obstruction. TRUS is also useful to evaluate for the presence or absence of the seminal vesicles. Those patients with ejaculatory duct obstruction are candidates for transurethral resection of the ejaculatory ducts.

LEVEL OF EVIDENCE

Ia. Systematic review and meta-analysis of randomized controlled trials.
Ib. At least one randomized controlled trial.
IIa. At least one well-designed controlled study without randomization.
IIb. At least one other type of well-designed quasi-experimental study.
III. Well-designed nonexperimental descriptive studies, such as comparative studies, correlation studies or case studies.
IV. Expert committee reports or opinions and/or clinical experience of respected authorities.

INFORMATION RESOURCES

1. Indian Council of Medical Research, National Academy of Medical Sciences (India). National guidelines for accreditation, supervision and regulation of ART clinics in India. New Delhi: Ministry of Health and Family Welfare, Government of India; 2005. [Guidelines for ART clinics in India]
2. www.icmr.nic.in/art/Chapter_4.pdf [consent forms for IUI/TDI and IVF]

REFERENCES

1. Thonneau P, Marchand S, Tallec A, et al. Incidence and main causes of infertility in a resident population (1,850,000) of three French regions (1988-1989). Hum Reprod. 1991;6:811-6.
2. Palermo G, Joris H, Devroey P, et al. Pregnancies after intracytoplasmic injection of single spermatozoon into an oocyte. Lancet. 1992;340:17-8.
3. World Health Organization. WHO Laboratory Manual for the Examination of Human Semen and Sperm Cervical Mucus Interaction.

Cambridge: Cambridge University Press, 2000.
4. Kruger TF, Menkveld R, Stander FS, et al. Sperm morphologic features as a prognostic factor in *in vitro* fertilization. Fertil Steril. 1986;46:1118-23.
5. World Health Organization. A double-blind trial of clomiphene citrate for the treatment of idiopathic male infertility. Int J Androl 1992;7:1067-72.
6. Gerris J, Comhaire F, Hellemans P, et al., Placebo controlled trial of high-dose Mesterolone treatment of idiopathic male infertility. Fertil Steril. 1991;55:603-7.
7. Mesterolone and idiopathic male infertility: a double-blind study. World Health Organization Task Force on the Diagnosis and Treatment of Infertility. Int J Androl. 1989;12:254-64.
8. Efficacy and safety of highly purified urinary follicle-stimulating hormone with human chorionic gonadotropin for treating men with isolated hypogonadotropic hypogonadism. European Metrodin HP Study Group. Fertil Steril. 1998;70:256-62.
9. Yamamoto M, Hibi H, Katsuno S, et al. Human chorionic gonadotropin adjuvant therapy for patients with Leydig cell dysfunction after varicocelectomy. Arch Androl. 1995;35:49-55.
10. Schill WB, Jungst D, Unterburger P, et al. Combined hMG/hCG treatment in subfertile men with idiopathic normogonadotrophic oligozoospermia. Int J Androl. 1982;5:467-77.
11. Scott R, MacPherson A, Yates RW, et al. The effect of oral selenium supplementation on human sperm motility. Br J Urol. 1998;82:76-80.
12. Suleiman SA, Ali ME, Zaki ZM, et al. Lipid peroxidation and human sperm motility: protective role of vitamin E. J Androl. 1996;17:530-7.
13. Lenzi A, Culasso F, Gandini L, et al. Placebo controlled, double-blind, cross-over trial of glutathione therapy in male infertility. Hum Reprod. 1993;8:1657-62.
14. Madgar I, Weissenberg R, Lunenfeld B, et al. Controlled trial of high spermatic vein ligation for varicocele in infertile men. Fertil Steril. 1995;63:120-4.
15. Matthews GJ, Matthews ED, Goldstein M. Induction of spermatogenesis and achievement of pregnancy after microsurgical varicocelectomy in men with azoospermia and severe oligoasthenospermia. Fertil Steril. 1998;70:71-5.
16. Baker HWG, Burger HG, de Kretser DM, et al. Testicular vein ligation and fertility in men with varicoceles. Br Med J. 1985;291:1678-80.
17. Kamischke A, Nieschlag E. Analysis of medical treatment of male infertility. Hum Reprod. 1999;14(Suppl 1):1-23.
18. Nilsson S, Edvinsson A, Nilsson B. Improvement of semen and pregnancy rate after ligation and division of the internal spermatic vein: fact or fiction? Br J Urol. 1979;51:591-6.
19. Breznik R, Vlaisavljevic V, Borko E. Treatment of varicocele and male infertility. Arch Androl. 1993;30:157-60.
20. Yamamoto M, Hibi H, Hirata Y, et al. Effects of varicocelectomy on sperm parameters and pregnancy rate in patients with subclinical varicocele: a randomized prospective controlled study. J Urol. 1996;155:1636-8.
21. Nieschlag E, Hertle L, Fischedick A, et al. Update on treatment of varicocele: counseling as effective as occlusion of the vena spermatica. Hum Reprod. 1998;13:2147-50.
22. Agarwal A, Deepinder F, Cocuzza M, et al. Efficacy of varicocelectomy in improving semen parameters: new meta-analytical approach. Urology. 2007;70:532-8.
23. Gerrard ER Jr, Sandlow JI, Oster RA, et al. Effect of female partner age on pregnancy rates after vasectomy reversal. Fertil Steril. 2007;87:1340-4.
24. Ransom MX, Blotner MB, Bohrer M, et al. Does increasing frequency of intrauterine insemination improve pregnancy rates significantly during superovulation cycles? Fertil Steril. 1994;61:303-7.
25. Alborzi S, Motazedian S, Parsanezhad ME, et al. Comparison of the effectiveness of single intrauterine insemination (IUI) versus double IUI per cycle in infertile patients. Fertil Steril. 2003;80:595-9.
26. Ragni G, Maggioni P, Guermandi E, et al. Efficacy of double intrauterine insemination

27. Cantineau AEP, Heineman MJ, Cohlen BJ. Single versus double intrauterine insemination (IUI) in stimulated cycles for subfertile couples. Cochrane Database Syst Rev 2003;(1):CD003854.
28. Sunde A, Kahn J, Molne K. Intrauterine insemination: A European collaborative report. Hum Reprod. 1988;3 (Suppl 2):69-73.
29. Guzick DS, Carson SA, Coutifaris C, et al. Efficacy of superovulation and intrauterine insemination in the treatment of infertility. for the National Cooperative Reproductive Medicine Network. New Engl J Med. 1999;340:177-83.
30. Botchan A, Hauser R, Gamzu R, et al. Results of 6139 artificial insemination cycles with donor spermatozoa. Hum Reprod. 2001;16:2298-2304.
31. Willott GM. Frequency of azoospermia. Forensic Sci Int. 1982;20:9-10.
32. Sharif K. Reclassification of azoospermia: the time has come? Hum Reprod. 2000;15:237-8.

CHAPTER 4

Recurrent Pregnancy Losses in Assisted Reproduction

HJA Carp

Chapter outline

- Causes of Recurrent Pregnancy Loss and Infertility
  - Abnormal Embryo
  - Antiphospholipid Syndrome
  - Alloimmune Factors
- Prognosis
  - Investigation Protocol
- Treatment
  - Progesterone Supplementation
  - hCG Supplementation
- Aspirin
- Heparin
- Immunoglobulin
- Assisted Reproductive Technology as Treatment of Recurrent Pregnancy Loss
  - Pregestational Screening
  - Gamete Donation
  - Surrogacy

INTRODUCTION

Although recurrent pregnancy loss (RPL) is a different condition to infertility, there is an association between the two conditions. There may be similar causes, one affects the prognosis of the other, and often treatment which is used for one may be used to treat the other. Concurrent infertility is found in 32% of RPL patients. In the author's database of 2500 patients with RPL, 74 patients were referred to assisted reproductive technology (ART) for subsequent infertility. Similarly, 182 ART patients have been assessed with RPL after ART. The incidence of missed abortion is 15 percent after ART (Schieve et al. 2003), which does not appear to be increased above that of the general population. This chapter will examine the influence of one condition on the other.

CAUSES OF RECURRENT PREGNANCY LOSS AND INFERTILITY

Both RPL and infertility may be caused by embryonic abnormalities or a hostile maternal environment. Table 4.1 shows the generally accepted causes of both conditions.

Abnormal Embryo

Structural malformations may cause pregnancy loss presenting as miscarriage. Embryoscopy has shown developmental defects in 200/233 missed abortions (85%) (Philipp et al., 2003), including: anencephaly, encephalocele, spina bifida, syndactyly, pseudosyndactyly, polydactyly, cleft hand and cleft lip. However, as 70% of miscarriages are blighted ova in which ultrasound only

Table 4.1: Causes of infertility and pregnancy loss.

Recurrent pregnancy loss	Implantation failure
Abnormal embryo	Abnormal embryo
Structural anomalies incompatible with life	Chromosomal anomalies
Chromosomal anomalies	
Hostile maternal environment	Hostile maternal environment
Uterine	Endocrine
APS	Defects in endometrial receptivity
Thrombophilia	
Alloimmune	
Infection	
Endocrine	

APS: antiphospholipid antibody syndrome

visualizes empty sac, it is often impossible to detect these malformations if present. In implantation failure, there can be no structural malformations.

Embryonic chromosomal aberrations may be responsible for both RPL and infertility. Five reports have assessed chromosomal aberrations in recurrent miscarriage and have reported that 19–60% of abortuses are chromosomally abnormal in women with recurrent miscarriage. The incidence is inversely proportional to the number of miscarriages, and rises with maternal age. The possibility of chromosomally aberrant chromosomes has also been assesses in ART using pregestational diagnosis (PGD) techniques. About 29% of embryos which appear morphologically normal have been found to be chromosomally abnormal (Munne et al., 1995). Even in those embryos developing to blastocysts, 29% have been reported to be mosaic.

Rubio et al. (2003) have described the effect of different chromosomal abnormalities on embryo development. Only 20.2% of autosomal monosomies developed into blastocysts, whereas embryos with monosomy X developed similarly to normal embryos. Trisomies also impaired embryo development, only 34.7% formed blastocysts. Most haploid embryos arrested before cavitation, and triploid and tetraploid embryos had lower rates of development to the blastocyst stage. Hence, the more severe cases of aneuploidy might be more likely to present clinically as infertility, and the less severe aneuploidies may present as recurrent miscarriage.

Antiphospholipid Syndrome

Antiphospholipid antibodies (aPL) such as lupus anticoagulant and anticardiolipin antibodies are associated with RPL. There is also evidence that additional antibodies may be associated with both pregnancy loss and infertility. In RPL, fetal demise is thought to be secondary to thrombosis in the small vessels of the placenta. Women with antiphospholipid antibody syndrome (APS) are at a high risk for pre-eclampsia, intrauterine growth retardation, fetal distress, stillbirth, and maternal autoimmune phenomena. Today, aPL are also known to have their effects by binding to trophoblast, inhibiting trophoblast differentiation "*in vitro*", invasiveness and human choriomic gonadotropin (hCG) secretion. Hence, the question arises whether aPL may also be involved in infertility. Bakimer et al. (1992), immunized BALB/c mice with human monoclonal anticardiolipin antibodies (aCA). Lower fecundity rate after immunization (21% vs. 48%) (P < .005). Shoenfeld et al. (2006) found a significantly higher prevalence of aPL in infertile patients (OR = 5.11, CI 1.18–25.35). Although there are reports of increased prevalences of aPL in prolonged infertility and IVF failure, the American Society of Reproductive Medicine has issued a practice bulletin in 1999 on this issue based on a systematic review. The clinical pregnancy and live birth rates were

57% and 46% respectively, in the aPL positive patients, compared with 49.2% and 42.9%, respectively, in the aPL negative patients. The bulletin concluded that aPL testing is not warranted in patients undergoing *in-vitro* fertilization (IVF), and treatment is not indicated in seropositive patients. The same conclusion was drawn by Hornstein et al. (2000), after a meta-analysis of studies which assessed aPL and IVF success.

However, there are other aPL in addition to anticardiolipin antibodies and lupus anticoagulant. Antiphosphatidyl ethanolamine and antiphosphatidyl serine antibodies may be relevant in IVF failure. Antiphosphatidyl ethanolamine antibodies may be risk factor for early fetal losses and infertility as they affect trophoblast formation. Antiphosphatidyl serine antibodies may be induced when phosphatidyl serine is exteriorized due to apoptosis.

Alloimmune Factors

Alloimmune factors such as cytokines and natural killer (NK) cells, have been linked to both RPL and infertility. NK cells physiologically accumulate in the decidua in the first trimester of pregnancy. Their role may be immunosurveillance, mediation of angiogenesis or remodeling of spiral arteries to uteroplacental arteries. NK cells are part of the innate immune system. Their response is not dependent on recognizing a specific antigen. Although the trophoblast is semi-allogeneic and contains foreign paternal antigens, NK cells do not normally attack the trophoblast. However, if NK cells become activated by cytokines, they can attack the trophoblast causing apoptosis. Increased numbers of NK cells have been found in the peripheral blood of patients with RPL (Emmer et al, 2000). Additionally, increased concentrations of NK cells have been found in luteal phase endometrial biopsies in RPL (Clifford et al., 2000). Aoki et al. (1995) first described the clinical relevance of NK cells in 68 women with 2 or more miscarriages, and compared them to 47 control patients. The patients with high NK activity had a 71% abortion rate compared to 20% in the low NK activity patients. They also tended to abort genetically normal embryos. Only 17% of aborted embryos had karyotypic aberrations, compared to 60% in women with low number of NK cells. Coulam and Beaman (1995) have reported that when NK cells are above 12% of total lymphocytes, there is an 87% predictive value for a pregnancy loss. These patients also tend to lose genetically normal embryos as opposed to the women with normal NK cells who lose genetically abnormal embryos.

Cytokines can mediate NK cell activity. TNFα can activate NK cells to attack the trophoblast. NK mediated attack can lead to implantation failure or pregnancy loss. TGFB$_2$ inhibits NK activation. In addition to the action on NK cells, cytokines affect each stage of implantation and embryonic development. There are cytokines preventing implantation such as IL-18, and cytokines which are essential for implantation, such as leukemia inhibitory factor (LIF). LIF also influences cytotrophoblast differentiation and invasion, as does IL-3. IL-15 increases trophoblast invasion, modulates MMP-1 and maintains uterine NK cells. Vascular endothelial growth factor (VEGF) is responsible for establishing the blood supply to the developing conceptus. There are cytokines affecting trophoblast proliferation such as GM-CSF, and TGFβ. Epidermal growth factor (EGF) affects hormone secretion (hPL and hCG) by the trophoblast. IFNγ influences the remodeling of spiral arteries to uteroplacental arteries. IL-4 and IL-10 inhibit coagulation. Coagulation is enhanced by TNFα and IL-6. Therefore, it can be seen that the right cytokine balance is essential for both implantation, hormonal secretion in pregnancy, maintenance of blood supply, and prevention of excessive coagulation. All of these may present as infertility or pregnancy loss.

Antiphospholipid antibodies also act through cytokines. IL-3 and IFNγ are decreased in automune polyendocrine syndrome (APS). TNFα and IL-6 are elevated in APS.

PROGNOSIS

As stated above, the incidence of missed abortion is 15% after ART (Schieve et al., 2003). This incidence is not greater to that of the general population; hence the prognostic factors affecting the outcome of pregnancy after RPL are the same as RPL without ART. The prognosis varies according to the following features, each of which increases the chance of another miscarriage—advanced maternal age, a higher number of previous miscarriages, primary (all pregnancies have terminated as miscarriage), as opposed to secondary abortions (live birth followed by a string of miscarriages), concurrent infertility, and a previous eukaryotypic abortion (Carp, 2001 a). The number of previous miscarriages seems to be the most important predictive factor. Concurrent infertility is a predictive factor, worsening the prognosis. Concurrent infertility refers to RPL patients who develop infertility, and who may or may not require ART. This is a different group of patients to those described by Schieve et al. (2003), who are ART patients who have one subsequent missed abortion.

Investigation Protocol

An investigation protocol should indicate the investigations required to reach a diagnosis. There is however, disagreement when investigation should commence. The American College of Obstetricians and Gynecologists practice bulletin states that women with two miscarriages should be investigated, however, the Royal College and ESHRE suggest that investigation be reserved for patients with three or more pregnancy losses. The author uses a different approach depending on whether the prognosis is good, medium or poor. The different approaches for different patients have been published elsewhere (Carp, 2007). In brief, "Good Prognosis Patients" refers to young women with two or three first trimester miscarriages. They probably require little investigation or treatment. However, they do require supportive care. In the event of another miscarriage, further investigations should be performed including fetal karyotyping. It is doubtful if "good prognosis" patients require pharmacological support.

"Medium Prognosis Patients" are those with three or four miscarriages. The prognosis is approximately 60% for a live birth after three miscarriages (40% after four miscarriages). Treatment should be based on the cause. However, despite extensive investigations, the cause may remain elusive. The author assesses the uterus by hysteroscopy or three dimensional ultrasound, if these investigations have not been performed for infertility. An autoantibody screen for antinuclear antibody, B_2-glycoprotein 1 dependent anticardiolipin antibody and lupus anticoagulant is performed, together with screening for the hereditary thrombophilias. Thyroid function and a glucose challenge test are ordered if indicated. Treatment is usually empiric. If there is a uterine septum, it can be resected. Ogasawara et al. (2009), showed in a case control study that uterine anomalies impacted on progression of normal pregnancies. If aPL or hereditary thrombophilias are present anticoagulants such as low molecular weight heparins are effective and safe. Hormone supplements such as hCG are also used empirically if there is no hyperstimulation after ART.

We define "Poor Prognosis Patients" as those with five or more miscarriages. They are poorly described in the literature, and have been assessed in few trials. These patients have usually had extensive investigations and empirical treatment. After five or more miscarriages, the likelihood of fetal chromosomal aberrations is less than after three miscarriages. In these patients, we perform alloimmune testing including a cytotoxic cross match between maternal serum and paternal cells to detect antipaternal complement dependent antibodies (APCA) and possibly assessment of NK cells. In poor prognosis patients in whom other forms of treatment have failed intravenous immunoglobulin can be effective (Carp et al., 2001 b).

TREATMENT

Similar treatment regimens are often used for both RPL and ART. Additionally ART is often used as a means of treatment for RPL. However, all forms of treatment are empirical if the karyotype of the embryo is unknown. Some of these treatment regimens are described below.

Progesterone Supplementation

Progesterone supplementation has been used for over fifty years to prevent miscarriage. The logic of progesterone support is based on the premise that lutectomy causes abortion if performed prior to seven weeks of gestation. Mifepristone blocks progesterone receptors, leading to fetal death and placental separation. Hence, a defective corpus luteum may produce insufficient levels of progesterone, for endometrial ripening, implantation or placentation. Progesterone enhances implantation and affects cytokine balance (inhibits IFNγ and TNFα production, and increases levels of IL-4). Additionally, progesterone inhibits NK activity at the fetomaternal interface, inhibits the release of arachidonic acid, favors the production of asymmetric, pregnancy-protecting antibodies and prevents myometrial contractility. Although progesterone supplementation is widely used routinely in most IVF programs, a large meta-analysis of data from 11 placebo controlled trials (Haas and Ramsey, 2009) concluded that there is no evidence to support routine use of progestogen to prevent miscarriage in early to mid-pregnancy. In RPL, Daya (1989) reported in a meta-analysis of three studies that progesterone supplementation was associated with a statistically significant increase in the live birth rate (OR = 3.09, CI, 1.28–7.52). However, the three trials in the meta-analysis were performed between 1953-1964. At that time there was no early ultrasound screening available; hence, progesterone may have been administered to patients with nonviable pregnancies, raising doubts about the meta-analysis' validity today.

There are also other arguments against progesterone supplementation. Diagnosis is usually by endometrial biopsy two days prior to menstruation and histologically dated. If the histology lags more than two days behind the chronological age luteal deficiency is thought to occur. However, if dating is determined by ultrasonic monitoring of follicular size and biopsy timed to 12 days later, the incidence is only 4% (Peters et al., 1992). Plasma progesterone levels are an unreliable test of luteal function as progesterone is secreted in a pulsatile fashion, and blood may be drawn at a pulse peak or nadir. Additionally, low progesterone levels may be a sign of failing pregnancy from chromosomal or other disorders. Progesterone is often used for luteal support in ART. If RPL follows ART, progesterone supplementation will not be appropriate treatment.

hCG Supplementation

Human chorionic gonadotropin (hCG) supplementation is often used in RPL. It is the only treatment for RPL described to have an effect in the Cochrane database (Scott and Pattison, 2000). When hCG supplementation is used, Scott and Pattison's systematic review (2000) showed a statistically significant benefit of 26.3%, (OR for miscarriage = 0.26, CI 0.14–0.52).

The hCG has numerous actions in pregnancy. Regular hCG stimulates the corpus luteum to secrete, progesterone, relaxin and prostaglandin E2 production. hCG influences TNFα and IL-6 secretion. The hyperglycosylated form of hCG is autocrine acting on the trophoblast to increase invasiveness. hCG is involved in differentiation of endometrial stromal cells to decidua, regulates smooth muscle cell gap junctions in the pregnant human myometrium inhibiting myometrial contractions, and hCG promotes angiogenesis via up regulation of VEGF. hCG also has immunoregulatory roles, including the prevention of T-cell activation at maternal-fetal interface. hCG influences the secretion of TNFα, IL-6, IL-1β and IL-2. However, it is interesting to note that all trials of hCG have used urinary derived hCG rather than the newer recombinant form. Urinary hCG contains Leukemia inhibitory bactor (LIF) which regulates trophoblast differentiation, and is essential for implantation. hCG is not usually used in ART cycles except for inducing luteinization of the follicle approximately 36 hours prior to ovum pick up. There are a few reports of using hCG for ovum ripening, but the effect has not been assessed on RPL. hCG supplementation cannot be used if ovarian hyperstimulation occurs after ART as hCG will worsen the effects of hyperstimulation.

In the authors series (unpublished), in "poor prognosis" patients with five or more recurrent miscarriages, there was an absolute benefit 34% after using hCG, which is statistically significant, (OR = 4.33, 95% CI 1.7–11.3).

Aspirin

Aspirin has been used as a fertility inducing agent. However, the literature is divided on the efficacy of aspirin in improving uterine blood flow or pregnancy rates. A recent meta-analysis by Daya et al. (2006), stated that, "Given the lack of efficacy and the potential for harmful effects to both the patient and her offspring, low-dose aspirin should not be administered to infertile women undergoing treatment with assisted reproduction". Aspirin is also in wide use for treating APS, where combined with heparin it forms standard treatment. However, there is not one single report in the literature which shows that aspirin has any beneficial effect. There are three papers which have compared the use of aspirin to placebo. Not one of the three papers showed aspirin to have any effect on the subsequent live birth rate. The three papers have been combined in a meta-analysis (Empson et al., 2002), which also showed aspirin to have no effect on the live birth rate. There is only one prospective randomized trial of aspirin for the prevention of miscarriage in unexplained RPL (Tulppala et al., 1997). Twenty seven women were randomized to receive aspirin, and 27 received placebo. There was no difference in the live birth rate, or the incidence of late obstetric complications. The authors concluded, "Low dose aspirin is ineffective in the prevention of miscarriage in recurrent spontaneous abortion".

Heparin

Heparin and the low molecular weight heparins have anticoagulant effects, and are therefore widely used in the antiphospholipid syndrome, and have come into use in hereditary thrombophilias when associated with RPL. In antiphospholipid syndrome a meta-analysis of three trials which compared the effect of aspirin to aspirin with the addition of heparin showed a common odds ratio of 2.63 in favor of heparin (95% CI 1.46–4.75) (Carp, 2004). Heparin also improves the live birth rate in hereditary thrombophilias (Carp et al., 2003).

In addition to the anticoagulant effects, heparins have anti-inflammatory effects. Heparins inhibit TNFα production, and increase serum TNFα binding protein, thereby protecting against the systemic harmful manifestations of TNFα. Heparin inhibits apoptosis of villous trophoblast induced by IFNγ and TNFα. Thrombosis results in vein wall inflammatory response. Heparin limits the anti-inflammatory response. *In vitro*, heparin restores ability of trophoblast to secrete hCG, which is inhibited by aPL. Due to the theoretical possibility that the anti-inflammatory effects of heparin may be relevant in unexplained RPL, heparin has been assessed in unexplained recurrent pregnancy loss. In the author's study (Dolitzky et al., 2006), 104 patients were randomized to receive either enoxaparin or aspirin. The live birth rate was similar in both groups of pateints (RR = 1.10; CI, 0.63-1.92). As aspirin is ineffective, enoxaparin offered no additional advantage.

Immunoglobulin

Intravenous immunoglobulin (IVIg) has been used for its immune modulating effects in both RPL and to increase the implantation rate after numerous cycles of ART. IVIg modulates antigen presentation, and B and T lymphocyte function. IVIg inhibits the action of antibodies by either the interaction of the Fc portion of immunoglobulin with Fc receptors, or the Fab receptors. IVIg can also itself act as an anti-idiotypic antibody. Additionally IVIg modulates cytokine effects, and depresses the killing activity of NK cells.

In RPL, IVIg has been used in aPL related pregnancy loss, and in unexplained pregnancy loss. In unexplained RPL a large meta-analysis (Porter et al., 2006) in the Cochrane database has not shown IVIg to confer benefit. However, the papers assessed in Porter et al. (2006), meta-analysis did not correct the results for fetal chromosomal aberrations. IVIg could not to be expected to benefit patients losing chromosomally abnormal embryos, or if administration commenced after fetal demise had occurred, which is the case in some of the randomized trials. A more recent meta-analysis by Hutton (2006), has found a statistically significant increase of 22% in the live birth rate when IVIg was administered prior to pregnancy, but not in the trials when IVIg was only administered in pregnancy (possibly after embryonic demise).

In recurrent implantation failure similar mechanisms may operate as in RPL. Hence IVIg has been used in an attempt to increase the pregnancy rate after previously failed ART. Again the literature is divided on the results. As stated above, *in vitro* karyotyping of the embryos of couples with implantation failure has shown that up to 66% may be chromosomally abnormal. As in RPL, IVIg cannot be expected to enhance the implantation of chromosomally abnormal embryos. Clark et al. (2006) have performed a meta-analysis of 3 randomized trials of IVIg in IVF failure. There was a significant increase in the live birth rate per woman (OR = 2.55, 95% CI 1.19-5.49), with a benefit of 16.7% ($P = 0.012$).

ASSISTED REPRODUCTIVE TECHNOLOGY AS TREATMENT OF RECURRENT PREGNANCY LOSS

Assisted reproductive technology (ART) techniques are often used to treat RPL. These techniques include pregestational screening (PGS) gamete donation and surrogacy. The first question is whether ART is required at all. As stated above, "good prognosis" patients probably require no active treatment. ART should probably be reserved for the patients with a poor prognosis. Some of the indications and pitfalls are described below.

Pregestational Screening

Pregestational screening (PGS) is based on the premise that RPL is due to chromosomal aberrations and that the patient should be given a eukaryotypic embryo. However, the current techniques used for PGS (FISH or PCR) can be applied to only five, possibly seven or a maximum of 9 DNA probes. Therefore, screening is performed for the most common chromosomal aberrations. Chromosomes 13, 16, 18, 21, and X and Y are the chromosomes which are most commonly assessed. Hence, PGS can exclude miscarriages due to 16 and 21 trisomies and XO. However, PGS could miss a chromosomal aberration in a chromosome which was not assessed. If a chromosomal aberration had been diagnosed in a previous miscarriage, PGD could be used for the specific chromosome which was associated with the previous miscarriage and PGS for the remaining chromosomes. In an ideal situation, the entire genome will be assessed. Microarrays using CGH techniques are becoming available to assess the entire genome, but at present the arrays are not sufficiently developed and too expensive to be used on a routine clinical basis. At the present time, the live birth rate per pregnancy does seem to be increased after PGS, saving the patient from further heartbreak from further miscarriages. RPL is probably only indication for which ART is used in fertile patients. However, the pregnancy rate is about 25–30 percent as in infertile patients. Additionally, the pregnancy rate is lowered after PGS (Mastenbroek et al., 2007). It seems that not all embryos survive the biopsy required for PGS; therefore many cases of RPL may be converted to implantation failure. Hence, the live birth rate per patient is certainly not increased. The author does however recommend pregestational diagnosis in cases of repeat fetal aneuploidy, or when there are parental chromosomal aberrations with an associated aberration in the fetus.

Gamete Donation

The series on ovum donation in the literature contain little information on ovum donation as treatmrnt for RPL. The Tel Hashomer registry shows 4 cases of egg donation if 2500 patients in the RPL registry. The author has used ovum donation for a patient age 46 years with no children and six previous miscarriages. Embryonic karyotyping had been performed on three of the abortuses. All three were karyotypically abnormal with different aberrations in each miscarriage. Ovum donation was chosen as the patient's age was thought to preclude a good outcome from IVF. Additionally, with three different embryonic chromosomal aberrations in the past, it was unclear which chromosomes should be screened. Ovum donation is probably indicated for only isolated patients with RPL. If all embryos are found to be abnormal at PGS, ovum donation may be indicated.

There are no series in the literature on the use of sperm donation for RPL. The Tel Hashomer registry shows 62 cases in which there was a change of male partner. Twenty-two patients had three partners, one patient had five partners. Changing the male partner did not prevent subsequent miscarriages. The logic of sperm donation is based on the fact that there is a significantly increased incidence of sperm diploidy and disomy for chromosomes 13, 18, 21, X, and Y in men whose partners had RPL compared to controls (0.84 vs 0.37%) (Rubio et al., 1999). Increases in disomy incidence have been related to increased aneuploidy in the offspring. However, in the current state of knowledge, sperm donation does not seem indicated for RPL.

Surrogacy

Surrogacy is also a technique which involves intensive treatment with ART techniques. Surrogacy is fraught with many legal and social problems, and is also only available in certain countries. The procedure is therefore only used for isolated patients with a "poor prognosis". The author has advised surrogacy in a secondary aborter with 12 consecutive miscarriages, and a primary aborter with 8 previous pregnancy losses. In both cases the surrogate delivered normal twins. Raziel et al (2000), reported a normal live birth in a patient with 24 prior pregnancy losses. The logic of surrogacy in patients with large numbers of miscarriages is due to the poor prognosis and low incidence of chromosomal aberrations.

CONCLUSION

Although there is an overlap between ART and RPL, both are distinct and different clinical entities. There may be similar causes of both conditions with more mild cases presenting with RPL whereas the more severe cases may present with infertility. Hence, some of the treatment modalities are similar. However, as RPL is not more common after ART, RPL patients should be investigated and treated as RPL patients who have not required ART. As many as one-third of RPL patients do have periods of subfertility, and some patients may require ART techniques. At present many treatment modalities used for ART failure and RPL are somewhat empiric, and will continue to be so, until patients are investigated accurately for either maternal or embryonic chromosomal aberrations as causes for RPL or infertility.

BIBLIOGRAPHY

1. American Society for Reproductive Medicine, a Practice Committee report. Antiphospholipid antibodies do not affect IVF success. Birmingham, Alabama, USA. American Society for Reproductive Medicine 1999; pp. 1-3.
2. Aoki K, Kajiura S, Matsumoto Y, et al. Preconceptional natural-killer-cell activity as a predictor of miscarriage. Lancet. 1995;345(8961):1340-42.
3. Bakimer R, Fishman P, Blank M, et al. Induction of primary antiphospholipid syndrome in mice by immunization with a human monoclonal anticardiolipin antibody (H-3). J Clin Invest. 1992;89:1558-63.
4. Carp HJA. Recurrent pregnancy loss: towards more accurate diagnosis and treatment. Isr Med Assoc J. 2001 a;3:528-32.
5. Carp HJA, Toder V, Gazit E, et al. Further experience with intravenous immunoglobulin in women with recurrent miscarriage and a poor prognosis. Am J Reprod Immunol. 2001. b;46:268-73.
6. Carp H, Dolitzky M, Inbal A. Thromboprophylaxis improves the live birth rate in women with consecutive recurrent miscarriages and hereditary thrombophilia. J Thromb Haemost. 2003;1:433-38.
7. Carp HJA. Antiphospholipid syndrome in pregnancy. Curr Opin Obstet Gynecol. 2004;16:129-33.
8. Carp HJA. Investigation protocol for recurrent pregnancy loss. In: Carp HJA (Ed). Recurrent Pregnancy Loss, Causes, Controversies and Treatment. Informa Healthcare Ltd. London, UK. 2007; pp. 269-80.
9. Clark DA, Coulam CB, Stricker RB. Is intravenous immunoglobulins (IVIg) efficacious in early pregnancy failure? A critical review and meta-analysis for patients who fail *in vitro* fertilization and embryo transfer (IVF). J Assist Reprod Genet. 2006;23:1-13.
10. Clifford K, Flanagan AM, Regan L. Endometrial CD56+ natural killer cells in women with recurrent miscarriage: a histomorphometric study. Hum Reprod. 1999;14:2727-30.
11. Coulam CB, Beaman KD. Reciprocal alteration in circulating TJ6+ CD19+ and TJ6+ CD56+ leukocytes in early pregnancy predicts success or miscarriage. Am J Reprod Immunol. 1995;34: 219-24.
12. Daya S. Efficacy of progesterone support for pregnancy in women with recurrent miscarriage. A meta-analysis of controlled trials. Br J Obstet Gynaecol. 1989;96:275-80.
13. Daya S. Is there a benefit of low-dose aspirin in assisted reproduction? Curr Opin Obstet Gynecol. 2006;18:313-18.
14. Dolitzky M, Inbal A, Segal Y, et al. A randomized study of thromboprophylaxis in women with unexplained consecutive recurrent miscarriages. Fertil Steril. 2006;86:362-66.

CHAPTER 5

Evaluation of Fertilizing Ability and DNA Damage in Spermatozoa

Suresh Kattera

Chapter outline

- Functional Tests
  - Hamster Penetration Test
  - Assessment of Acrosome Reaction
  - Sperm Morphology Assessment using Kruger's strict criteria
  - Assessment of Motility and Sperm Survival Test
  - Computer Assisted Semen Analyzer
  - Newer Sperm Function Tests
- Recent Technological Advances

INTRODUCTION

Male contributes exclusively to about 40% of infertility and in about 30% in combination with female factor infertility. Semen analysis remains the cornerstone of male infertility evaluation. Many studies have shown how a paternal effect can cause repeated assisted reproductive techniques (ART) failures (Vanderzwalmen et al., 1991, Perinaud et al., 1993, Janny and Menezo 1994, Hammadeh et al., 1996, Sanchez et al., 1996 and Shoukir et al., 1998). Numerous studies have explored a key factor(s) that would be predictive for male fertility potential, including sperm count, motility, and/or sperm heads and integrity of nuclear chromatin. However, to date, no single laboratory test can assess male fertility potential (Amann 1989).

It is important to identify viable and functional spermatozoa that have the ability to fertilize and make viable embryos. Apart from fertilization failure, spermatozoon can contribute to poor quality embryos. Oocytes fertilized by non-viable spermatozoa may result in fragmented and arrested embryos resulting in miscarriage; hence it is important to identify viable spermatozoa for insemination during intrauterine insemination (IUI), *in vitro* fertilization (IVF) or intracytoplasmic sperm injection (ICSI). Thus, spermatozoa play two important roles; fertilization and contribution to the formation of embryos.

Standard semen analysis has limited predictive value for assessing the sperm fertilizing potential (Polansky and Lamb, 1988). Functional parameters of spermatozoa are important for fertilization. Several sperm function tests, such as acrosome reaction, hemizona binding assay, sperm morphology, creatine kinase have been proposed to explore sperm fertilization ability and to predict the rate of fertilization *in vitro* (Katsuki et al., 2005, Makkar et al., 2003, Mahutte and Arici 2003, Sidhu et al., 1998). Various factors in spermatozoa include motility, membrane integrity, ability to bind to the zona pellucida, acrosin activity and membrane fusion ability, and also the acrosome reaction (Mortimer, 1985). Fertilization failure due to male factors occurs in 5-10% of IVF cycles and 2-3% of intracytoplasmic sperm injection cycles, in those patients with normal seminal parameters (Lui and Baker 2002, Mahutte and Arici 2003). For these reasons, several functional tests have been proposed to explore and predict fertilizing ability of spermatozoa.

FUNCTIONAL TESTS

Hamster Penetration Test

One of the most studied in the early nineties was the zona-free hamster egg sperm penetration assay (SPA). Although good correlation with IVF have been reported, SPA is not a clinically relevant test because it cannot be performed routinely, it is expensive and time-consuming, it gives some false-negative responses, and it explores together several functions (capacitation, acrosome reaction and fusion to the oolemma) (Gould et al., 1983). The ideal test would be to human oocytes, however due to ethical constraints, cannot be used for diagnostic purpose. Other tests such as hemizona assay, creatine kinase (Coddington 1994 and Sidhu et al., 1998) were developed but were not practical to perform routinely.

Assessment of Acrosome Reaction

The acrosome reaction test (AR) is another parameter of sperm function (Calvo et al., 1994 and Henkel et al., 1993) which was used to predict fertilization success. The test is based on sperm physiology, and involves capacitation and acrosome reaction. Capacitation prepares the sperm to undergo the acrosome reaction with the accompanying release of lytic enzymes and exposure of membrane receptors, which are required for sperm penetration through the zona pellucida and for fusion with the oolemma (Mortimer, 1985). Integrity of acrosomal function seems to be of crucial importance to normal fertilization. Round-headed spermatozoa, which lack acrosome, cannot fertilize oocytes, and increased percentages of morphologically abnormal acrosomes were related to IVF failure. Several techniques have been used to differentiate acrosome—intact from acrosome—reacted spermatozoa, including cytochemical staining techniques (Talbot and Chacon 1981 and Viggiano et al., 1996), indirect immunofluorescence using monoclonal antibodies (Sanchez et al., 1991), labeling with fluoresceinated lectins (Aitken et al., 1993, Cross et al., 1986) and phase-contrast microscopy to examine partial head decondensation (Silverstroni et al., 2004). However, acrosome reaction test remained a research tool but not employed routinely.

Sperm Morphology Assessment using Kruger's Strict Criteria

During the late eighties, Kruger et al. (1988) introduced strict morphology criteria that can predict fertilization outcome of oocytes. A cut off level of 14% of spermatozoa was used to predict fertilization outcome. Sperm morphology assessed by strict criteria has been shown by multiple authors to have a high predictive value for the outcome of advanced assisted reproductive technologies. Recent work (unpublished) has shown that morphology can predict fertilization outcome in almost all the patients with a lowest cut off value of 5%. However, in spite of having normal morphology, in about 10% of the cases, fertilization failure occurs during IVF. Thus, strict morphology does not predict fertilization outcome in all the patients. Sperm morphology must only be considered as an indicator of fertilization potential, not as an absolute indicator of sterility.

Assessment of Motility and Sperm Survival Test

Motility is one of the key parameters in the assessment of male infertility. Motility is assessed routinely in wet preparations and the percentage of total motile spermatozoa is calculated using a laboratory counter. Any sample that has more than 40% motility is considered as normal.

Apart from total motility, sperm progression is assessed routinely. Progression has been classified into 4 types. Fast forward progression, slow forward progression, non-progression and non-motile. In any normal given sample, the ratio of fast forward progressive spermatozoa is higher than slow progressive spermatozoa. A reversal in ratio affects fertilizing ability of spermatozoa. This is reflected in the classical swim-up method where recovery of motile spermatozoa would be poor when the ratio of slow progressive spermatozoa is higher compared to fast progressive spermatozoa. In addition, the recovered motile spermatozoa do not survive longer when observed at 24 and 4 have poor survival when observed for 24h and 48h. It has been observed that either a partial or total fertilization failure of oocytes occurs when sperm survival is poor. Thus, sperm survival test is a valuable tool in the prediction of fertilizing ability of spermatozoa. Thus, it is important to perform routinely sperm survival test which predicts fertilization outcome.

Computer-assisted Semen Analyzer

In the nineties, to overcome the labor intensive semen analysis and interobserver variations, computer-assisted sperm analysis (CASA) systems were introduced for analysis of motility and sperm concentration. However, the disadvantage of this system is that it counts artifacts and gives erroneous results about total sperm count. CASA measures the velocity of spermatozoa, which may be predictive of fertilizing ability. However, it did not become a routine tool and the cost is prohibitive.

Newer Sperm Function Tests

Hyaluronan Binding Assay

For many years, interest in sperm function test diminished and during the last few years again there is a renewed interest in assessing the viability of spermatozoa. Two new commercial tests have been introduced, one is hyaluronan binding assay (HBA) and the other Sperm DNA fragmentation test. HBA test assesses the ability of spermatozoa to bind beads coated with hyaluronan and the percentage of bound spermatozoa is calculated. The percentage of bound sperms within 10 minutes indicates the percentage of mature sperms with normal DNA. However, after 10 minutes, majority of sperms bind to the beads which gives false positive results. Hence, this test is not relevant clinically to predict outcome of fertilization (Ye et al., 2006).

Sperm DNA Fragmentation Test

Several tests have been introduced to assess the DNA integrity of spermatozoa during the last several years. However, recently, a commercial kit (Halosperm) has been introduced which is being used frequently in many laboratories to assess the sperm DNA fragmentation (Fernandez et al. 2005). This test involves staining the spermatozoa after denaturation. Normal spermatozoa show larger halo around the sperm head while DNA fragmented spermatozoa have smaller halo or no halo around them (Fig. 5.1). The percentage of DNA fragmented spermatozoa is then calculated as DNA fragmentation index. Any sample with >30% fragmentation is considerd to have low fertility potential. A higher DNA fragmentation index is associated in about 10% of normospermic samples and in

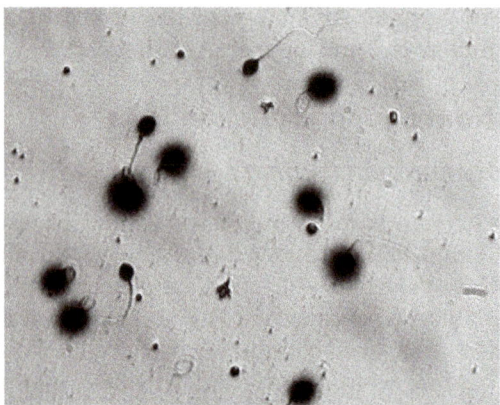

Fig. 5.1: Spermatozoa head with large halo (normal DNA) and small halo or no halo (DNA fragmented).

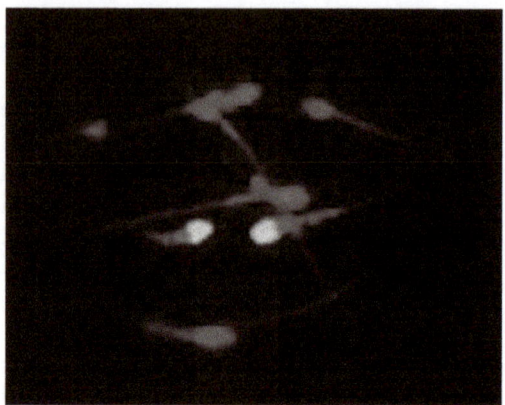

Fig. 5.2: Comet assay: Healthy DNA in male sperm nuclei resembles bright stars, while defective DNA looks more diffuse and appears to trail comet like tails.

majority of oligospermic samples. Samples with higher DNA fragmented spermatozoa that fertilize oocytes results in fragmented embryos leading to higher miscarriage rates. Thus, DNA fragmented spermatozoa results in fragmented embryos but do not result in fertilization failure. Comet assay for sperms is described in Figure 5.2.

RECENT TECHNOLOGICAL ADVANCES

Fertilization of oocytes with viable and functionally normal spermatozoa results in viable embryos. However, particularly during ICSI, it is difficult to identify viable spermatozoa. Currently, spermatozoa for ICSI are being chosen based on strict sperm morphology. However, subtle defects are not identified with magnification using the current models of microscopes. Recent studies have demonstrated that intracytoplasmic morphologically selected sperm injection (IMSI), based on sperm normality as defined by motile sperm organelle morphology examination (MSOME), improves ICSI pregnancy rates. However, MSOME is not a commonly used method to classify sperm morphology. Despite the high positive correlation, MSOME is a much stricter criterion of sperm morphology classification since it identifies vacuoles and chromatin abnormalities that are not evaluated with the same precision by the analysis of Kruger (1986). The MSOME should be included among the routine criteria for selection of patients for ART cycles.

CONCLUSION

The two most important roles of spermatozoa are to fertilize oocytes and contribute to the formation of viable embryos. In order to achieve this, it is important to identify the fertilizing ability of spermatozoa and the normal DNA complement. Several tests have been developed during the last several years. Of these, strict sperm morphology predicts fertilization outcome in majority of patients except in about 10% and in those cases, sperm progression seems to affect the fertilizing ability. Hence, it is important to assess the progression of spermatozoa by means of sperm survival test routinely. Sperm DNA fragmentation test using Halosperm kit is a useful test that predicts embryo quality outcome as higher DNA fragmentation indicates fragmentation in the embryos.

Further, IMSI will assist in the selection of spermatozoa with less morphological defects at higher magnification which results in better embryos and pregnancy outcomes in ICSI.

BIBLIOGRAPHY

1. Aitken RJ, Buckingham DW, Fang HG. Analysis of the responses of human spermatozoa to A23187 employing a novel technique for assessing the acrosome reaction. J Androl. 1993;14:132-41.
2. Amann RP. Can the fertility potential of a seminal sample be predicted accurately? J Androl. 1989;10:89-98.
3. Calvo L, Dennison-Lagos L, Banks SM, et al. Acrosome reaction inducibility predicts fertilization success at in vitro fertilization. Hum Reprod. 1994;9:1880-6.
4. Cross NL, Morales P, Overstreet JW, et al. Two simple methods for detecting acrosome-reacted human sperm. Gam Res. 1986;15:213-26.
5. Coddington CC, Oehninger SC, Olive DL, et al. Hemizona index (HZI) demonstrates excellent predictability when evaluating sperm fertilizing capacity in in vitro fertilization patients. J Androl. 1994;15:250-4.
6. Fernandez JL, Muriel L, Goyanes V, et al. Halosperm® is an easy, available, and cost-effective alternative for determining sperm DNA fragmentation Fertil Steril. 2005;84:860-6.
7. Gould JE, Overstreet JW, Yanagimachi H, et al. What functions of the sperm cell are measured by in vitro fertilization of zona-free hamster eggs? Fertil Steril. 1983;40:344-52.
8. Henkel R, Muller C, Miska W, et al. Determination of the acrosome reaction in human spermatozoa is predictive of fertilization in vitro. Hum Reprod. 1993;8:2128-32.
9. Hammadeh ME, al-Hasani S, Stieber M, et al. The effect of chromatin condensation (aniline blue staining) and morphology (strict criteria) of human spermatozoa on fertilization, cleavage and pregnancy rates in an intracytoplasmic sperm injection programme. Hum Reprod. 1996;11:2468-71.
10. Janny L, Menezo YJR. Evidence for a strong paternal effect on human preimplantation embryo development and blastocyst formation. Mol Reprod Dev. 1994;38:36-42.
11. Katsuki T, Hara T, Ueda K, et al. Prediction of outcomes of assisted reproduction treatment using the calcium ionophore-induced acrosome reaction. Hum Reprod. 2005;20:469-75.
12. Kruger, TF, Menkveld R, Stander FSH. et al. Sperm morphologic features as a prognostic factor in in vitro fertilization. Fertil Steril. 1986;46:1118-23.
13. Kruger TF, Acosta AA, Simmons KF, et al. Predictive value of abnormal sperm morphology in in vitro fertilization. Fertil Steril. 1988;49:112-17.
14. Kumi-Diaka J, Townsend J. Toxic potential of dietary genistein isoflavone and beta-lapachone on capacitation and acrosome reaction of epididymal spermatozoa. J Med Food. 2003;6:201-8.
15. Liu DY, Baker HW. Evaluation and assessment of semen for IVF/ICSI. Asian J Androl. 2002;4:281-5.
16. Makkar G, Ng EH, Yeung WS, et al. The significance of the ionophore-challenged acrosome reaction in the prediction of successful outcome of controlled ovarian stimulation and intrauterine insemination. Hum Reprod. 2003;18:534-9.
17. Mahutte NG, Arici A. Failed fertilization: is it predictable? Curr Opin Obstet Gynecol. 2003;15: 211-8.
18. Mortimer D. From the semen to oocyte: the long route in vivo and in vitro short cut. In: Testart J, Frydman R. Eds Human In Vitro Fertilization: Actual Problems and Prospects. Amsterdam: Elsevier Science Publishers. 1985; p. 93.
19. Perinaud J, Mieusset R, Vieitez G, et al. Influence of sperm parameters on embryo quality. Fertil Steril. 1993;60:888-92.
20. Polansky FF, Lamb EJ. Do the results of semen analysis predict future fertility? A survival analysis study. Fertil Steril. 1988;49:1059-65.
21. Shoukir Y, Chardonnens D, Campana A, et al. Blastocyst development from supernumerary embryos after intracytoplasmic sperm injection: a paternal influence? Hum Reprod. 1998;13:1632-37.

22. Sanchez R, Stalf T, Khanaga O, et al. Sperm selection methods for intracytoplasmic sperm injection (ICSI) and andrological patients. J Assist Reprod Genet. 1996;13:228-33.
23. Sanchez R, Toepfer-Petersen E, Aitken RJ, et al. A new method for evaluation of the acrosome reaction in viable human spermatozoa. Andrology. 1991;23:197-203.
24. Sidhu RS, Sharma RK, Agarwal A. Relationship between creatine kinase activity and semen characteristics in subfertile men. Int J Fertil Womens Med. 1998;43:192-7.
25. Suri A. Contraceptive vaccines targeting sperm. Expert Opin Biol Ther. 2005;5:381-92.
26. Talbot P, Chacon RS. A triple–stain technique for evaluating normal acrosome reactions of human sperm. J Exp Zool. 1981;215:201-8.
27. Vanderzwalmen P, Berin-Segal G, Geertz L, et al. Sperm morphology and IVF pregnancy rate: comparison between percoll gradient centrifugation and swim-up procedures. Hum Reprod. 1991;6:581-88.
28. Viggiano JM, Herrero MB, Martinez SP, et al. Analysis of the effect of nitric oxide synthase inhibition on mouse sperm employing a modified staining method for assessment of the acrosome reaction. J Androl. 1996;17:692-8.
29. Ye H, Huang G, Gao Y et al. Relationship between human sperm-hyaluronan binding assay and fertilization rate in conventional *in vitro* fertilization: Hum Reprod. 2006;21:1545-50.

CHAPTER 6

The Role of Semen Analysis in the Investigation of Infertility

Peter Sjoblom

Chapter outline

- Semen Analysis
- Semen Analysis Variables and their Physiological Significance
  - Semen Volume
  - Sperm Count
  - Sperm Motility
  - Morphology
- Antisperm Antibodies
- Postwash Motile Sperm Count
- Inflammatory Cells
- Sperm DNA Integrity Tests
- Diagnostic Use of Semen Analysis: Threshold Values

INTRODUCTION

Once it has been established that the couple are experiencing difficulties in achieving pregnancy, the infertility investigation, of both the female and the male, tries to answer three fundamental questions.

Are there Gametes?

In the female the presence of gametes can only be determined through a medical intervention, so, instead, one has to rely on surrogate indicators, i.e. menstrual cycle patterns. The situation in the male is obviously easier and in most instances, a semen sample will tell whether gametes are produced. The semen analysis will also give an indication of the functional capacity of the sperm. If there are no sperm in the ejaculate, a testicular biopsy needs to be done, to ascertain whether spermatogenesis occurs. In cases of retrograde ejaculation, an analysis of the urine is required.

Can the Gametes Meet?

For gametes to be able to meet, the male and the female must be capable of normal sexual function and the man must not experience any disturbance, such erectile or ejaculatory dysfunction. Furthermore, there should not be obstructions in the internal genitals ducts in the male or the female. Finally, the sperm must be motile in order to reach the oocyte and penetrate the oocyte's investments.

Do the Gametes Function?

To answer this question, *in vitro* fertilization must be performed. If there is a failure of fertilization or development, the gametes are obviously not functional. However, it may be difficult to decide with certainty which gamete is malfunctioning. It is also difficult to precisely ascertain what the specific problem is and even harder to address it.

Thus, the semen analysis is a critical step in the infertility investigation and the findings determine further diagnostic interventions and therapeutic options.

SEMEN ANALYSIS

This chapter will not describe how the various analytical procedures are to be performed. Instead it will discuss their utility and possible limitations.

This chapter will also not discuss sperm function tests, like the hemizona binding assay or the hamster oocyte penetration test, as they require resources beyond those available to most clinics. A borderline case, which is briefly commented on, is sperm DNA damage assessment.

In order to increase the validity of the semen analysis, certain parameters need to be standardized, such as time of abstinence (Mortimer and Templeton, 1982 and Amann et al., 2009), and the time between ejaculation and analysis (Elzanaty and Malm, 2007). The results of the analysis can also be affected by the handling of the sample, like exposure to extreme temperatures.

It is also important to record the occurrence of fever in the preceding three months period, as elevated body temperature does affect spermatogenesis (Carlsen et al., 2003, Jung and Schuppe, 2007 and Sergerie et al., 2007).

Certain medicines are known to affect sperm function, e.g. sulfasalazine (Levi et al., 1979), and calcium channel blockers (Benoff et al., 1994), and therefore the patient's history of medication must be explored. Similarly, smoking is clearly detrimental to male fertility (Practice committee of ASRM, 2006) as is exposure to environmental contaminants (Jensen et al., 2006).

Many infertility clinics work on the basis that if a couple have failed to conceive after one to two years of unprotected intercourse, then there is an infertility factor present and the couple could be helped by assisted reproduction. The diagnostic question is then "Which treatment method is the most appropriate?", rather than "Could this couple conceive by natural means?" The diagnostic procedure for judging a man's fertility potential through natural conception would be different from a procedure that aims to determine whether or not ICSI is indicated. For the latter case, less than ten sperm are sufficient, and these do not even have to be of normal (Lundin et al., 1997), as they can be injected directly into the cytoplasm. On the other hand, millions of sperm are required for natural conception, and these sperm have to overcome a number of hurdles before they can fertilize an egg. For this reason, the semen analysis is often simplified in IVF clinics.

Today, most clinics consider that, if findings are normal, a single semen analysis is sufficient for the diagnostic work-up of the couple. However, if there are significant abnormal findings, a second semen analysis will ensure that there is a good basis for the informing the patient of the diagnosis of male factor infertility.

The investigtion into the semen quality is shown as an algorithmic approach in Flowhart 6.1.

SEMEN ANALYSIS VARIABLES AND THEIR PHYSIOLOGICAL SIGNIFICANCE

The minimal set of variables in the semen analysis comprises of semen volume, total count, proportion of motile sperm and sperm morphology, although the latter is sometimes excluded. In addition, sperm antibody tests can be performed as well as documentation of the presence of inflammatory cells. Some laboratories assess postwash motile sperm count in order to determine which fertilization method to use, in case the couple is undergoing assisted reproduction treatment.

Semen Volume

The volume of the ejaculate is determined using a graduated pipette and it adequate to

Flowchart 6.1: Semen analysis.

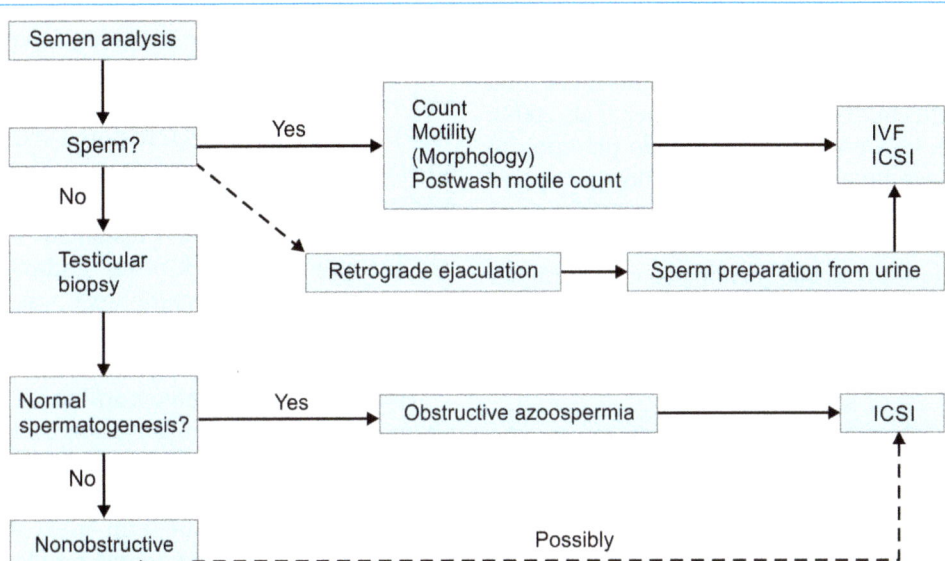

(ICSI: intracytoplasmic sperm injection; IVF; *in vitro* firtility)

measure it in steps of 0.5 mL. It reflects the function of the accessory glands, since the spermatocrit is only about 5–10%. Exposure to seminal plasma is not required for sperm to function, as evidenced from the success of using epididymal and testicular sperm in intracytoplasmic sperm injection (ICSI) over the last 15 years. However, an abnormally low volume could impair the chances natural conception by not protecting the sperm against the acidic vaginal environment (Fox et al., 1973).

Sperm Count

The sperm count is determined using a hemocytometer or computerized assisted semen analysis, CASA. Hemocytometer counts are considered to be Poisson distributed and thus the accuracy of the determination is dependent on the total number counted. However, a significant proportion of the variance in the count is attributable to operator variability. With adequate training, this variability can be greatly reduced (Bjorndahl et al., 2002).

The total sperm count indicates the level of spermatogenic activity (Amann, 2009). Many papers report sperm concentration, a variable which not only depends on spermatogenic activity, but also on the function of the accessory glands, and this makes this variable less useful for assessing spermatogenic capacity.

The biological significance of sperm counts is that only a minute fraction of the inseminated spermatozoa reaches the Fallopian tube, a fraction estimated to be just over one in a million (Mortimer and Templeton, 1982). Therefore, the actual number of sperm in the Fallopian tube will be in the order of 10^2 (Williamson et al., 1993), assuming that a normal ejaculate contains 10^8 sperm. If the number of sperm in the ejaculate is only 10^6–10^7 it follows that only occasional sperm will find their way into the tube and fertilization is less likely to occur. The validity of this theoretical relationship is confirmed by observations that 95% of men who had had a time to pregnancy of ≤12 months had a total sperm count of $\geq 15 \times 10^6$ (Cooper et al., 2009). Also, in a population of couple planning to achieve pregnancy it was found that sperm count was a significant predictor of time to pregnancy if the total count was below 40 million sperm, but not if the count was higher than that (Bonde et al., 1998).

Sperm Motility

The proportion of motile sperm can be estimated by CASA or by 'eyeballing'. The accuracy of the estimate depends on the number of sperm observed, and with 'eyeballing' it is commonly estimated in steps of 10% or possibly 5%. The swimming speed is graded into categories from fast to nonprogressive. Again, training and repeated interobserver comparisons will lead to improved reproducibility. With CASA, a better assessment of swimming speed is achievable.

Motility is obviously needed for fertilization under natural conditions, as sperm need to migrate to the oocyte and then exert enough force to penetrate the zona pellucida after facilitation by enzymatic degradation (Green, 1987 and Baltz et al., 1988). Motility is also an indicator of vitality, although immotile sperm may well be viable, and the hypo-osmotic swelling test (Jeyendran et al., 1984) can be used to differentiate between viable and nonviable immotile sperm.

The proportion of motile sperm may be multiplied by the total sperm count to give the total motile count, which supposedly gives a better indication than total sperm count of the chances of achieving pregnancy (Badawy et al., 2009, Merviel et al., 2010 and Wainer et al., 2004). The swimming speed of the spermatozoa may be indicative of the fertilizing potential (Bollendorf et al., 1994).

Morphology

Assessment of sperm morphology requires strict adherence to methodology of staining and criteria of assessment (Barroso et al., 1999). A significant effort is required to obtain an acceptable level of between- and within-assessor variability. Various staining methods are available, including prestained slides, which simplify the work of the andrologist. Image analysis using computers was first described by Jagoe et al. (1987) and has since been refined.

Human sperm are pleomorphic, as they often seem to be in monogamous species (for review, see Short 1997). Thus, the "normal" forms, as in the most common forms, are not the norm, and instead the term 'ideal' forms could be used. A fundamental problem in using morphology as a predictor of fertilizing capacity is the choice of end point, which is usually the proportion of sperm that show 'normal' morphology. This is problematic, as it is difficult to describe the morphology of the individual sperm that actually fertilizes the egg. However, Liu and Baker (1992) suggested that the morphology of sperm that were bound to the zona pellucida could be used as physiological standard against which sperm should be compared.

Kruger et al. (1987) reported that assessment using strict morphological criteria has a reasonable power of predicting failed fertilization in IVF. The latest version of the WHO manual for semen analysis, proposes the use of these strict criteria for assessing male fertility, although this has been criticized (Eliasson, 2010). Many IVF units, though, do not use morphology assessment for deciding on whether to use ICSI or conventional IVF for fertilization, as it they feel that it is of little utility (Lundin et al., 1997). On the other hand, Bonde et al. (1998) observed in a study of pregnancy planners that sperm morphology was an independent predictor of time to pregnancy by natural conception.

Antisperm Antibodies

The presence of antisperm antibodies (ASAB) is usually assessed with the mixed agglutination reaction (Grobler et al., 1987) and the presence of ASAB is indicated by the binding of immunoglobulin-coated latex beads to the sperm, particularly to the head and midpiece.

Binding of ASAB to sperm may impair fertilization by agglutinating spermatozoa, by causing sterical interference with molecular interactions at fertilization, or, in combination with complement activation, by causing sperm immobilization through disruption of the membrane potential (Chiu et al., 2004).

As a rule of thumb, it seems that if 70% of the sperm have latex beads bound, there will be an effect on the probability of achieving fertilization by intercourse or by IVF (for review, see Chui et al., 2004). About 10% of men presenting at infertility clinics have significant levels of ASAB (Collins et al., 1993). ICSI results are rarely affected by ASAB (Nagy et al., 1998), and ICSI is therefore the treatment method of choice.

Immunosuppressive treatment is no longer used, as it is not only ineffective, but also carries a significant risk of serious side effects (for review, see Naz, 2004).

Postwash Motile Sperm Count

Total count after sperm preparation is capable of predicting failure to achieve pregnancy by intrauterine insemination (van Weert et al., 2004) or IVF (Rhemrev et al., 2001). In the author's clinic, morphology assessment is not used in semen analysis for patients presenting with failure to conceive after 12 months unprotected intercourse. Instead, sperm preparation using gradient centrifugation is performed, using the methodology recommended by the supplier of the gradient product. A strict cut-off level of postprepared total motile count of 1 million is used, and below this level ICSI is recommended. If the postprepared total motile count is between 1 to 2 million, ICSI is recommended if either the percentage motile sperm or the motility grade is low. This approach seems to produce a reasonable outcome, since the failed fertilization rate was 2.1% after IVF, while it was 1.6% after ICSI.

Inflammatory Cells

The definition of leukocytosis is >1×10^6/mL leukocytes in the ejaculate. The presence of inflammatory cells is obviously indicative of an inflammatory process, but in most cases it is not caused by an infection, so, unless a specific bacterial cause has been identified, treatment with antibiotics is not called for (for review, see Krause et al., 2003). Chronic prostatitis with high levels of inflammatory cells may cause intermittent or partial obstruction of the ejaculatory ducts, causing oligozoospermia or azoospermia (Dohle, 2003). In such cases, a second semen analysis should always be done before discussing implications with the patient. Chronic prostatitis is suspected of being associated with a higher risk of prostate cancer (MacLennan et al., 2006) and it may be worthwhile to monitor such patients more closely.

Sperm DNA Integrity Tests

Tests of DNA integrity have been developed and applied in clinical practice. The most commonly studied DNA integrity tests are the sperm chromatin structure assay (SCSA), the deoxynucleotidyl transferase-mediated dUTP nick end labeling assay (TUNEL) the single-cell gel electrophoresis assay (COMET), and the sperm chromatin dispersion (SCD) test. Each of these tests provides a semi-quantitative estimate of the general state of DNA but does not provide an indication of specific DNA sequences that might be affected. For example, the SCSA utilizes flow cytometry of fluorescently labelled sperm to determine the proportion of sperm susceptible to DNA damage (red fluorescence) compared with normal sperm (green fluorescence). The TUNEL assay utilizes flow cytometry of sperm fluorescently labelled at DNA strand breaks to determine the degree of DNA damage where fluorescence intensity is proportional to the number of strand breaks. In the COMET assay, fluorescently labelled sperm cells are embedded in agarose gel, lysed to relax DNA, and electrophoresed. DNA damage is proportional to displacement between the nuclear material and the tail material. The SCD test utilizes fluorescence microscopy to distinguish cells with intact DNA (large halo) from sperm cells with damaged DNA (small or absent halo).

Numerous studies utilizing the above techniques for assessing sperm DNA integrity support the existence of a significant association between sperm DNA damage and pregnancy outcomes in both humans and non-human species. Fertile men with normal semen parameters usually have high levels of DNA integrity, whereas infertile men, especially those with abnormal semen parameters, often have decreased DNA integrity. Moreover, a significant number of infertile men will have abnormal DNA integrity despite normal semen parameters.

There is insufficient evidence to recommend the routine use of sperm DNA integrity tests in the evaluation and treatment of the infertile couple (Level C) ASRM.

DIAGNOSTIC USE OF SEMEN ANALYSIS: THRESHOLD VALUES

There is a finite probability of conception (however small) as long as there are motile sperm in the ejaculate. Therefore, there cannot be a strict cut-off limit (except for the zero value) of any variable, below which fertility is impossible. Instead, one could approach the problem by analyzing time to pregnancy in different situations. In the latest WHO standard (Cooper et al., 2010), the reference values are based on findings in men with a time to pregnancy of ≤12 months, since failure to conceive within 12 months is a commonly used medical definition of infertility. The lowest 5th percentile is used as the lower end of the normal range, and values below that are considered to be indicative of a male infertility factor. However, one cannot exclude the possibility of achieving pregnancy by intercourse if the result is below that limit. The latest reference values for semen analysis are shown in Table 6.1.

To conclude, the semen analysis, although indispensable in the work-up of the infertile couple, is not a perfect diagnostic tool and the published guidelines are only just that. The findings must be considered together with the male medical history as well that of the female and the interpretation of results requires experience.

Table 6.1: Lower reference values for men with a time to pregnancy of ≤12 months (Cooper et al., 2010)

Variable	5th percentile	95% CI
Semen volume (mL)	1.5	1.4–1.7
Sperm concentration (10^6/mL)	15	12–16
Total sperm number (10^6/ejaculate)	39	33–46
Total motility [progressive (grade a+b) and nonprogressive (grade c); %]	40	38–42
Progressive motility (grade a+b; %)	32	31–34
Normal forms (%)	4	3.0–4.0
Vitality (%)	58	55–63

BIBLIOGRAPHY

1. Amann RP. Considerations in evaluating human spermatogenesis on the basis of total sperm per ejaculate. J Androl. 2009; 30(6):626-41.

2. Badawy A, Elnashar A, Eltotongy M. Effect of sperm morphology and number on success of intrauterine insemination. Fertil Steril. 2009; 91(3):777-81.
3. Baltz JM, Katz DF, Cone RA. Mechanics of sperm-egg interaction at the zona pellucida. Biophys J. 1988;54(4):643-54.
4. Barroso G, Mercan R, Ozgur K, et al. Intra- and inter-laboratory variability in the assessment of sperm morphology by strict criteria: impact of semen preparation, staining techniques and manual versus computerized analysis. Hum Reprod. 1999;14(8):2036-40.
5. Benoff S, Cooper GW, Hurley I, et al. The effect of calcium ion channel blockers on sperm fertilization potential. Fertil Steril 1994;62(3):606-17.
6. Björndahl L, Barratt CL, Fraser LR, et al. ESHRE basic semen analysis courses 1995-1999: immediate beneficial effects of standardized training. Hum Reprod. 2002;17(5):1299-305.
7. Bollendorf A, Check JH, Lurie D. Evaluation of the effect of the absence of sperm with rapid and linear progressive motility on subsequent pregnancy rates following intrauterine insemination or in vitro fertilization. J Andrology. 1996;17(5):550-7.
8. Bonde JP, Ernst E, Jensen TK, et al. Relation between semen quality and fertility: a population-based study of 430 first-pregnancy planners. Lancet. 1998;352(9135):1172-7.
9. Carlsen E, Andersson AM, Petersen JH, et al. History of febrile illness and variation in semen quality. Hum Reprod. 2003;18(10):2089-92.
10. Collins JA, Burrows EA, Yeo J, et al. Frequency and predictive value of antisperm antibodies among infertile couples. Hum Reprod. 1993;8:592-8.
11. Dohle GR. Inflammatory-associated obstructions of the male reproductive tract. Andrologia. 2003; 35(5):321-4.
12. Eliasson R. Semen analysis with regard to sperm number, sperm morphology and functional aspects. Asian J Androl. 2010;12(1):26-32.
13. Fox CA, Meldrum SJ, Watson BW. Continuous measurement by radio-telemetry of vaginal pH during human coitus. J Reprod Fertil. 1973; 33(1):69-75.
14. Green DP. Mammalian sperm cannot penetrate the zona pellucida solely by force. Exp Cell Res. 1987;169(1):31-8.
15. Grobler S, Franken DR, Pretorius E. IgG-coated latex particles and the identification of sperm antibodies. S Afr Med J. 1984;66(3):97-8.
16. Hershlag A, Cooper GW, Benoff S. Pregnancy following discontinuation of a calcium channel blocker in the male partner. Hum Reprod. 1995; 10(3):599-606.
17. Jagoe JR, Washbrook NP, Pratsis L, et al. Sperm morphology by image analysis compared with subjective assessment. Br J Urol. 1987;60(5):457-62.
18. Jensen TK, Bonde JP, Joffe M. The influence of occupational exposure on male reproductive function. Occup Med (Lond). 2006;56(8):544-53.
19. Jeyendran RS, Van der Ven HH, Perez-Pelaez M, et al. Development of an assay to assess the functional integrity of the human sperm membrane and its relationship to other semen characteristics. J Reprod Fertil. 1984; 70(1):219-28.
20. Jung A, Schuppe HC. Influence of genital heat stress on semen quality in humans. Andrologia. 2007;39(6):203-15.
21. Krause W, Bohring C, Gueth A, et al. Cellular and biochemical markers in semen indicating male accessory gland inflammation. Andrologia. 2003;35(5):279-82.
22. Kruger TF, Acosta AA, Simmons KF, et al. New method of evaluating sperm morphology with predictive value for human in vitro fertilization. Urology. 1987;30(3):248-51.
23. Levi AJ, Fisher AM, Hughes L, et al. Male infertility due to sulphasalazine. Lancet. 1979;2(8137):276-8.
24. Liu DY, Baker HW. Morphology of spermatozoa bound to the zona pellucida of human oocytes that failed to fertilize in vitro. J Reprod Fertil. 1992;94(1):71-84.
25. Lundin K, Söderlund B, Hamberger L. The relationship between sperm morphology and rates of fertilization, pregnancy and spontaneous abortion in an in-vitro fertilization/intracytoplasmic sperm injection programme. Hum Reprod. 1997; 12(12):2676-81.
26. MacLennan GT, Eisenberg R, Fleshman RL, et al. The influence of chronic inflammation

in prostatic carcinogenesis: a 5-year follow-up study. J Urol. 2006;176(3):1012-6.
27. Merviel P, Heraud MH, Grenier N, et al. Predictive factors for pregnancy after intrauterine insemination (IUI): an analysis of 1038 cycles and a review of the literature. Fertil Steril. 2010;93(1):79-88.
28. Mortimer D, Templeton AA, Lenton EA, et al. Influence of abstinence and ejaculation-to-analysis delay on semen analysis parameters of suspected infertile men. Arch Androl. 1982;8(4):251-6.
29. Mortimer D, Templeton AA. Sperm transport in the human female reproductive tract in relation to semen analysis characteristics and time of ovulation. J Reprod Fertil. 1982;64(2):401-8.
30. Nagy ZP, Verheyen G, Tournaye H, et al. Special applications of intracytoplasmic sperm injection: the influence of sperm count, motility, morphology, source and sperm antibody on the outcome of ICSI. Hum Reprod. 1998;13(Suppl 1):143-54.
31. Naz RK. Modalities for treatment of antisperm antibody mediated infertility: novel perspectives. Am J Reprod Immunol. 2004;51(5):390-7.
32. Practice Committee of the American Society for Reproductive Medicine. Smoking and infertility. Fertil Steril. 2006;86(5 Suppl 1):S172-7.
33. Rhemrev JP, Lens JW, McDonnell J, et al. The postwash total progressively motile sperm cell count is a reliable predictor of total fertilization failure during in vitro fertilization treatment. Fertil Steril. 2001;76(5):884-91.
34. Sergerie M, Mieusset R, Croute F, et al. High risk of temporary alteration of semen parameters after recent acute febrile illness. Fertil Steril. 2007;88(4):970.e1-7.
35. Short RV. The testis: the witness of the mating system, the site of mutation and the engine of desire. Acta Paediatr (Suppl.) 1997;422:3-7.
36. Cooper TG, Noonan E, von Eckardstein S, et al., World Health Organization reference values for human semen characteristics. Human Reproduction Update Advance Access. 2009.
37. van Weert JM, Repping S, Van Voorhis BJ, et al. Performance of the postwash total motile sperm count as a predictor of pregnancy at the time of intrauterine insemination: a meta-analysis. Fertil Steril. 2004;82(3):612-20.
38. Wainer R, Albert M, Dorion A, et al. Influence of the number of motile spermatozoa inseminated and of their morphology on the success of intrauterine insemination. Hum Reprod. 2004;19(9):2060-5.
39. Williams M, Hill CJ, Scudamore I, et al. Sperm numbers and distribution within the human fallopian tube around ovulation. Hum Reprod. 1993;8(12):2019-26.
40. World Health Organization. WHO Laboratory Manual for the Examination of Human Semen and Sperm-cervical Mucus Interaction, 4th edn). Cambridge: Cambridge University Press. 1999; p. 128.
41. Zini A, Boman JM, Belzile E, et al. Sperm DNA damage is associated with an increased risk of pregnancy loss after IVF and ICSI: systematic review and meta-analysis. Hum Reprod. 2008;23(12):2663-8.
42. Zini A, Sigman M. Are tests of sperm DNA damage clinically useful? Pros and cons. J Androl. 2009;30(3):219-29.

CHAPTER 7

Optimizing Ovulation Induction: Back to Basics

Niranjana Jayakrishnan, K Jayakrishnan

Chapter outline

- Excess Body Weight
- Clomiphene Citrate
  - Dosage
  - Complications
- Metformin
  - Dosage
- Thiazolidinediones
- Aromatase Inhibitors
  - Letrozole
  - AI and Unexplained infertility
  - AI and Endometriosis
  - Safety of Aromatase Inhibitors
- Gonadotropins

INTRODUCTION

Polycystic ovary syndrome (PCOS) is the most common cause of anovulatory infertility. Although many options are available for ovulation induction in these patients, there is currently no evidence-based algorithm to guide the initial and subsequent choices of medical ovulation induction methods. In obese women with PCOS, mild to moderate weight loss results in improvement of ovulatory dysfunction and should be advocated at the onset of the evaluation.

Clomiphene citrate is currently the first-line pharmacological therapy for ovulation induction, although metformin appears to also be a promising agent for first-line therapy, at least in some patients. Studies are currently ongoing to address which first-line agent (clomiphene or metformin) is of greater benefit and/or which subpopulations of patients with PCOS will benefit from either treatment alone or in combination. Alternatively, glucocorticoids do not result in consistent ovulation and have significant side effects, although they may have a role in the treatment of the patient who is clomiphene resistant. These patients may also benefit from the addition of metformin. In this setting, exogenous pulsatile gonadotropin-releasing hormone (GnRH) treatment has also been advocated, although overall it has low ovulation and pregnancy rates, with a high risk of miscarriage. The most commonly used medical agents for ovulation induction in clomiphene-resistant women with PCOS, or those who fail to conceive following treatment with first-line agents and their adjuvants, are parenteral gonadotropins.

Various gonadotropin preparations and different protocols are available; however, the risk of multiple pregnancy and ovarian hyperstimulation is high with gonadotropin therapy in the patient with PCOS. As such, various investigators advocate proceeding first to laparoscopic ovarian drilling, possibly combined with retreatment with clomiphene and/or metformin or, in an effort to control more aggressively the number of multiples, to *in vitro* fertilization.

EXCESS BODY WEIGHT

Excess body weight is a common problem of modern society, reaching epidemic proportions in some countries. For women with PCOS, an excess of body fat accentuates insulin resistance and its associated clinical sequelae. Central obesity and body mass index (BMI) are major determinants of insulin resistance, hyperinsulinemia and hyperandrogenemia. The rate of insulin resistance in women with PCOS is 50-80% and a large majority of these women are obese.

They almost inevitably have the stigmata of hyperandrogenism and irregular or absent ovulation.[1] Insulin stimulates luteinizing hormone (LH) and ovarian androgen secretion and decreases sex hormone binding globulin concentrations.

The successful treatment of obesity and hyperinsulinemia is capable of reversing their deleterious effects, of which there are several, on the outcome of treatment. More gonadotrophins are required to achieve ovulation in insulin resistant women. Obese women being treated with low dose gonadotropin therapy have inferior pregnancy and miscarriage rates. Both obese and insulin resistant women with PCOS, even on low dose follicle-stimulating hormone (FSH) stimulation, have a much greater tendency to a multifollicular response and thus a relatively high cycle cancellation rate in order to avoid hyperstimulation.[2]

Just as obesity expresses and exaggerates the signs and symptoms of insulin resistance, then loss of weight can reverse this process by improving ovarian function and the associated hormonal abnormalities. Loss of weight induces a reduction of insulin and androgen concentrations and an increase in sex hormone binding hormone concentrations. Curiously, in obese women with PCOS, a loss of just 5-10% of body weight is enough to restore reproductive function in 55-100% within 6 months of weight reduction. Weight loss has the undoubted advantages of being effective and cheap with no side effects and should be the first line of treatment in obese women with anovulatory infertility associated with PCOS.

CLOMIPHENE CITRATE

Clomiphene citrate has long been the first-line of treatment for those with absent or irregular ovulation.

Dosage

It is given in a dose of 50-250 mg per day for 5 days starting from day 2-5 of spontaneous or induced bleeding starting with the lowest dose and raising the dose in increments of 50 mg/day each cycle until an ovulatory cycle is achieved.

In practice, it is used, at a starting dose of 100 mg per day from day 4 or 5 and no advantage has been found in using a daily dose of more than 150 mg which seems neither to significantly increase the ovulation rate nor follicular recruitment.

This sort of regimen will cut down the number of 'superfluous' cycles of treatment until ovulation is achieved and until those resistant to clomiphene are identified.

Some clomiphene citrate-resistant anovulatory women may require higher doses of 200-250 mg for an extended period of time, usually 8-10 days. This can be considered prior to second-line agents such as exogenous gonadotropins, but may delay time to ovulation and conception. Antiestrogenic side effects become more common at higher doses.

A course of 3-6 ovulatory cycles is usually sufficient to know whether pregnancy will be achieved using clomiphene citrate before moving on to more complex treatment as approximately 75% of the pregnancies achieved with clomiphene occur within the first three cycles of treatment.[2]

The Practice Committee of the American Society of Reproductive Medicine (ASRM) has stated that clomiphene citrate treatment should be limited to the minimum effective dose and to no more than 6 ovulatory cycles.

Ovulation is restored in approximately 80% but will result in pregnancy in only about 35-40% of patients who are given clomiphene.

The timing of sexual intercourse in relation to ovulation has been shown to influence the chance of conception in the general population. Some clinicians advise couples to have intercourse a minimum of twice a week or every other day during the week of ovulation; however, no supporting data exist regarding a specific coitus schedule for women taking clomiphene citrate. Coitus should ideally be planned to coincide with the expected time of ovulation. In properly selected women, approximately 46% will ovulate while using the 50 mg per day dosage, and approximately another 21% will ovulate if the dosage is increased to 100 mg. Additionally, around 20-25% of anovulatory women with PCOS will not respond at all to clomiphene citrate and are considered to be 'clomiphene resistant'.[3]

Patients who do not respond to clomiphene are likely to be more obese, insulin resistant and hyperandrogenic than those who do respond. As clomiphene citrate induces a discharge of LH as well as FSH and elevated LH concentrations are believed to impede conception, those with high basal LH levels are also less likely to respond to clomiphene treatment. The most probable factor involved in this large discrepancy between ovulation and pregnancy rates in patients treated with clomiphene is the antiestrogenic effects of clomiphene at the level of the endometrium and cervical mucus. While the depression of the cervical mucus, occurring in about 15% of patients, may be overcome by performing intrauterine insemination (IUI), suppression of endometrial proliferation, unrelated to dose or duration of treatment but apparently idiosyncratic, indicates a poor prognosis for conception when endometrial thickness never reaches 8 mm.

Monitoring of the clomiphene treated cycle by ultrasound evaluation of follicular growth, endometrial thickness and even estradiol and progesterone concentrations on day 12-14 of the cycle is justified by the identification of those who are not responding or have depressed endometrial thickness and is helpful in the timing of natural intercourse or IUI. Although this monitoring implies added expense, this is neutralized by the prevention of protracted periods of possibly inappropriate therapy and delay in the inception of more efficient treatment.

The results of clomiphene treatment may be improved by cotreatment with several proposed adjuvants. The addition of an ovulatory dose of human chorionic gonadotropin (hCG), 5,000-10,000 IU is only theoretically warranted when the reason for a nonovulatory response is that the LH surge is delayed or absent despite the presence of a well developed follicle. Although the routine addition of hCG at midcycle seems to add little to the improvement of conception rates it has been found to be useful, given when an ultrasonically demonstrated leading follicle attains a diameter of 18-24 mm, for the timing of intercourse or IUI.

Daily doses of dexamethasone, 0.5 mg at bedtime, as an adjunct to clomiphene therapy, suppress the adrenal androgen secretion and may induce responsiveness to clomiphene in previous nonresponders, mostly hyperandrogenic women with PCOS with elevated concentrations of dehydroepiandrosterone sulfate. Although this method meets with some success, medium to long-term glucocorticoid steroid therapy often induces side effects including increased appetite and weight gain which is not an appealing proposition for women with PCOS.[4]

Complications

Clomiphene citrate is generally a well-tolerated drug. Side effects include vasomotor flushes (13.6% prevalence), abdominopelvic discomfort/distention/bloating (5.5%), nausea and vomiting (2.2%), headache (1.3%), and visual symptoms such as blurred eyesight (<1%). Because the half-life of clomiphene citrate is 5 days, symptoms may persist long after the last dose; however, they usually abate after the treatment cycle ends. Treatment should be discontinued and other alternative methods of ovulation induction should be considered in women with clomiphene-induced visual changes.

The main contraindications to the use of clomiphene citrate are pregnancy, hypersensitivity to the medication, and the presence of significant ovarian cysts. As previously discussed, antiestrogenic effects of clomiphene citrate in the endometrium and endocervix may interfere with sperm survival and transport and may affect implantation.

There is a modest increase in the risk of multiple gestation with clomiphene citrate use, most of which are twins (6-9%) and, very rarely, triplets (0.3-0.5%). No evidence has been found of increased risk of spontaneous abortion in pregnancies resulting from clomiphene citrate treatment.

Ovarian hyperstimulation syndrome is a known complication of clomiphene citrate usage; however, most cases are usually mild and patients rarely develop severe manifestations, which include abdominal pain, hypovolemia, nausea, vomiting, and oliguria.

A few studies have associated infertility treatment with an increased risk for neoplasms, particularly ovarian tumors. Rossing et al. examined the risk of ovarian tumors in a cohort of infertile women. Among those who had taken clomiphene citrate, the adjusted relative risk ratio of developing an ovarian tumor compared with that among infertile women who had not taken this drug was 2.3 (95% CI, 0.5-11.4). Of note, the majority of the women who developed ovarian tumors had taken the drug during 12 or more monthly cycles, suggesting increased risk with prolonged use.

Subsequent studies have not shown an increased risk of neoplasm. In a meta-analysis of 3 cohort and 7 case-control studies by Kashyap et al.[5] cases of ovarian cancer did not appear to increase in treated infertile patients compared with untreated infertile patients (OR, 0.99; 95% CI, 0.67-1.45). The studies examined in this meta-analysis included such treatments as clomiphene citrate, gonadotropins, human chorionic gonadotropin, and gonadotropin-releasing hormone (GnRH) agonists. Ness et al., in a pooled analysis of 8 case-control studies, concluded that neither fertility drug use nor use for more than 12 months was associated with invasive ovarian cancer. Infertility was noted to be an independent risk factor for developing ovarian cancer.

METFORMIN

The basic etiology behind the anovulation associated with PCOS is mainly insulin resistance and hyperinsulinemia.[6] This strong association between hyperinsulinemia and anovulation would suggest that a reduction of insulin concentrations could be of great importance. Weight loss for the obese can reverse this situation as mentioned above but for those who fail to lose weight or are of normal weight but hyperinsulinemic, an insulin sensitizing agent such as metformin is indicated. However, the indications for the administration of metformin to anovulatory women with PCOS in an ovulation induction program have widened as it seems to be difficult to predict which individuals will respond well with this medication.

Metformin is an oral biguanide, well established for the treatment of hyperglycemia, that does not cause hypoglycemia in normoglycemic patients. The sum total of its actions is a decrease in insulin levels and, as a consequence, a lowering of circulating total and free androgen levels with a resulting improvement of the clinical sequelae of hyperandrogenism.

Dosage

There are now a large number of studies published on the effect of metformin in a dose of 1500–2550 mg/day in women with PCOS. The vast majority of these studies have demonstrated a significant improvement in insulin concentrations, insulin sensitivity, and serum androgen concentrations accompanied by decreased LH and increased sex hormone-binding globulin (SHBG) concentrations.[7] The restoration of regular menstrual cycles by metformin has been reported in the large majority of published series and the reinstatement of ovulation occurred in 78–96% of patients.

Fleming et al.,[8] in the largest randomized controlled trial published to date, demonstrated a significantly increased frequency of ovulation with metformin as compared to placebo in a group of 92 oligomenorrheic women with PCOS. This was achieved without any significant changes in the insulin response to glucose challenge after 14 weeks of metformin treatment in a dose of 850 mg, twice a day.

In a randomized controlled trial (RCT) performed on clomiphene resistant infertile patients with PCOS, compared with placebo, metformin markedly improved ovulation and pregnancy rates with clomiphene treatment. In a large study, 46 anovulatory obese women with PCOS who did not ovulate on metformin or placebo for 35 days were given 50 mg of clomiphene daily for 5 days while continuing metformin or placebo. Of those on metformin, 19 of 21 ovulated compared with 2 of 25 on placebo.[9]

When women with clomiphene resistant PCOS were administered FSH with or without pretreatment with metformin for one month in an RCT, those receiving metformin developed significantly less large follicles, produced less estradiol and had fewer cycles cancelled due to excessive follicular development. The reduction of insulin concentrations induced by metformin seemed to favor a more orderly follicular growth in response to exogenous gonadotropins for ovulation induction.

In the one published study on the effects of metformin on clomiphene resistant patients undergoing IVF/ICSI, the results of cycles preceded by treatment with metformin were compared retrospectively to those in which metformin was not given. Those receiving metformin had a decreased total number of follicles but no difference in the mean number of oocytes retrieved. There were more mature oocytes, embryos cleaved, increased fertilization and clinical pregnancy rates (70% vs 30%) in the metformin group. These latter two studies would seem to confirm that both obese and insulin resistant women with PCOS have a much greater tendency to a multifollicular response and thus a relatively high cycle cancellation rate on low dose FSH stimulation.

The evidence so far is encouraging concerning the efficiency and safety of metformin as a single agent or in combination with clomiphene citrate or gonadotropins for induction of ovulation in women with hyperinsulinemic PCOS. It remains to be seen whether metformin, which probably also has a direct androgen lowering action on the ovary, will be of help to all women with PCOS wishing to conceive. Not only does metformin seem to be safe when continued throughout pregnancy but preliminary data strongly suggest that this strategy can severely decrease the high miscarriage rate usually associated with PCOS.[10] It is hoped that the apparent lack of teratogenicity and beneficial effect of metformin on miscarriage rates will be confirmed by future studies.[11]

Other compounds with the property of lowering insulin concentrations, the glitazones rosiglitazone and pioglitazone, and d-chiro-inositol, are under investigation and may also prove useful for women with anovulatory PCOS.

THIAZOLIDINEDIONES

The thiazolidinediones are insulin-sensitizing agents that improve insulin resistance by acting on the intranuclear hormone receptor peroxisome proliferator activated receptor. Enhanced insulin sensitivity is noted particularly in the liver, adipose tissue, and muscle, reducing insulin resistance and improving pancreatic-cell function.

Troglitazone was the first member of this category used in the treatment of PCOS. In a large, multicenter, double-blind placebo-controlled dose-determining study of 305 patients with PCOS, 60% of "expected" cycles were ovulatory on troglitazone 600 mg/day after 6 months of treatment, compared with a baseline rate of 30% in the placebo group. In addition to increasing the rates of ovulation, troglitazone has been shown to improve androgen levels and insulin sensitivity. However, troglitazone was withdrawn from the market because of an increased, albeit minimal, risk of hepatotoxicity and fulminant liver failure.

The more recently introduced thiazolidinediones, rosiglitazone and pioglitazone, appear not to have the same degree of hepatic side effects observed for troglitazone. However, only a few studies are available, with small numbers of participants, that address the effects of these new agents in the treatment of PCOS. In an uncontrolled study of rosiglitazone and clomiphene vs clomiphene for ovulation induction in PCOS, the rates of improvement in menstrual pattern were 92 and 68%, respectively. In a randomized, double-blind, placebo-controlled study of 25 clomi-phene-resistant PCOS patients, ovulation rates of 33 and 77%, respectively, were observed after rosiglitazone alone vs rosiglitazone and clomiphene. In another randomized, controlled double blind trial, Baillargeon and colleagues randomized 100 nonobese PCOS women with normal indices of insulin sensitivity to receive metformin (850 mg twice a day), rosiglitazone (4 mg twice a day), the combination of both drugs, or at least one placebo for 6 months. The ovulatory response was higher after treatment with an insulin-sensitizing drug compared to placebo, and the ovulatory frequency was significantly greater with metformin than rosiglitazone, while the combination was not more effective (ovulations per subject in 6 months: metformin 3.3, rosiglitazone 2.4, combination 3.4, and placebo 0.4).

Overall, insulin-sensitizing agents appear to improve the ovulatory response of PCOS, regardless of weight. Several points remain to be addressed in further studies regarding use of these agents for ovulation induction in women with PCOS, including the optimum dose and duration of therapy, the pregnancy and neonatal outcome, and the variability in ovarian response. Current evidence suggests that insulin-sensitizing agents may be beneficial in a subset, but probably not all PCOS patients. Of particular importance is whether therapy with insulin-sensitizing agents should be limited to patients with documented insulin resistance. Needless to say, the greatest challenge remains to predict who will benefit and who will not.

AROMATASE INHIBITORS

Aromatase inhibitors have been suggested as an alternative treatment to clomiphene as the discrepancy between ovulation and pregnancy rates with clomiphene citrate has been attributed to its antiestrogenic action and estrogen receptor depletion. The aromatase inhibitors do not possess the adverse antiestrogenic effects of clomiphene but, by suppressing estrogen production, mimic the central reduction of negative feedback through which clomiphene works. Letrozole, the most prevalently used anti-aromatase for this indication, has been shown to be effective, in early trials, in inducing ovulation and pregnancy in women with anovulatory PCOS and inadequate clomiphene response and improving ovarian response to FSH in poor responders.

Letrozole

The first papers on the use of the aromatase inhibitor (AI) letrozole for ovulation induction were published over 10 years ago. Two early randomized trials in women with PCOS compared CC to letrozole, first showed comparable ovulation rates, live birth rates, and endometrial thickness, with a lower estradiol level in the letrozole group, whereas the second showed a significantly thicker endometrium, higher ovulation and pregnancy rate, with a lower number of mature follicles in the letrozole group. More recent studies in women with PCOS resistant to CC have shown that treatment with letrozole produced a significantly higher ovulation rate and comparable endometrial thickness when compared to both combined CC and metformin or placebo.[12]

Letrozole has also recently been compared to laparoscopic ovarian diathermy (LOD) for ovulation induction in women with PCOS and CC resistance.[13] In this study, 260 women were randomized to either letrozole daily for 5 days for up to 6 cycles (n = 128) or with 6 months of follow-up. Ovulation occurred in 335 of 512 cycles (65.4%) in the letrozole group and 364 of 525 cycles (69.3%) in the laparoscopy group without significant difference between the groups. Resumption of regular menstruation was similar in both treatment groups. A significant increase in midcycle endometrial thickness was observed in the letrozole group (8.8 ± 1.1 vs 7.9 ± 1.2 mm) (P <.05). Pregnancy rate was similar in both groups (15.6 vs 17.5%). There were no statistically significant differences with regard to miscarriage and live birth rates between the groups. No multiple pregnancy or ovarian hyperstimulation occurred in either group. This study concluded that letrozole and LOD are equally effective for inducing ovulation and achieving pregnancy in CC-resistant PCOS patients.[13]

Another recent prospective, randomized, nonblinded trial compared the effectiveness of letrozole and CC in induction of ovulation in 64 anovulatory women with PCOS who failed to ovulate when taking 100 mg/d of CC in previous cycles.[14] Patients were randomly divided into 2 groups, then treated with either 7.5 mg/d letrozole or 150 mg/d CC for 5 days starting from day 3 of the menstrual cycle. Twenty (62.5%) patients from the letrozole group and 12 (37.50%) patients from the CC group ovulated during the observation period, and this difference was statistically significant. This study found that there was a significantly lower estradiol level but greater endometrial thickness in the letrozole group on the day of human chorionic gonadotropin (hCG) administration. The pregnancy rate was also higher in the letrozole group (n = 13; 40.62%) in comparison with the CC group (n = 6; 18.75%), although this was not statistically significant. No multiple pregnancies occurred in either group.

Letrozole has also been compared to anastrozole for ovulation induction in CC-resistant women with PCOS.[15] In this prospective randomized trial, a total of 220 infertile women (574 cycles) were randomized to treatment with 2.5 mg/d of letrozole (111 patients, 295 cycles) or 1 mg/d of anastrozole

(109 patients, 279 cycles) for 5 days starting on menstrual cycle day 3. Both the total number of follicles and mature follicles were significantly higher in the anastrozole group. The endometrial thickness at the time of hCG administration was also significantly higher in the anastrozole group. Ovulation occurred in 183 of 295 cycles (62%) in the letrozole group and 177 of 279 cycles (63.4%) in the anastrozole group, whereas pregnancy occurred in 36 of 295 cycles (12.2%) in the letrozole group and 42 of 279 cycles (15.1%) in the anastrozole group, and these differences were not statistically significant. This study concluded that there were no significant differences in pregnancy or miscarriage rates between anastrozole and letrozole when used for ovulation induction in women with CC-resistant PCOS.

A recent meta-analysis of 4 trials showed a significant advantage for both pregnancy and delivery rates when AIs were compared to CC in women with PCOS. The odds ratio for pregnancies per patient was 2.0 (95% confidence interval, 1.1-3.8). Further, randomized trials comparing letrozole and CC as first-line treatment for ovulation induction in women with PCOS are needed.

AI and Unexplained Infertility

Fouda and Sayed[16] published a recent RCT comparing the efficacy of extended letrozole regimen with CC in 214 women with unexplained infertility undergoing superovulation and IUI. Women were randomized to either letrozole 2.5 mg/d from cycle days 1-9 (211 cycles) or CC 100 mg/d from cycle days 3-7 (210 cycles). Both groups were comparable with regard to the number of mature follicles and the day of hCG administration. Serum estradiol was significantly greater in the CC group, and the endometrial thickness was significantly greater in the extended letrozole group. Both the pregnancy rate per cycle (18.96 vs 11.43%) and the cumulative pregnancy rate were significantly greater in the extended letrozole group (37.73 vs 22.86%). This study concluded that the extended letrozole regimen had a superior efficacy compared to CC in patients with unexplained infertility undergoing superovulation and IUI.

Overall pregnancy rates are similar for women with unexplained infertility being treated with either CC or AIs. There may be a benefit to the use of an extended letrozole regimen. Further randomized trials are needed to assess the efficacy of AIs for superovulation for the treatment of unexplained infertility.

AI and Endometriosis

Many studies have found that the combination of AI with conventional therapy can be used to alleviate endometriosis-related pain. However, few studies have been done using AI to treat endometriosis-related infertility. One recent study by Abu Hashim et al.[17] evaluated pregnancy rates with IUI combined with either letrozole or CC for superovulation in women who had recently undergone surgical treatment for minimal to mild endometriosis. A total of 136 women with primary infertility because of minimal to mild endometriosis who did not achieve pregnancy 6-2 months after laparoscopic treatment were randomized to 5 mg/d letrozole (69 women, 220 cycles) or 100 mg/d CC (67 women, 213 cycles) for 5 days, combined with IUI for up to 4 cycles. The clinical pregnancy rate per cycle and the cumulative pregnancy rate after 4 cycles were comparable in both groups. Two twin pregnancies occurred in the CC/IUI group. Miscarriage and live birth rates were also comparable between both groups. The total number of follicles and serum estradiol on the day of hCG administration were significantly increased in the CC group. This study concluded that superovulation with letrozole was equally as effective as CC for women with minimal to mild endometriosis who did not achieve pregnancy 6–12 months after laparoscopic treatment. Interestingly, pregnancy rates were similar between the groups, although follicular development was greater in the CC group.[17]

Molecular studies have found that eutopic endometrium of women with endometriosis as well as ectopic endometriotic lesions express aromatase. Perhaps this inhibition of aromatase expression improved pregnancy potential in patients with endometriosis, explaining why there were equal pregnancy rates in both groups, despite a decrease in follicular development.

Safety of Aromatase Inhibitors

Safety is a major concern in the use of AIs for ovulation induction or superovulation. There was a study presented and published only in abstract form that suggested an increase in congenital cardiac and bone malformations in pregnancies achieved using letrozole.[18] This report was never fully published in a peer-reviewed journal, likely because of issues relating to the control group. Specifically, the control group used was not comparable to the treated group in terms of the patients' age and background risk of congenital malformations. Other studies failed to find an increased teratogenicity in pregnancies conceived using AIs. A large multicenter retrospective study by Tulandi et al.[19] found a significantly higher rate of congenital cardiac anomalies in the CC group compared to the AI-treated group. A recent randomized trial by Badawy et al. to assess the outcome of pregnancies after treatment with AIs also failed to detect a difference in malformation rate after treatment with either letrozole or anastrozole when compared with CC. More studies are needed to assess the safety of using AIs for either ovulation induction or superovulation.

Early studies suggested a lower multiple pregnancy rate, with more cycles resulting in monofollicular growth in women treated with letrozole 2.5 or 5 mg/d compared to CC. However, a more recent randomized trial has questioned this finding, showing a comparable twin pregnancy rate between CC and letrozole (8.3% vs 9.1%) in women with unexplained infertility. In addition, a case report has been published describing the first reported case of a triplet pregnancy after using letrozole for ovulation induction in a woman with PCOS and primary infertility. Taken together, these studies suggest that the use of an AI does not eliminate the risk of either twins or higher order multiples, although it is associated with a higher rate of monofollicular growth.

GONADOTROPINS

Exogenous gonadotropins have traditionally been used in PCOS patients who are resistant to ovulation induction with clomiphene and more recently those not responding to the addition of metformin or laparoscopic ovarian drilling. Gonadotropin preparations derived from human menopausal gonadotropin (hMG), a mixture that contains FSH, LH, and large quantities of urinary proteins, have been in use since the early 1960s. Other gonadotropin preparations in use today include purified urinary FSH (uFSH) and recombinant FSH (rFSH). Highly purified uFSH contains a reduced amount of LH and very small amounts of urinary proteins. The lack of urinary proteins in this preparation reduces adverse reactions such as local allergy or hypersensitivity. Preparations of rFSH were recently developed with a complete absence of LH and copurified proteins, giving high specific bioactivity. These preparations share similar pharmacokinetic characteristics with purified uFSH. Whereas hMG is administered intramuscularly, uFSH and rFSH can be given by subcutaneous injection, which can be self-administered and appear to be better tolerated by the patient. There are no data suggesting a higher pregnancy rate in PCOS with the use of one product compared with another.

In general, ovulation induction with gonadotropins in clomiphene-resistant PCOS patients is less successful than in patients with hypogonadotropic hypogonadism. However, women with PCOS are more sensitive to gonadotropin stimulation compared with spontaneously cycling women. This increased sensitivity appears to result from a larger pool of small antral follicles available for recruitment, rather than on differences in the FSH threshold level. Women with PCOS receiving gonadotropins for ovulation induction are particularly prone to a higher risk of overstimulation, multiple pregnancy, and ovarian hyperstimulation syndrome (OHSS) rates.

Inappropriately elevated serum LH levels are found in up to 70% of women with PCOS. This persistent elevation in serum LH during the follicular phase has been correlated with decreased pregnancy and increased spontaneous abortion rates. These complications were also related to the higher LH levels commonly seen in women with PCOS. Consequently, it has been suggested that purified uFSH would be more effective than hMG for ovulation induction in PCOS. However, a recent meta-analysis including 14 randomized, controlled trials did not find any differences in pregnancy rates between women with PCOS receiving uFSH or hMG. The incidence of OHSS was lower, however, in women using uFSH compared with hMG (OR: 0.20; 95% CI 0.08–0.46). In this study no conclusions could be drawn regarding the relative effect of these preparations on miscarriage and multiple pregnancy rates because of insufficient reporting of these outcomes in the trials.

The conventional regimen of ovulation induction with gonadotropins begins with a starting dose of 75–150 IU/day, with an increase of 75–150 IU/day every 3–5 days in those women with an inadequate response. Regardless of the specific gonadotropin preparation used, this regimen generally induces multiple follicular development, resulting in high rates of multiple pregnancy and OHSS.[20] Administration of lower doses of gonadotropins in a stepwise fashion (low-dose step-up or step-down, or sequential step-up, step-down) has generally replaced the conventional regimen and is reported to be effective in significantly reducing risks. The low-dose step-up protocol generally involves starting with a dose of 75 IU/day or less, which is increased after 14 days by 37.5 IU/day and every 7 days thereafter if no response is observed. The goal of the low-dose step-up protocol is to achieve the development of a single dominant follicle, rather than the development of multiple large follicles. This regimen is based on the concept of a follicular FSH threshold. The rationale is not to exceed the critical FSH concentration above which multiple follicles develop and result in increased risks of OHSS and multiple gestation.

The step-down protocol usually begins with a dose of 150–225 IU/day for 2 days, which is decreased to 75 IU/day for 7 days and increased to 150 IU/day after the seventh day if there is inadequate follicular response. More recently, a "sequential step-up, step-down" protocol has been used, in which the FSH dose is reduced by half when the leading follicle has reached 14 mm. The purpose of the sequential step-up, step-down protocol is to mimic the normal menstrual cycle, in which the normal early follicular phase FSH elevation is followed by a decline until a small FSH peak accompanies the normal LH surge.[21]

Low-dose regimens appear to be a promising approach when using gonadotropins for ovulation induction in clomiphene-resistant women with PCOS. The mono-ovulatory cycle rate is approximately 70%. The cumulative pregnancy rate is approximately 40%, and can be as high as

20% per cycle, comparable with conventional regimens. However, a multiple pregnancy rate of 6% and a low rate of OHSS (<1%) with low-dose regimens make these protocols more attractive than conventional gonadotropin regimens.

CONCLUSION

There are many options for ovulation induction in anovulatory women with PCOS, although treatment should be individualized to the patient. Weight loss through lifestyle modification in obese women with PCOS has the beneficial effect of frequently restoring regular ovulation. When pharmacological agents are required, clomiphene citrate remains the first-line therapy for ovulation induction, pending studies evaluating its effectiveness to metformin. Approximately 20% of women with PCOS fail to ovulate on the maximum clomiphene dose, and therapeutic alternatives include extending the duration of clomiphene administration, generally with the addition of midcycle hCG; the addition of midcycle hCG, an insulin sensitizer, or glucocorticoids as adjuvants; or proceeding to gonadotropin or pulsatile GnRH therapy. The use of hCG as an adjuvant to clomiphene is generally not needed. Glucocorticoids are used with some success, particularly in clomiphene-resistant patients, but side effects are significant. Ovulatory response to insulin sensitizers is modest, but may not be much lower than that in response to clomiphene. Pulsatile GnRH has overall low rates of ovulation and pregnancy and high risk of miscarriage and is not generally used in PCOS. The most promising medical treatment option for the clomiphene-resistant women with PCOS is low-dose gonadotropin therapy, although it has an increased risk of multiple pregnancy and OHSS.

Despite significant advances in the field of PCOS, induction of ovulation in women with PCOS remains a challenge for the clinical investigator and practicing physician.

Future studies should address the alternative approaches to achieve and maintain weight loss in obese women with PCOS

REFERENCES

1. Greenblatt RB. Chemical induction of ovulation. Fertil Steril. 1961;12:402-4.
2. Roy Homburg. Management of infertility associated with polycystic ovarian syndrome. Reproductive Biology and Endocrinology. 2003;1:109.
3. Imani B, Eijkemans MJ, te Velde ER, et al. Predictors of patients remaining anovulatory during clomiphene citrate induction of ovulation in normogonadotropic oligomenorrheic infertility. J Clin Endocrinol Metab. 1998;83:2361-5.
4. Parsanezhad ME, Alborzi S, Motazedian S, et al. Use of dexamethasone and clomiphene citrate in the treatment of clomiphene citrate-resistant patients with polycystic ovary syndrome and normal dehydroepiandrosterone sulfate levels: a prospective, double-blind, placebo-controlled trial. Fertil Steril. 2002;78(5): 1001-4.
5. Kashyap S, Moher D, Fung MF, et al. Assisted reproductive technology and the incidence of ovarian cancer: a meta-analysis. Obstet Gynecol. 2004;103(4):785-94.
6. Velazquez EM, Acosta A, Mendoza SG. Menstrual cyclicity after metformin therapy in polycystic ovary syndrome. Obstet Gynecol. 1997;90:392-5.
7. Nestler JE, Stovall D, Akhter N, et al. Strategies for the use of insulin-sensitizing drugs to treat infertility in women with polycystic ovary syndrome. Fertil Steril. 2002;77: 209-15.
8. Fleming R, Hopkinson ZE, Wallace AM, et al. Ovarian function and metabolic factors in women with oligomenorrhea treated with metformin in a randomized double blind placebo-controlled trial. J Clin Endocrinol Metab. 2002;87:569-4.
9. Nestler JE, Jakubowicz DJ, Evans WS, et al. Effects of metformin on spontaneous and clomiphene-induced ovulation in the polycystic ovary syndrome. N Engl J Med. 1998;338:1876-80.

10. Glueck CJ, Wang P, Goldenberg N, et al. Pregnancy outcomes among women with polycystic ovary syndrome treated with metformin. Hum Reprod. 2002;17:2858-64.
11. Homburg R. Should patients with polycystic ovary syndrome be treated with metformin?. Hum Reprod. 2002;17:853-6.
12. Kamath MS, Aleyamma TK, Chandy A et al. Aromatase inhibitors in women with clomiphene citrate resistance: a randomized, double-blind, placebo-controlled trial Fertil Steril. 2010;94:2857-9.
13. Abu Hashim H, Mashaly AM, Badawy A. Letrozole versus laparoscopic ovarian diathermy for ovulation induction in clomiphene-resistant women with polycystic ovary syndrome: a randomized controlled trial. Arch Gynecol Obstet. 2010;282:567-71.
14. Begum MR, Ferdous J, Begum A. Comparison of efficacy of aromatase inhibitor and clomiphene citrate in induction of ovulation in polycystic ovarian syndrome. FertilSteril. 2009;92:853-7.
15. Badawy A, Mosbah A, Shady M. Anastrozole or letrozole for ovulation induction in clomiphene-resistant women with polycystic ovarian syndrome: a prospective randomized trial. Fertil Steril. 2008;89:1209-12.
16. Fouda UM, Sayed AM. Extended letrozole regimen versus clomiphene citrate for superovulation in patients with unexplained infertility undergoing intrauterine insemination: a randomized controlled trial. Reprod Biol Endocrinol. 2011;9:84.
17. Abu Hashim H, El Rakhawy M, Abd Elaal I. Randomized comparison of superovulation with letrozole vs. clomiphene citrate in an IUI program for women with recently surgically treated minimal to mild endometriosis. Acta Obstet Gynecol Scand. 2012;91:338-45.
18. Biljan M, Hemming R, Brassard N. The outcome of 150 babies following the treatment with letrozole or letrozole with gonadotropins. Fertil Steril. 2005;84(suppl 1):S95.
19. Tulandi T, Martin J, Al-Fadhli R, et al. Congenital malformations among 911 newborns conceived after infertility treatment with letrozole or clomiphene citrate. Fertil Steril. 2006;85:1761-5.
20. Wang CF, Gemzell C. The use of human gonadotropins for the induction of ovulation in women with polycystic ovarian disease. Fertil Steril: 1980;33:479-86.
21. Fauser BC, Donderwinkel P, Schoot DC. The step-down principle in gonadotrophin treatment and the role of GnRH analogs. Baillieres Clin Obstet Gynaecol. 1993;7:309-30.

CHAPTER 8

Polycystic Ovarian Syndrome: Diagnosis, Management and Recent Advances

Praveena Pai, Pratap Kumar

Chapter outline

- Pathophysiology
- Clinical Features and Diagnosis
- Diagnosis of PCOS in Adolescence
- Management
  - Menstrual irregularity
  - Hyperandrogenism
  - Metabolic Syndrome
  - Subfertility

INTRODUCTION

Polycystic ovarian syndrome (PCOS) is a heterogeneous condition with hyperandrogenism, insulin resistance and chronic anovulation as the hallmark features. It is the most common endocrinopathy to affect women of reproductive age. The common presentations are menstrual irregularities, hirsutism/acne, obesity, subfertility, and long-term implications such as diabetes and endometrial cancer.

This heterogeneity seems to be affected by multiple factors, such as prenatal androgen exposure, nutritional status in the uterus, genetic factors, ethnicity and the insulin resistance of puberty.[1-3]

PATHOPHYSIOLOGY

Puberty is heralded with the maturation of the hypothalamic-pituitary-ovarian axis and secretion of gonadotropin-releasing hormone (GnRH), which was suppressed during childhood. Varying GnRH pulse frequencies trigger the pituitary to release luteinizing hormone (LH) and follicle-stimulating hormone (FSH), which stimulate ovarian theca and granulosa cells, respectively. Theca cells produce androstenedione, which is aromatized in the granulosa cells to estradiol. This causes estrogenic changes including breast development, bone growth, and fat deposition. At the same time, adrenal gland also releases increasing amounts of androgens, such as dehydroepiandrosterone (DHEA) and DHEA sulfate (DHEAS), which are responsible for the development of pubic and axillary hair, also causing acne. The ovarian androgen also brings about the development of sexual hair growth.[4]

Although the exact etiology of PCOS is still a mystery, increased androgen level is the main problem. Androgen is mainly produced by the ovaries (with a smaller contribution from the adrenals and peripheral adipose tissue) and interferes with hypothalamic sensitivity to negative feedback from the ovary, thereby increasing GnRH pulse frequency.[5] This persistent and rapid pulse frequency favors increased LH secretion[6] resulting in overproduction of androgens from the ovarian theca cells. The relative decrease in FSH secretion means less aromatization of androgens to estradiol resulting in impaired follicular development and hence prolonged periods of oligomenorrhoea—a hallmark of PCOS.

CLINICAL FEATURES AND DIAGNOSIS

The symptoms may vary—some women presenting with mild symptoms, while others with more severe range of symptoms.

In its fully developed form, PCOS is characterized by menstrual abnormalities, hirsutism, obesity, hyperandrogenemia, impaired blood glucose, subfertility, and ultrasonographic evidence of polycystic ovaries.

Various diagnostic criteria have evolved over the decades as shown in Box 8.1. PCOS as it is popularly known was first defined by National Institute of Child Health and Human Development (NICHD) in 1990, as the combination of androgen excess and oligoanovulation in the absence of all other causes for anovulatory infertility.[7] The primary etiology was believed to be androgen excess leading to menstrual derangements. Polycystic appearance of the ovaries was not considered a prerequisite for diagnosis. This was an important first step but the criteria were based on opinions rather than evidence. In 2003, European Society of Human Reproduction and Embryology (ESHRE) and American Society for Reproductive Medicine (ASRM) met in Rotterdam and introduced polycystic ovaries as a third diagnostic criterion, allowing a diagnosis of PCOS if 2 of the 3 criteria were met.[8] The syndrome was thus deemed to be more a problem of ovarian dysfunction (reflected as menstrual irregularities or polycystic ovarian morphology).[9]

The freedom to choose 2 out of the 3 criteria meant that this syndrome could be diagnosed in the absence of hyperandrogenism or menstrual dysfunction—both of which had been the etiopathological basis for the previous classifications![10] The idea of dropping androgen excess as a prerequisite was difficult to digest for many. In 2006, the Androgen Excess Society Task Force came up with their new diagnostic criteria which acknowledged androgen excess as key and coupled it with menstrual irregularity/polycystic morphology to diagnose this condition. Having gone around in full circle, the National Institute of Health (NIH) Evidence-based Methodology Workshop on PCOS in December 2012 recommended that Rotterdam classification was the most

Box 8.1: A comparison of diagnostic criteria for polycystic ovary syndrome.

1990 National Institute of Child Health and Human Development (NICHD) Guidelines

Patients demonstrates both:
1. Clinical and/or biochemical signs of hyperandrogenism
2. Oligo-or chronic anovulation

Exclusion of other etiologies of androgen excess and anovulation infertility is necessary.

2003 European Society of Human Reproduction and Embryology and American Society for Reproductive Medicine (ESHRE/ASRM or Rotterdam) Guidelines

Patient demonstrates two of three criteria:
1. Oligo- or chronic anovulation
2. Clinical and/or biochemical signs of hyperandrogenism
3. Polycystic ovaries

Exclusion of other etiologies of androgen excess and anovulatory infertility is necessary.

2006 Androgen Excess Society (AES) Guidelines

Patient demonstrates both:
1. Hirsutism and/or hyperandrogenemia
2. Oligo-anovulation and/or polycystic ovaries

Exclusion of other etiologies of androgen excess and anovulatory infertility is necessary.

inclusive in the global context, but suggested that a less 'ovary focused' name should be sought.[11] This workshop proposed classifying PCOS patients into 4 distinct phenotypes in any future research so, as to get more meaningful information for comparison between various ethnicities. The phenotypes proposed were:
- Androgen excess + ovulatory dysfunction
- Androgen excess + polycystic ovarian morphology
- Ovulatory dysfunction + polycystic ovarian morphology
- Androgen excess + ovulatory dysfunction + polycystic ovarian morphology.

With huge improvements in ultrasound machines, it is not uncommon to detect higher number of follicles in absence of any other features suggesting PCOS. Consequently, it has been suggested that we should increase the number of follicles required per ovary (FNPO) to fulfill the criteria of being 'polycystic'. Based on receiver operating curve analysis, recent studies have suggested an FNPO of ≥19 or ≥26, but the jury is still out over this matter.[12,13] The ESE recommends that situations where imaging facilities do not allow FNPO estimation, ovarian volume must be used.[14]

It should be noted that the diagnosis of PCOS can only be made when other etiologies have been excluded. The recommended baseline screening tests are free androgen index, thyroid function tests, prolactin and glucose tolerance test.

It is usually the free testosterone that is increased in PCOS. However, in the absence of robust methods to measure this, total testosterone is recommended as the first simple test. Free Androgen Index (FAI) is nothing but the ratio between total testosterone and sex hormone binding globulin (SHBG) multiplied by 100. Though currently the recommended method, FAI is not completely foolproof as the SHBG levels are reduced in obese women.[15] Testosterone level in PCOS is usually <150 ng/dL (5.2 nmol/L). A value of >200 ng/dL (6.9 nmol/L) raises suspicion of ovarian or adrenal tumor.[10] Dehydroepiandrosterone-sulphate (DHEA-S) should then be requested. A value >800 μg/dL (21.7 mSmol/L) is highly suggestive of adrenal tumor. If the DHEAS is normal then androgen secreting tumour of ovarian origin or ovarian hyperthecosis may be responsible. Imaging of the ovaries is essential. Late onset 21-hydroxylase deficiency must be ruled out. A morning, fasting 17-hydroxyprogesterone of <200 ng/mL (6 nmol/L) reliably rules out this condition. A higher value warrants adrenocortico-tropic hormone (ACTH) stimulated 17-hydroxyprogesterone testing. If Cushing's syndrome is suggested by clinical examination, a dexamethasone suppression test is advised. All these values can be affected by oral contraceptive pills, which should therefore be ideally stopped at least 3 months prior to evaluation.

Total testosterone may also increase due to increase in SHBG levels either due to estrogenic effects of drugs (e.g. tamoxifen) or due to liver dysfunction (portal hypertension with biliary cirrhosis) or hyperthyroidism.[16]

Routine assessment of FSH and LH and for diagnosis of PCOS is no longer recommended. However, LH, FSH measurements do help in ruling out premature ovarian failure as a cause for oligo/amenorrhea and hence should be advised if deemed necessary.

Impaired blood glucose or overt diabetes is not an uncommon occurrence in PCOS. Hence, the local protocol should be followed to assess and treat this.

Anti-Müllerian hormone (AMH), secreted by small antral follicles is increased in women with PCOS. Increasing number of papers are discussing its use as a diagnostic test in PCOS.[17,18] It is a particularly attractive option given that currently a debate is raging about the ultrasound parameters that should be used for diagnosis of polycystic ovarian morphology.[13,19,20] Moreover, ultrasound imaging quality may be compromised in obese women, particularly if transabdominal scans need to be done (such as in sexually nonactive adolescents). Standardization of AMH assays and a consensus on AMH threshold to diagnose PCOS is however still awaited.[21]

DIAGNOSIS OF PCOS IN ADOLESCENCE

Diagnosis of PCOS is particularly challenging as characteristics of normal puberty often overlap with signs and symptoms of PCOS. Certain metabolic changes associated with PCOS are also physiologic during puberty. Hyperinsulinemia is common in healthy adolescents; insulin sensitivity decreases with a compensatory rise in insulin secretion, which later returns to prepubertal levels in adulthood.[4] Interestingly, both insulin resistance and hyperinsulinemia are more severe in adolescents likely to develop PCOS compared with the general adolescent population.[11] Insulin stimulates ovarian theca cell synthesis of androgens and inhibits hepatic production of sex hormone–binding globulin, together resulting in increased circulating free androgen levels. In addition, insulin resistance promotes release of nonesterified fatty acids from the liver and adipose tissue due to decreased lipoprotein lipase activity, which contributes to the dyslipidemia that is associated with PCOS.

Adult criteria cannot be applied to diagnose PCOS in adolescence as irregular cycles, slight hirsutism and acne are seen in a majority as a part of the physiological changes of puberty. International Pediatric Subspecialty Societies have recently reached a consensus that unexplained persistent hyperandrogenic anovulation using age—and stage-appropriate standards—are appropriate diagnostic criteria for PCOS in adolescents.[17] Simply put, the criteria include abnormal uterine bleeding pattern (for >2 years) along with evidence of hyperandrogenism (persistent testosterone elevation or moderate-severe hirsutism or moderate-severe inflammatory acne vulgaris). Ultrasound appearance of ovaries has not been given importance in diagnosis as this morphology is not uncommon during adolescence and moreover, transabdominal scanning (preferred in this age-group) coupled with obesity may yield suboptimal images. Though the diagnosis should not be made earlier than 2 years, a diagnostic evaluation has been recommended at the end of 1 year to avoid delay in treatment.

MANAGEMENT

Menstrual Irregularity

There is a 2.7-fold increased risk of endometrial cancer in women with PCOS due to the associated oligomenorrhea and prolonged exposure to unopposed estrogen.[18] It is recommended that women should have atleast 4 bleeds per year to reduce this risk.[19] Weight loss (whether with lifestyle changes or combined with pharmacotherapy such as orlistat) of as little as 5% is associated with resumption of normal menstruation, ovulation and improvement in metabolic disturbances.[20]

Combined hormonal contraception remains the next line treatment in those not desiring to conceive. The progestin component decreases LH, which suppresses androgen production and estrogen decreases the SHBG production, decreasing the free androgen levels. The estrogen content of most of the preparations is fairly similar. Differences are seen in the progestogens, some with lesser androgenic effects (desogestrel, norgestimate, and gestodene) and some such as drospirenone having antiandrogenic effects.

Hyperandrogenism

Hyperandrogenism my manifest as hirsutism, acne, androgenic alopecia, acanthosis nigricans, and skin tags. Hirsutism, considered the best marker, occurs when androgens change normally vellous hair to terminal hair in androgen-sensitive areas, most commonly on facial areas. Treatments try to decrease the production or circulation of androgens. Contraceptives decrease SHBG, thus reducing the free testosterone. As the terminal hair turnover is slow, the treatment should be continued for at least 6 months to see a difference.[21] Antiandrogen treatment includes aldosterone antagonist such as spironolactone, androgen receptor antagonist such as flutamide and 5-α reductase type 2 inhibitor such as finasteride. These prevent new terminal hair growth but are fetotoxic and hence a reliable contraception should be used. Flutamide can also be hepatotoxic. Another agent, eflornithine (the only topical agent), acts by irreversibly binding to ornithine decarboxylase, thus preventing the natural substrate from binding to its active site. It has been shown to slow down facial hair growth considerably at the end of 1 year.[22] Insulin sensitizers do not ameliorate this condition. The other treatment modalities include electrolysis and laser. Combined oral contraceptive also work well for acne as do antiandrogens. Severe acne may require isotretinoin, though this may itself cause alopecia. Moreover, this agent is highly teratogenic and child bearing should be avoided for atleast 3 months postcessation of the medication.[23]

Metabolic Syndrome

Polycystic ovarian syndrome is linked to metabolic syndrome most of which are due to the associated obesity. Insulin resistance leading to compensatory hyperinsulinemia, causes androgen excess by stimulating ovarian theca cells and by decreasing the hepatic synthesis of SHBG. This results in impaired blood sugars or overt type 2 diabetes. Visceral obesity and dyslipidemias are not uncommon. Cornerstone of treatment remains weight loss with lifestyle interventions along with the use of insulin sensitizers such as metformin and thiazolidinediones such as pioglitazone. Metformin's efficacy is well proven in this regard. It acts mainly in the liver, by suppressing gluconeogenesis and hepatic glucose output. It also enhances peripheral insulin action, and reduces glucose absorption from the digestive tract. Metformin also directly inhibits thecal androgen production.[24] Bariatric surgery may be helpful in cases of morbid obesity or obesity with severe metabolic syndrome.

Subfertility

Subfertility in women with PCOS may be due to anovulation, suboptimal oocyte quality or suboptimal endometrial receptivity. The approach to the patient with PCOS should involve the use of progressively more aggressive treatment strategies until ovulation is established and pregnancy can be achieved. Obesity is a common association with PCOS. The PPCOS II (Pregnancy in Polycystic Ovarian Syndrome II) trial has shown an inverse correlation between body mass index (BMI) and live births.[25] Lifestyle measures for weight loss hence remain the first line intervention in those who are overweight/obese. The next step is ovulation induction with clomiphene citrate, a selective estrogen receptor modulator. This is associated with a live birth rate of 23%.[25] However, a small risk of ovarian hyperstimulation syndrome (OHSS) and multiple gestations (4–8%) is seen with this agent. Usually 3–4 cycles with increasing doses of clomiphene (50–150 mg in the event of no ovulation) are tried. Fifty-two percent of women will ovulate in response to 50 mg of clomiphene, and an additional 22% will respond to 100 mg.[26] Though US Food and Drug Administration (FDA) has approved doses only up to 150 mg, many bodies including American College of Obstetricians and Gynecologists (ACOG) approve doses of 250 mg particularly in women with high BMI. Another selective estrogen receptor modulator (SERM) tamoxifen, can be tried in clomiphene resistant cases. Lack of superiority data and side effects like hot flushes has limited its use.[27]

In the event of clomiphene resistance (no ovulation), a combination with metformin has been shown to yield better results.[28] The largest single trial comparing live birth rates in patients who took the 2 medications individually or in combination found that clomiphene alone or in combination with metformin resulted in significantly higher birth rates (22.5% and 26.8%, respectively) than did metformin alone as a single agent (7.2%).[29] Metformin is usually administered at 1500–2000 mg daily, starting with a dose of 500 mg daily, titrating upwards.

On the other hand, aromatase inhibitors (AIs) such as letrozole are making a comeback as agents for ovulation induction (perhaps even first line) due to the associated higher live births, lower risk of OHSS and lower multiple pregnancy rates as demonstrated in a landmark trial by Legro et al.[30] India has recently permitted the use of this agent once again. These act by competitive inhibition of aromatase. When aromatase is blocked, androgens cannot be converted to estrogens, resulting in a low estrogen state, releasing the hypothalamic-pituitary axis from the negative feedback of estrogen (similar to clomiphene). After cessation of AI, estrogen levels increase immediately. This leads to a more abrupt decrease in FSH. This decrease makes gonadotropin support of multiple pregnancies less likely, and the associated increase in estrogen enhances the production of cervical mucus and endometrial proliferation. This is how AI differ from clomiphene.[27] In clomiphene resistant cases, 60% ovulation rates and between 12% and 40% pregnancy rates have been quoted in another small study.[31]

If none of the above agents fail to elicit ovulation, one is left with options of using gonadotropins or ovarian drilling to improve the response of the ovaries to pharmacotherapy. Both are equally efficacious.[32] Gonadotropins increase the risk of OHSS and multiple pregnancies as against ovarian drilling. Laparoscopic ovarian drilling restores ovulation in about 50% of women with conception rates of 50% over the first year.[33]

SUMMARY

Polycystic ovarian syndrome is characterized by a complex set of symptoms and remains a fascinating subject for reproductive endocrinologists. This chapter has touched upon the pathophysiology and dealt with diagnosis and management of its varied presentations. However, the last word has not yet been said on many issues such as the most comprehensive method of classification, ultrasound thresholds for diagnosis or the role of AMH in diagnosis. Hence, we need to watch the space with keen interest.

REFERENCES

1. Abbott DH, Tarantal AF, Dmesic DA. Fetal, infant, adolescent and adult phenotypes of polycystic ovary syndrome in prenatally androgenized female rhesus monkeys. Am J Primatol. 2009;71:776-84.
2. Oberfield SE, Sopher AB, Gerken AT. Approach to the girl with early onset of pubic hair. J Clin Endocrinol Metab. 2011;96:1610-22.
3. Zhang HY, Guo CX, Zhu FF, et al. Clinical characteristics, metabolic features, and phenotype of Chinese women with polycystic ovary syndrome: a large-scale case control study. Arch Gynecol Obstet. 2013;287:525-31.
4. Roe AH, Dokras A. The diagnosis of polycystic ovary syndrome in adolescents. Rev Obstet Gynecol. 2011;4(2):45-51.
5. Waldstreicher J, Santoro NF, Hall JE, et al. Hyperfunction of the hypothalamic-pituitary axis in women with polycystic ovarian disease: indirect evidence for partial gonadotroph desensitization. J Clin Endocrinol Metab. 1988;66:165-72.
6. Venturoli S, Porcu E, Fabbri R, et al. Longitudinal evaluation of the different gonadotropin pulsatile patterns in anovulatory

cycles of young girls. J Clin Endocrinol Metab. 1992;74:836-41.
7. Zawadski JK, Dunaif A. Diagnostic criteria for polycystic ovary syndrome: towards a rational approach. In: Dunaif A, Givens JR, Haseltine FP, Merriam GR (Eds). Polycystic Ovary Syndrome. Boston: Blackwell Scientific Publications; 1992. pp. 377-84.
8. Rotterdam ESHRE/ASRM-Sponsored PCOS Consensus Workshop Group. Revised 2003 consensus on diagnostic criteria and long-term health risks related to polycystic ovary syndrome. Fertil Steril. 2004;81(1):19-25.
9. Azziz R. Diagnostic criteria for polycystic ovary syndrome: a reappraisal. Fertil Steril. 2005;83(5):1343-6.
10. Azziz R, Carmina E, Dewailly D, et al. Position statement: criteria for defining polycystic ovary syndrome as a predominantly hyperandrogenic syndrome: an Androgen Excess Society Guideline. J Clin Endocrinol Metab. 2006;91(11):4237-45.
11. Final Report National Institute of Health. Evidence-based Methodology Workshop on Polycystic Ovary Syndrome December 3-5, 2012. Executive summary at http://prevention.nih.gov/workshops/2012/pcos/resources.aspx.
12. Dewailly D, Gronier H, Poncelet E, et al. Diagnosis of polycystic ovary syndrome (PCOS): revisiting the threshold values of follicle count on ultrasound and of the serum AMH level for the definition of polycystic ovaries. Hum Reprod. 2011;26(11):3123-9.
13. Lujan ME, Jarrett BY, Brooks ED, et al. Updated ultrasound criteria for polycystic ovary syndrome: reliable thresholds for elevated follicle population and ovarian volume. Hum Reprod. 2013;28(5):1361-8.
14. Conway G, Dewailly D, Diamanti-Kandarakis E, et al. ESE PCOS Special Interest Group. The polycystic ovary syndrome: a position statement from the European Society of Endocrinology. Eur J Endocrinol. 2014;171(4):1-29.
15. Pai PJ, Sahoo P, Kumar P. New insights into infertility associated with polycystic ovarian syndrome. Int J Infertil Fetal Med. 2015;6(2):43-50.
16. Pugeat M, Dechaud H, Raverot V, et al. Recommendations for investigation of hyperandrogenism. Ann Endocrinol. 2010;71(1):2-7.
17. Sahmay S, Atakul N, Aydogan B, et al. Elevated serum levels of anti-Mullerian hormone can be introduced as a new diagnostic marker for polycystic ovary syndrome. Acta Obstet Gynecol Scand. 2013;92(12):1369-74.
18. Wiweko B, Maidarti M, Priangga MD, et al. Anti-mullerian hormone as a diagnostic and prognostic tool for PCOS patients. J Assist Reprod Genet. 2014;31(10):1311-6.
19. Chen Y, Li L, Chen X, et al. Ovarian volume and follicle number in the diagnosis of polycystic ovary syndrome in Chinese women. Ultrasound Obstet Gynecol. 2008;32:700-3.
20. Kösüs N, Kösüs A, Turhan NÖ, et al. Do threshold values of ovarian volume and follicle number for diagnosing polycystic ovarian syndrome in Turkish women differ from western countries? Eur J Obstet Gynecol Reprod Biol. 2011;154:177-81.
21. Singh AK, Singh R. Can anti-Mullerian hormone replace ultrasonographic evaluation in polycystic ovary syndrome? A review of current progress. Indian J Endocrinol Metab. 2015;19(6):731-43.
22. Balfour J, McClellan K. Topical eflornithine. Am J Clin Dermatol. 2001;2:197-201.
23. Choi JS, Koren G, Nulman I. Pregnancy and isotretinoin therapy. CMAJ. 2013;185(5):411-3.
24. Spritzer PM. Polycystic ovary syndrome: reviewing diagnosis and management of metabolic disturbances. Arq Bras Endocrinol Metabol. 2014;58(2):182-7.
25. Legro R, Kunselman A, Brzyski R, et al. The Pregnancy in Polycystic Ovary Syndrome II (PPCOS II) trial: rationale and design of a double-blind randomized trial of clomiphene citrate and letrozole for the treatment of infertility in women with polycystic ovary syndrome. Contemp Clin Trials. 2012;33:470-81.
26. Gorlitsky GA, Kase NG, Speroff L. Ovulation and pregnancy rates with clomiphene citrate. Obstet Gynecol. 1978;51(3):265-9.

27. Von Hofe J, Bates GW. Ovulation induction. Obstet Gynecol Clin North Am. 2015;42(1):27-37.
28. Practice Committee of the American Society for Reproductive Medicine. Use of clomiphene citrate in infertile women: a committee opinion. Fertil Steril. 2013;100(2):341-8.
29. Legro RS, Barnhart HX, Schlaff WD, et al. Clomiphene, metformin, or both for infertility in the polycystic ovary syndrome. N Engl J Med. 2007;356(6):551-66.
30. Legro RS, Brzyski RG, Diamond MP, et al. Letrozole versus clomiphene for infertility in the polycystic ovary syndrome. N Engl J Med. 2014;371(2):119-29.
31. Begum MR, Ferdous J, Begum A, et al. Comparison of efficacy of aromatase inhibitor and clomiphene citrate in induction of ovulation in polycystic ovarian syndrome. Fertil Steril. 2009;92(3):853-7.
32. The Thessaloniki ESHRE/ASRM- Sponsored PCOS Consensus Workshop Group. Consensus on infertility treatment related to polycystic ovary syndrome. Hum Reprod. 2007;23:462-77.
33. Farquhar C, Brown J, Marjoribanks J. Laparoscopic drilling by diathermy or laser for ovulation induction in anovulatory polycystic ovary syndrome. Cochrane Database Syst Rev. 2012;(6):CD001122.

CHAPTER 9

Ovarian Hyperstimulation Syndrome: Newer Concepts

Ameet Patki, Abhimanyu Shinde

Chapter outline

- Early and Late Forms of OHSS
- Classification of OHSS
- Risk Factors Associated with OHSS
- Pathophysiology
- Management of OHSS
- Prevention
  - Primary Prevention
  - Secondary Prevention
- OHSS and Pregnancy

INTRODUCTION

Ovarian hyperstimulation syndrome (OHSS) is a potentially fatal iatrogenic condition resulting from excessive stimulation of the ovaries. The vast majority of OHSS occurs in the setting of injectable like gonadotropins in IVF although in the absence of proper monitoring oral clomifene and other drugs can result in massive ovarian hyperstimulation. In anovulatory women treated with different preparations for ovulation induction the incidence of mild OHSS is 5-10%, moderate OHSS is 2-4% and severe forms of OHSS occur in 0.5-5.0% of IVF cycles (Alvarez et al., 2007).

EARLY AND LATE FORMS OF OHSS

The early form of OHSS is due to human chorionic gonadotropin (hCG) and is related to an exaggerated ovarian response to gonadotropin stimulation whereas the late form is mainly related to secretion of placental hCG. The early form is within days after the ovulation triggering injection of hCG and the late form within 10 days after hCG. The early cases particularly constitute the serious and long lasting morbidity.

CLASSIFICATION OF OHSS

Several schemes have been developed for classifying the severity of OHSS, with no clear agreement between investigators. The scheme in Table 9.1 is based on the

Table 9.1: Classification of OHSS as per its severity.

Sl No.	Grade	Signs and Symptoms
1.	Mild	• Abdominal bloating • Mild abdominal Pain • Ovarian size < 8 cm
2.	Moderate	• Moderate abdominal pain • Nausea and vomiting • Ovarian size 8–12 cm
3.	Severe	• Ascites, pleural effusion • Oliguria (< 30 mL/hr) • Hematocrit (> 45%) • Hypoproteinemia (Albumin < 3.5 mg/dL) • Ovarian size > 12 cm
4.	Critical	• Tense ascites or large pleural effusion • Hematocrit (> 55%) • Oliguria/anuria • Thromboembolism • Respiratory distress

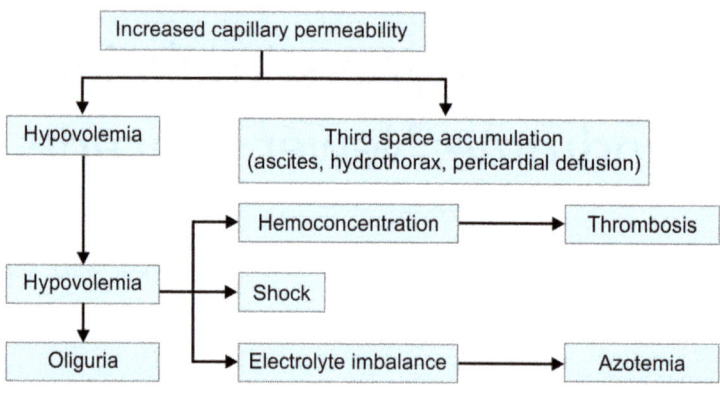

Flowchart 9.1: Severe and critical OHSS.

(OHSS: ovarian hyperstimulation syndrome)

classification of OHSS severity proposed as per RCOG guidelines combined with useful features from previous classifications (Flowchart 9.1).

RISK FACTORS ASSOCIATED WITH OHSS

Several risk factors young age (<35 years of age), polycystic ovary like patients, asthenic habitus, pregnancy and hCG luteal supplementation. Different protocols of ovarian stimulation in ART affects incidence and severity of OHSS. Risk of OHSS is observed in patients having higher number of immature follicles (<12 mm) and large follicles (>18 mm) on the day of hCG administration.

PATHOPHYSIOLOGY

The pathophysiology of this condition is characterized by ovarian enlargement, massive extra, vascular exudates accumulation in combination with profound intravascular volume depletion and hemoconcentration. The underlying cause of these pathophysiological changes remain unknown, but there are evidences that vascular endothelial growth factor (VEGF), tumor necrosis factor alpha (TNFα), interleukin 2 (IL 2) and interleukin 6 (IL 6) contribute to the development of OHSS. (Elchalal et al., 1997). The angiogenic properties of human follicular fluid combined with high prorenin, high plasma rennin like activity, angiotensin II like immunoreactivity and angiotensinogen converting enzyme raised the hypothesis on possible involvement of renin-angiotensin system in pathogenesis of OHSS through new vessel formation and increased capillary permeability (Navot D et al., 1987).

MANAGEMENT OF OHSS

Relevant history from a woman suspected to be suffering from OHSS should be taken.

History:
- Time of onset of symptoms relative to trigger
- Medication used for trigger (hCG or GnRH agonist)
- Number of follicles on final monitoring scan
- Number of eggs collected
- Were embryos replaced and how many?
- Polycystic ovary syndrome diagnosis.

Symptoms:
- Abdominal bloating
- Abdominal discomfort/pain, need for analgesia
- Nausea and vomiting

- Breathlessness, inability to lie flat or talk in full sentences
- Reduced urine output
- Leg swelling
- Vulval swelling
- Associated comorbidities such as thrombosis.

Examination and investigations of women with suspected OHSS
- **Examination**
  - **General:** Assess for dehydration, edema (pedal, vulval and sacral); record heart rate, respiratory rate, blood pressure, body weight
  - **Abdominal:** Assess for ascites, palpable mass, peritonism; measure girth
  - **Respiratory:** Assess for pleural effusion, pneumonia, pulmonary edema
- **Investigations**
  - Full blood count
  - Hematocrit (hemoconcentration)
  - C-reactive protein (severity)
  - Urea and electrolytes (hyponatremia and hyperkalemia)
  - Serum osmolality (hypo-osmolality)
  - Liver function tests (elevated enzymes and reduced albumin)
  - Coagulation profile (elevated fibrinogen and reduced antithrombin)
  - hCG (to determine outcome of treatment cycle) if appropriate
  - **Ultrasound scan:** Ovarian size, pelvic and abdominal free fluid. Consider ovarian Doppler if torsion suspected

Other tests that may be indicated
- Arterial blood gases
- D-dimers
- Electrocardiogram (ECG)/echocardiogram
- Chest X-ray
- Computerized tomography pulmonary angiogram (CTPA) or ventilation/perfusion (V/Q) scan.

After history and examinations severity should be graded as per standard classification system and treated accordingly.

All patients of OHSS does not require in patient management. Mild and moderate OHSS should be managed on out-patient basis (Lincoln SR et al., 2002; Smith LP et al., 2009).

- **Mild and Moderate OHSS:-**
  - Patient should be appropriately counseled and provided with information regarding fluid intake and output monitoring.
  - Paracetamol and oral opiates including codeine can be offered to women for pain relief.
  - Nonsteroidal anti-inflammatory drugs (NSAIDs) should be avoided as they may compromise renal function in women with OHSS. (Balasch J et al., 1990)

Clinicians and patients should be vigilant for signs that the severity of OHSS is worsening (RCOG guidelines, 2015).

These include:
- Increasing abdominal distension and pain
- Shortness of breath
- Tachycardia or hypotension
- Reduced urine output (<1000 mL/24 hours) or positive fluid balance (>1000 mL/24 hours)
- Weight gain and increased abdominal girth
- Increasing hematocrit (greater than 45%).

- **Severe and critical OHSS:**
  - Patients with severe and critical OHSS must be hospitalized
  - Women with severe OHSS are at increased risk of thromboembolism. Although there are no trials on this subject, thromboprophylaxis should be provided for these women in view of the serious nature of this complication.
  - GnRH antagonist administration and Dopamine agonist help in quicker regression of established OHSS (Baumgarten M et al., 2013).

Indications for paracentesis include the following:
- Severe abdominal distension and abdominal pain secondary to ascites
- Shortness of breath and respiratory compromise secondary to ascites and increased intra-abdominal pressure
- Oliguria despite adequate volume replacement, secondary to increased abdominal pressure causing reduced renal perfusion.

Paracentesis should be carried out under ultrasound guidance and can be performed abdominally or vaginally.

Intravenous colloid therapy should be considered for women who have large volumes of fluid removed by paracentesis

PREVENTION

This can be basically primary or secondary. Mechanism and management of ohss has been described in Figure. 9.1.

Primary Prevention

Patients who have a primary risk of OHSS should be exposed to gonadotropins as little as possible. That means all other safer options like lifestyle changes to include diet and exercises, oral ovulation induction drugs, use of insulin sensitizers and laparoscopic ovarian drilling should be kept in mind. This holds true especially for young women and those with history of OHSS in the past.

Careful history regarding thromboembolism in family, thrombophilia and antiphospholipid antibodies should be identified earlier to treatment with gonadotropins. Lowest possible doses of gonadotrophins should be used with frequent monitoring with transvaginal scans and serum estradiol measurements. Prophylactic heparin can be used in selected cases.

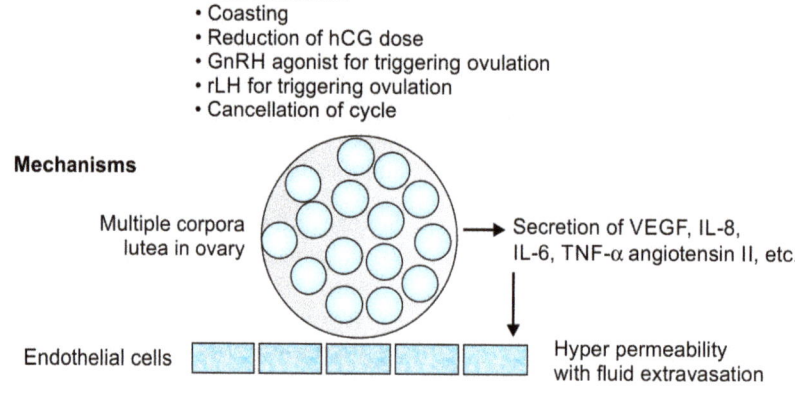

Fig. 9.1: Mechanisms and management of ovarian hyperstimulation syndrome.
(rLH: recombinaut luteinizing hormone; hCG: human chorionic gonadotropin; VEGF: vascular endothelial growth factor)

Secondary Prevention

Withholding ovulatory hCG reduces incidence of both early and late OHSS. However, the cycle is wasted and can cause both financial and emotional trauma to the couple.

Cycle Cancellation

In high-risk patients the dose of hCG can be reduced from 5000 to 3000 IU.

Reducing hCG Dosage

In high-risk patients the dose of hCG can be reduced from 5000 to 3000 IU.

Coasting

In high-risk patients with serum estradiol levels more than 3000 pg/mL and/or more than 20 follicles per ovary, stimulation with gonadotropins can be stopped while continuing the GnRH agonist administration. The principle behind this management is that the larger follicles continue to grow while the intermediate and small follicles undergo atresia (FSH threshold theory). Coasting also causes a downregulation of VEGF gene expression and protein production as a result of increased apoptosis in granulose cells of all, but mainly immature follicles, but does not influence oocyte quality and endometrial receptivity. Although, there are no clear guidelines when coasting should be started and stopped, this method is very popular with acceptable pregnancy rates. Based on studies coasting can be started when follicles are 14 mm in size and the estradiol levels are more than 3000 IU. Coasting should not be more than 4 days since it can affect implantation rates (Chen et al., 2003).

Modification of the Ovulation Trigger Agent

Replacement of hCG by exogenous or endogenous LH:

An endogenous LH surge can be provoked by administration of a short acting GnRH agonist (Triptorelin 0.2 mg). This is only possible in cycles without pituitary desensitization by a GnRH agonist, it significantly reduces chances of OHSS (Humaidan et al. 2010).

A single dose of recombinant LH can also be used. The development of recombinant LH (rLH) may offer an opportunity to replace hCG. The European rLH study performed a prospective and comparative study on the effective dose of rLH to induce oocyte maturation and luteinization in patients undergoing IVF. A dose of 15,000–30,000 IU rLH compares to 5,000 iu hCG resulting in similar number of oocytes, embryos and pregnancies (European Study Group, 2001).

Administration of Macromolecules

Prophylactic administration of 20% albumin is supposed to reduce the incidence of severe OHSS by preventing the fluid shift to the third space and binding factors responsible for the development of this syndrome.

The Cochrane review also shows that intravenous administration at the time of oocyte retrieval has a preventive effect in at-risk cycles. However, two studies have shown a reduced pregnancy rate after IV albumin. Albumin infusion has side effects like nausea, vomiting, and febrile reactions. Risk of viral transmission is also possible.

Hydroxyethyl starch solution (HES): Works as effective as albumin, is cheaper and safer alternative.

Cryopreservation of All Embryos

Instead of canceling the cycle it is also possible to administer hCG as trigger, retrieve the oocytes and freeze all the resulting embryos. Although this can exclude late form of OHSS, the early form can still occur and must be noted.

Dopamine Agonists/Cabergoline

Most recent suggested strategy to prevent the development of OHSS is the use of low dose dopamine agonists such as cabergoline. It inhibits the phosphorylation of the VEGF receptor thereby preventing increased capillary permeability, the main action of VEGF. In a study by Alvarez et al. 2007, cabergoline was given in the dose of 0.5 mg daily for 8 days starting from the day of hCG. This was randomized with placebo. All patients underwent evaluation for OHSS. There was a statistically significant difference in the third space fluid collection in the cabergoline group. No difference was detected between groups in the fertilization, implantation, or pregnancy rates.

Early Aspiration

Early aspiration of the follicles in patients at risk after four to seven days of gonadotropin stimulation can be an effective therapy for prevention of OHSS.

GnRH Antagonist Administration

Studies done by Lainas et al., in 2009 showed that GnRH antagonist administration combined with cryopreservation of embryos for use in subsequent cycles might represent an effective approach for management of patients with severe OHSS. In the study the antagonist was administered daily for one week after retrieval. More recent studies have shown that the GnRH antagonist lowers the VEGF concentrations in human granulosa lutein cell cultures (Freiden 2005), as well as the expression of VEGF and VEGF-R in the ovaries of hyperstimulated rats (Taylor 2004).

OHSS AND PREGNANCY

Controlled studies do not show an increase in miscarriage in pregnancy after ART complicated by OHSS. But pregnancies complicated by OHSS showed higher incidence of pre-eclampsia and pre-term delivery (Courbiere 2011).

CONCLUSION

It is very important to identify high-risk patients prior to ART and choose appropriate therapy. Identification of all risk factors and its correlation with clinical features require more large randomized studies but can be the key to preventing and managing this rather dangerous condition.

BIBLIOGRAPHY

1. Alvarez C, Marti-Bonmati L, Novella-Maestre E, et al. Dopamine agonist cabergoline reduces hemoconcentration and ascites in hyprestimulated women undergoing assisted reproduction. J Clin Endocrinol Metab. 2007;92:2931-7.
2. Balasch J, Carmona F, Llach J, et al. Acute prerenal failure and liver dysfunction in a patientwith severe ovarian hyperstimulation syndrome. Hum Reprod. 1990;5:348-51.
3. Baumgarten M, Polanski L, Campbell B, et al. Do dopamine agonists prevent or reduce the severity of ovarian hyperstimulation syndrome in women undergoing assisted reproduction? A systematic review and meta-analysis. Hum Fertil (Camb). 2013;16:168-74.
4. Alvarez C, Alonso-Muriel I, Garcia G. Implantation is apparently unaffected by dopamine agonist cabergoline when administered to prevent OHSS in women undergoing ART. A pilot study. Hum Reprod. 2007;22:3210-4.
5. Chen CD, Chao KH, Yang JH. Comparison of coasting and intravenous albumin in the prevention of ovarian stimulation syndrome. Fertil Steril. 2003;80:86-90.
6. Elchalal U, Schenkar JG. The pathophysiology of ovarian hyperstimulation syndrome—views and ideas. Hum Reprod. 1997;12:1129-37.
7. European Recombinant LH Study. Recombinant human luteinizing hormone is as effective as, but safer than, urinary human chorionic gonadotropin in inducing

final follicular maturation and ovulation in vitro fertilization procedure: results of a multicentric double blind study. J Clin Endocrinol Metab. 2001; 86:2607-18.
8. Lainas TG, Sfontouris IA, Kolibianakis EM. Management of severe OHSS using GnRH antagonist and blastocyst cryopreservation in PCOS patients treated with long protocol. Reprod Biomed Online. 2009;18(1): 15-20.
9. Lincoln SR, Opsahl MS, Blauer KL, et al. Aggressive outpatient treatment of ovarian hyperstimulation syndrome with ascites using transvaginal culdocentesis and intravenous albumin minimizes hospitalization. J assist Reprod Genet. 2002;19:159-63.
10. Smith LP, Hacker MR, Alper MM. Patients with severe ovarian hyper stimulation syndrome can be managed safely with aggressive outpatient transvaginal paracentesis. Fertil Steril. 2009;92:1953-9.
11. Navot D, Margalioth EJ, et al. Direct correlation between plasma renin activity and severity of ovarian hyperstimulation syndrome. Fertil Ster. 1987;48(1);57-61.
12. Royal College of Obstetricians and Gynaecologists. Reducing the Risk of Venous Thromboembolism during Pregnancy and the Puerperium. Green-top Guideline No. 37a. London: RCOG;2015.
13. Practice Comittee of the American Society for Reproductive Medicine. Ovarian hyperstimulation Syndrome. Fertil Steril. 2008;90 (Suppl 5):S188-93.
14. Humaidan P, Ejdrup Bredkjaer H, Westergaard LG, et al. 1,500 IU human chorionic gonadotropin administered at oocyte retrieval rescues the luteal phase when gonadotropin-releasing hormone agonist is used for ovulation induction: a prospective, randomized, controlled study. Fertil Steril. 2010;93(3):847-54.
15. Friden BE, Nilsson L. Gonadotropin-releasing hormone-antagonist luteolysis during the preceding mid-luteal phase is a feasible protocol in ovarian hyperstimulation before in vitro fertilization. Acta Obstet Gynecol Scand. 2005;84(8):812-6.
16. Taylor PD, Hillier SG, Fraser HM. Effects of GnRH antagonist treatment on follicular development and angiogenesis in the primate ovary. J Endocrinol. 2004;183(1):1-17.
17. Courbiere B, Oborski V. Obstetric outcome of women wih in vitro fertilization pregnancies hospitalized for OHSS: a case control study. Am J Obstet Gynecol. 2014;210.

CHAPTER 10

GnRH Agonist Versus GnRH Antagonist in *In Vitro* Fertilization and Embryo Transfer

Raffaella Depalo, Gabriella Garruti

Chapter outline

- Gonadotropin-releasing Hormone Analogs
- Treatment Regimens with GnRH Agonist
  - GnRH Agonist: Long versus Short and Ultrashort Protocol
  - GnRh Agonists: Low and Long Acting Doses
- Treatment Regimens with GnRH Antagonist
  - Single versus Multiple Dose GnRH Antagonist Protocol
  - Fixed versus Flexible Antagonist Administration
  - Dose of Exogenous FSH in GnRH Antagonist Cotreatment Cycles
- LH Supplementation in GnRH Antagonist Cotreatment Cycles
- Oral Contraceptive Pill Pretreatment in Ovarian Stimulation with GnRH Antagonists
- GnRH Antagonist in IUI Cycles
- Long Acting Gonadotropins
- GnRH Agonist versus GnRH Antagonist Regimens
  - GnRH Antagonist versus GnRH Agonist in Poor Ovarian Responders
  - GnRH Agonist Trigger for Final Oocyte Maturation

INTRODUCTION

Controlled ovarian hyperstimulation (COH) is a key procedure of assisted reproductive technique as it induces coordinated multifollicular development, leading to a high yield of oocytes and, consequently, to a high number of embryos. The possibility to select those with the highest implantation dynamics increases the chance of clinical pregnancy.[1,2] High doses of gonadotropins are commonly used to achieve multiple follicular development. However, a premature surge of LH is known to occur in 20% of cycles stimulated with gonadotropins.[3] Luteinizing hormone (LH) surge, defined as LH rise with concomitant P rise is associated with a decreased probability of pregnancy, owing to spontaneous ovulation before oocyte retrieval. Moreover, LH surge may lead to premature secretory transformation of the endometrium, which causes asynchrony between the embryos and the endometrium at the time of embryo transfer.[4]

GONADOTROPIN-RELEASING HORMONE ANALOGS

After being identified and synthesized in 1971, gonadotropin-releasing hormone (GnRH) analogs (agonists and antagonists) in combination with gonadotropins, have been used in ovarian stimulation for in vitro fertilization (IVF) with the aim to reduce the incidence of premature luteinizing hormone (LH) surge.[4] Native GnRH binds selectively the highly specific receptors of the anterior pituitary gonadotropic cells, and activates intracellular signalling pathaways that regulate both the production and the release of FSH and LH.[5] The GnRH agonists, which have greater potency and a longer half-life than native GnRH, produce an initial stimulation of pituitary gonadotrophins that results in a secretion of follicle-stimulating hormone (FSH) and luteinizing hormone (LH) followed by down-regulation and inhibition of the pituitary-gonadal axis. Porter et al., first reported that exogenous gonadotropins associated with gonadotropin-releasing hormone agonists (GnRH-a) were used for ovarian stimulation in IVF cycles.[4-6]

The major benefits of GnRH-a include decreased cancellation rate through prevention of premature LH surge and luteinization,[7] enhancement of follicular recruitment, recovery of a larger number of oocytes,[8] improvement in routine patient treatment schedule[9] and increased pregnancy rate.

On the other hand, the use of GnRH agonists is characterized by some disadvantages for the patients. The standard long GnRH agonist protocol has the drawback of a long treatment period (two to three weeks) until desensitization occurs; and the desensitization period may be associated with side effects such as hot flushes, headache, bleeding and ovarian cyst development. Moreover, an increased risk of ovarian hyperstimulation syndrome (OHSS) has been documented with the addition of GnRH-a in ovarian stimulation.[10,11]

In 1999, the introduction of GnRH antagonists in assisted reproductive technologies (ART), to prevent LH surge, seemed to open up new pathways towards a more "friendly IVF". Unlike GnRH-a, GnRH antagonist administration causes immediate and dose-related inhibition of gonadotropins release by competitive occupancy of the GnRH receptors in the pituitary gland and allow flexibility in the degree of pituitary-gonadal suppression. Discontinuation of GnRH antagonist treatment leads to a rapid and predictable recovery of the pituitary-gonadal axis.[11]

Several advantages for the use of GnRH antagonists in IVF have been reported: GnRH antagonists act within a few hours after their administration lowering the risk for an LH surge; GnRH antagonists are not associated with an acute stimulation of gonadotropins and steroid hormones, which occurs with GnRH agonist administration, avoiding the risks of flare up; their use does not result in profound hypoestrogenemia observed with GnRH agonists eliminating the side effects of desensitization; requirements for exogenous gonadotropins are reduced, and duration of ovarian stimulation protocols is shortened, improving patient discomfort.[10]

A disadvantage for the use of GnRH antagonists consists in less flexibility regarding cycle programming as compared with the long GnRH agonist protocol, although this can be improved by using the oral contraceptive pill (OCP).[10]

TREATMENT REGIMENS WITH GnRH AGONIST

Different GnRH agonists drugs, routes of administration and protocols of controlled ovarian hyperstimulation (COH) have been used in ART.

1. GnRH agonist long protocol: This protocol induces profound suppression of endogenous gonadotropins, avoiding a premature LH surge, and allowing the early antral follicles to grow coordinately in response to exogenous gonadotropins and to accomplish simultaneous maturation, leading to an extended widening of the FSH window and more retrieved oocytes.[12]

   GnRHa is administered at least two weeks before starting stimulation (to achieve suppression of the ovarian activity),

starting from either the second day of the menstrual cycle (long follicular protocol) or the mid-luteal phase (21st day) of the previous cycle (long luteal protocol), and continued up until human Chorionic gonadotropin (hCG) is given.
2. GnRH agonist short protocol: In this protocol GnRHa is administered on day 1-3 of the menstrual cycle followed by gonadotropin treatment started on day 3. This regimen exploits the initial rise (flare up effect) of FSH and LH on recruitment of growing follicles, whereas pituitary desensitization will occur several days later while the patients are still on gondatropin treatment. Then, GnRHa is stopped when the follicular maturity is obtained and ovulation triggering is planned with hCG.[2,5]
3. GnRH agonist ultrashort protocol: A shorter period of GnRH-a administration for 3 days or for 7 days, was also suggested and was termed "Ultra-Short GnRH-a Protocol". This protocol is based on the assumption that suppression of the endogenous LH surge may be obtained through a very short course of GnRH-a administration.[2,5]

GnRH Agonist: Long versus Short and Ultrashort Protocol

The long GnRH-a protocol is the most popular regimen in IVF-ET/ICSI treatment. The short GnRH-a protocol was suggested as an alternative protocol. Because GnRH agonist can induce an initial "flare-up" effect, the short GnRH-a protocol is usually provided to poor responders to avoid excessive pituitary suppression.[1-5]

There is no consensus on which protocol is the best treatment for all patients. Two meta-analyses exhibited different results. A first, a meta-analysis concluded that there was no difference between the short and long protocols.[12] The other meta-analysis, a systematic overview of twenty-six trials comparing different GnRH-a protocols for pituitary desensitization in *in vitro* fertilization, demonstrated the superiority of the long protocol over the short and ultrashort protocol ones (OR 1.32 for clinical pregnancy rate per cycle started), either when GnRH analog was commenced in follicular phase or in luteal phase.[13]

Most recently, a retrospective analysis of 5662 IVF-ET/ICSI cycles performed with long protocol and short protocol, showed that, if the patients were of the same age range, the number of oocytes retrieved, the proportion of mature (MII) oocytes, the high-quality embryos and the clinical pregnancy rate in the long protocol group were all significantly higher than in the short protocol group ($P < 0.05$). The same trend was also found in the implantation rates and clinical pregancy rates when patients were stratified in age ranges. However, as the age increased, the clinical pregnancy and implantation rates, as well as the number of oocytes retrieved, MII oocytes, and high-quality embryos, in the long protocol group, significantly decreased ($P < 0.05$).[1]

On the other hand, a meta-analysis of 37 RCTs (3872 women) evaluates the effectiveness of the different GnRHa protocols in women undergoing ART cycles showing that there was no conclusive evidence of a difference between a long protocol and a short protocol in live birth and ongoing pregnancy rates (OR 1.30, 95% CI 0.94-1.81). Moreover, there was no evidence of a difference between the groups in terms of live birth and ongoing pregnancy rates when the following GnRH a protocols were compared: long versus ultrashort protocol (OR 1.78, 95% CI 0.72-4.36), long luteal versus long follicular phase protocol (OR 1.89, 95% CI 0.87-4.10), when GnRH-a was stopped versus when it was continued (OR 0.75, 95% CI 0.42-1.33), when the dose of GnRH-a was reduced versus when the same dose was continued (OR 1.02, 95% CI 0.68-1.52), when GnRH-a was discontinued versus continued after human chorionic gonadotropin (hCG) administration in the long protocol (OR 0.89, 95% CI 0.49–1.64), and when administration of GnRH-a lasted for two versus three weeks before stimulation (OR 1.14, 95% CI 0.49– 2.68).[2]

In conclusion, there was no conclusive evidence that GnRHa-long protocol was associated with an increase in live birth and ongoing clinical pregnancy rates in comparison with the GnRHa-short protocol. However, in normoresponders women, the luteal long protocol may result in a better follicular synchronization, in an increased cohort of the growing follicles recruited , and than in more oocytes harvested.

GnRh Agonists: Low and Long Acting Doses

There are two types of GnRH agonist administration that can be used to lead to hypophysis desensitization in the long protocol: one consisting of daily GnRH-a low doses (0.1 mg), and another consisting of the administration of analogs in higher long-acting doses (depot 3.75 mg). Albuquerque et al.,[14] in a meta-analysis of six RCTs, found that the pregnancy rates were similar in long protocol using depot or daily GnRH-a. However, the use of analogs long-acting is associated with an increasing requirements for gonadotropins and a longer time of ovarian stimulation compared to the daily GnRH-a low dose. In normal-weighted patients with respect to over-weighted, it was demonstrated that low doses of triptorelin (triptorelin daily half dose, 0.05 mg) are adequate to prevent a premature LH rise, reducing gonadotropic consumption and increasing clinical outcome. It was suggested that as GnRH receptors are expressed in human ovary, high doses of GnRH agonist may induce over-suppression of ovarian receptors in normal or underweight patients. In contrast, in overweight women, as fat tissue is both a steroid reservoir and site of steroid metabolism, peripheral conversion of androgens may sustain serum E2 levels even when ovarian steroidogenesis is suppressed.[15]

TREATMENT REGIMENS WITH GnRH ANTAGONIST

Single versus Multiple Dose GnRH Antagonist Protocol

Two GnRH antagonist (GnRH-ant) protocols have been developed for controlled ovarian stimulation, involving either single administration[16] or multiple.[17]

In the single dose protocol, a 3 mg dose of GnRH antagonist given on day 7 during ovarian stimulation was shown to prevent a premature LH surge.[18] In case of the need to delay hCG, low daily doses of GnRH antagonists could be added 4 days after the single antagonist dose.

In the multiple dose protocol, the GnRH antagonist was administered continuously until the day of hCG, starting 5 days after stimulation with gonadotropins. 0.25 mg cetrorelix was identified as the minimal effective dose to prevent the occurrence of a premature LH rise in the great majority of patients.[19,20]

No significant difference in pregnancy rates was shown in a randomized controlled trial which compared single injection of cetrorelix acetate (3 mg) and daily dose of ganirelix (0.25 mg) in the inhibition of premature LH surge. However, the single dose GnRH antagonist protocol has the advantage to reduce the number of injections, although in 10% of the cycles additional daily doses of antagonist are necessary.[21] Moreover, in some cases 3 mg dose may result in an excessive and potentially harmful suppression of endogenous LH.[22]

Fixed versus Flexible Antagonist Administration

The most appropriate time to start GnRH antagonist administration has been the subject of several studies. Theoretically, GnRH antagonist could be administered anytime during the early or mid-follicular phase of a treatment cycle to prevent a premature

LH surge. In the *fixed protocol*, the decision to start antagonist administration at the day six of ovarian stimulation was based on the concept of preventing the premature LH rise without causing any harmful effect on oocyte maturation.[17] On a physiological basis, GnRH antagonist administration should commence when there is follicular development and/or production of estradiol (E2) by the developing follicles, which may cause a premature elevation in pituitary LH release, due to positive feedback mechanisms. These considerations lead to introduce a *flexible regimen*, in which the GnRH antagonist administration was delayed until the dominant follicle reached >12 mm in diameter, leading to simplification of the multiple dose protocol.

A meta-analysis by Al Inany (2005) evaluated four RCTs that have been performed to compare a fixed protocol (on day 6) versus flexible (by a follicle diameter of 14-15 mm) ones of GnRH antagonist administration. The study showed that there was no significant difference in pregnancy rate per woman randomized (OR = 0.7 95% CI = 0.47-1.05), and no significant difference in incidence of premature LH surge in both protocols.[23]

Similar results were observed in a more recent RCT comparing flexible versus fixed GnRH-antagonist protocols. No significant differences were observed between the flexible (23.3%) and fixed (24.7%) groups (mean difference -1.4%; 95% CI -5.1% to +12.4%) regarding ongoing pregnancy rates per started cycle. A lower incidence of LH rise was observed in the flexible group compared with the fixed group (11.0% vs 15.1%, difference -4.1%, 95% CI -15.4% to +7.1%), which, however, was not statistically significant.[4]

GnRH-antagonist flexible protocol allows to tailor stimulation to patients' needs and to reduce the amount of antagonist administered, without compromise the clinical outcome of the IVF cycle. However, implementation of this protocol is dependent on the dose and the timing of gonadotropin administration and on the criteria for antagonist initiation (i.e. ultrasound data, hormonal parameters or both). Starting patient evaluation early in the follicular phase (i.e. day 3 of stimulation) can avoid the possibility that an LH rise/ surge has already occurred.

Dose of Exogenous FSH in GnRH Antagonist Cotreatment Cycles

On a physiological basis, the required starting dose of FSH in GnRH antagonist cycles may be lower compared to GnRH agonist long protocol, due to the presence of higher endogenous FSH levels during the intercycle phase.[24]

Two RCTs have shown that a higher starting dose of FSH results in an increased number of cumulus-oocytes complex (COC) retrieved but it does not appear to be associated with higher pregnancy rates.[25,26]

LH Supplementation in GnRH Antagonist Cotreatment Cycles

An abrupt suppression of endogenous LH by GnRH antagonist administration occurs in the mid-follicular phase, at a critical stage for follicular development. In view of the decreased probability of pregnancy associated with low LH levels, which was observed using high GnRH antagonist doses[20] and of the increased pregnancy loss observed with low LH levels in GnRH agonist cycles,[27] it was assumed that LH supplementation might improve pregnancy outcome in GnRH antagonist cycles.

A meta-analysis was performed to assess whether combination of r-LH with r-FSH for COH benefits the pregnancy outcomes in general women undergoing IVF/ICSI with GnRH antagonist protocol. The study did not show differences on ongoing pregnancy per ET between the r-LH supplementation group and the r-FSH alone group (OR 0.80; 95% CI 0.49-1.31). But, a significantly higher number of retrieved oocytes per oocyte retrieval in the rFSH alone group was observed (−1.3, 95% CI −2.29 to −0.32).[28]

A multicenter observational analysis of 21,212 COH antagonist cycles for autologous IVF/ICSI, found that the addition of LH—either rLH or hMG—to rFSH does not seem to improve or worsen the outcome of autologous IVF/ICSI cycles in terms of the mean number of oocytes recovered or inseminated or miscarriage or delivery rate, regardless of the age of the female.[29]

Oral Contraceptive Pill Pretreatment in Ovarian Stimulation with GnRH Antagonists

The use of OCP has been considered as a mean for programming IVF cycles using GnRH antagonists, and it has been speculated that the use of OCP pretreatment may result in improved synchronization of the recruitable cohort of ovarian follicles.[30] A RCT by Kolibianakis et al 2006 showed no significant effect of OCP pretreatment on the probability of pregnancy in GnRH antagonist cycles; however easier scheduling of the cycle, an increase of gonadotropin requirement, and a longer duration of treatment has been observed with the use of OCP. Moreover, administration of OCP might be emotionally disturbing, since OCP is mainly used to prevent conception.[31]

GnRH Antagonist in IUI Cycles

GnRH antagonists can be used for preventing the premature LH surge in combination of ovarian stimulation with IUI. In addition, they may be helpful in cycle programming and avoidance of inseminations during weekends. The potential beneficial effect of GnRH antagonist on pregnancy rate in IUI cycles, has been assessed in a recent meta-analysis conducted by Kosmas on six studies with 521 women.[32] Higher pregnancy rate was found (16.9% in the antagonist group and 11.5% in the control group) when GnRH antagonist was administered. Moreover, a trend for multiple pregnancies and an increased duration for gonadotropins administration was observed in the GnRH antagonist group compared with the control-group.

Long Acting Gonadotropins

Chimeric rFSH, corifollitropin alfa, by a combination of the human FSH α-subunit with the carboxy terminal peptide (CTP) β-subunit of human chorionic gonadotropin (hCG), has longer elimination time (~68 hours) and shorter time to reach the peak serum concentration (25~45 hours after injection). A single dose of corifollitropin alfa is able to initiate and sustain the growth of multiple follicles for the first 7 days of ovarian stimulation.[33]

Recently, a widely used protocol involves a single injection of corifollitropin alfa followed by fixed GnRH antagonist suppression and short-acting gonadotropin supplementation.

In a systematic review and meta-analysis including 4 randomized trials, Mahmoud Youssef et al.[34] concluded that corifollitropin alfa in combination with daily GnRH antagonist seemed to be an alternative for daily rFSH injections in view of efficiency and safety profile among normoresponder patients undergoing controlled ovarian hyperstimulation in IVF/ICSI treatment cycles.

Most recently, a meta-analysis was conducted by Griesinger et al.[35] to evaluate the overall efficacy and safety of corifollitropin alfa compared with recombinant FSH, from the Engage, Ensure and Pursue clinical trials (3292 patients). The results of the study showed that the difference (corifollitropin alfa versus rFSH) in the number of oocytes retrieved was +1.0 (95% CI: 0.5–1.5); vital pregnancy rate: −2.2% (95% CI: −5.3%–0.9%); ongoing pregnancy rate: −1.7% (95% CI:

−4.7%–1.4%); and live birth rate: −2.0% (95% CI: −5.0%–1.1%). The odds ratio for overall OHSS was 1.15 (95% CI: 0.82–1.61), and for moderate-to-severe OHSS: 1.29 (95% CI: 0.81–2.05). The study concluded that a single dose of corifollitropin alfa for the first 7 days of ovarian stimulation is a generally well-tolerated and similarly effective treatment compared with daily rFSH.

GNRH AGONIST VERSUS GNRH ANTAGONIST REGIMENS

The debate regarding the efficacy and safety of GnRH antagonists and agonists for *in vitro* fertilization-embryo transfer (IVF-ET) continues even today. With the aim to effectively resolve the dispute by evaluating the differences in the effects of the GnRH antagonist and GnRH agonist protocols, several studies have been published.

A systematic review of 27 RCTs, conducted by Al-Inany in 2006,[36] showed that the clinical pregnancy rate was significantly lower with GnRH antagonist treatment than with the GnRH agonist long protocol, while the differences in the ongoing pregnancy and live birth rates did not significantly differ between the 2 groups; however, the incidence of severe OHSS was significantly lower in the GnRH antagonist group.

The live birth rate in a systematic review of 22 RCTs, conducted by Kolibianakis,[37] was consistent with the findings reported by Al-Inany 2006.[36]

Another systematic review of 45 RCTs, conducted by Al-Inany in 2011,[38] reaffirmed the earlier results by the same author regarding to the ongoing pregnancy and live birth rates and the incidence of severe OHSS. However, a review by Orvieto[39] stated that the ongoing pregnancy and live birth rates were significantly higher in the group treated according to the GnRH agonist long protocol compared to those treated with the GnRH antagonist and that the agonist protocol remained significantly better than the GnRH antagonist protocol.

A more recent a meta-analysis of 23 RCTs evaluated the effectiveness and safety of the GnRH antagonist and GnRH agonist long protocols for IVF in normal ovarian responders. The study demonstrated that the number of stimulation days, the amount of gonadotropins, E2 levels on the day of hCG administration, number of oocytes, clinical pregnancy rate, and ovarian hyperstimulation syndrome (OHSS) incidence were significantly lower in GnRH antagonist protocol than GnRH agonist protocol. However, ongoing pregnancy rate, live birth rate, miscarriage rate, and cycle cancellation rate did not significantly differ between the 2 groups.[40]

In 2016, Al Inany et al.[41] updated the Cochrane review including seventy-three RCTs (12,212 women) to evaluate the efficacy and safety of GnRH antagonists compared to GnRH agonists long protocol. The findings showed that there was no evidence of a difference in live birth rates following GnRH antagonist compared with GnRH agonist (OR 1.02, 95% CI 0.85–1.23) per women randomized. However, there was evidence of a lower OHSS rate in women who received GnRH antagonist compared with those were treated with GnRH agonist (6% versus 11%;OR 0.61, 95% CI 0.51–0.72), and of a higher cycle cancellation rates due to poor ovarian response in GnRH antagonist groups compared with GnRH agonist groups (OR 1.32, 95% CI 1.06–1.65).

The last meta-analysis includes 29 RCTs (6399 patients with normal ovarian reserve). The findings show that stimulation days, gonadotrophin dosage, estradiol (E2) level on the day of human chorionic gonadotropin (hCG) administration, the number of oocytes retrieved, the embryos obtained, and incidence of ovarian hyperstimulation syndrome (OHSS) were statistically significantly lower in GnRH-ant protocol than GnRH-a long protocol. However, the clinical pregnancy rate, ongoing pregnancy rate, live birth rate, miscarriage rate, and cycle cancellation rate showed no significant differences between the two groups.[42]

GnRH Antagonist versus GnRH Agonist in Poor Ovarian Responders

Poor ovarian response is defined as reduced follicle/oocyte production after controlled ovarian hyperstimulation for IVF treatment according to the "Bologna Criteria".[43] In comparison to normal responders, these patients have impaired fertilization rates and lower embryo quality. Moreover, the poor response to ovulation induction results in high cancellation and failure rates, which thus influences the overall IVF success rates as well as cost-effectiveness significantly. Therefore, the management of poor responders has been one of the most difficult challenges in assisted reproductive technology (ART), with disappointing overall IVF success rates. Various treatment regimens and interventions have been investigated in an effort to improve ovarian response and IVF outcome including high doses of gonadotropins, 'flare-up' GnRH-a protocol with OC pretreatment, and use of growth hormone or growth hormone-releasing factor or aspirin as adjunct therapies. However, most of these interventions have only limited success in poor responders. The availability of effective GnRH antagonists has offered an alternative protocol for poor responders. Since GnRH-ant avoids suppression of endogenous gonadotropin secretion at the stage of follicular recruitment, it appears rational to use antagonists in patients with expected or proven decreased ovarian response to exogenous gonadotropins.[44]

A meta-analysis of 14 RCTs involving 1127 poor responders patients treated with GnRH-a or GnRH-ant for ovarian stimulation demonstrated that the duration of stimulation was significantly lower in GnRH-ant than in GnRH-a cycles, there was no significant difference in the number of oocytes retrieved and in the number of mature oocytes retrieved and in clinical pregnancy rate although it appears lower in the antagonist than in the agonist group.[35]

GnRH Agonist Trigger for Final Oocyte Maturation

Human chorionic gonadotropin (hCG) has been used as a surrogate for midcycle LH peak to induce final oocyte maturation before oocyte retrieval in IVF/ICSI cycles. The relatively long elimination half time of hCG obtains a luteotrophic effect during the luteal phase, but also increases the OHSS risk. During the last decade, the introduction of gonadotropin-releasing hormone agonist (GnRHa) trigger has provided a tool to minimize the risk of OHSS without compromising the reproductive outcome. GnRH-a trigger is only possible in GnRH antagonist cotreated IVF/ICSI cycles: instead of hCG the administration of a bolus of GnRH-a will displace the GnRH antagonist from the receptors, inducing a flare-up of gonadotropins (LH and FSH), which activates oocyte maturation.[45]

GnRH-a trigger effectively reduces OHSS rates due to the shorter half-life of the endogenous LH compared to the long acting LH activity after an hCG trigger – approximately 33 h versus 6–10 days respectively, which results in a defective corpora lutea (CL) formation and a decrease in the release of vasoactive peptides such as VEGF.[46]

The early GnRH-a trigger studies with the use of a standard luteal phase support (LPS) found significantly lower implantation rates and significantly higher early pregnancy loss rates compared to hCG triggered cycles.[47-49]

In fact, despite the achievement of a stimulus for final oocyte maturation, ovulation triggering with GnRH-a has no beneficial effect on endometrial receptivity and oocyte quality. During the luteal phase of ART cycles triggered with GnRH-a, the relative shortstanding LH surge and central inhibition of gonadotropin secretion, due to the supraphysiological serum estradiol levels, causes depletion of LH support and consequently lower secretion of progesterone by the corpora lutea.[45]

Youssef et al. (2014) performed a Cochrane meta-analysis to evaluate the differences between GnRH agonists and hCG in terms of safety and effectiveness for triggering final oocyte maturation in IVF-ICSI among women undergoing a GnRH antagonist protocol. The authors concluded that when GnRH agonists were used for final oocyte maturation in fresh autologous cycles, lower live birth rates, lower ongoing pregnancy rates, and a higher rates of early miscarriage were achieved. Youssef et al.[50] recommended the use of GnRH agonists trigger for women who are spared for fresh transfers, who are oocyte donors, and who demand to freeze autologous oocytes for fertility preservation.[50]

As the luteal phase after GnRH-a trigger is impaired, it is crucial to modify the luteal phase support (LPS) after fresh transfer. Two main policies have been suggested. One of these approaches has been called the "European approach" in which endogenous steroid support is obtained by adding LH activity either in the form of a small bolus of hCG after the initial trigger or by adding daily recombinant LH injections during the luteal phase, aiming at rescuing the CL function. The other approach has been called the "American approach" in which luteal progesterone and estradiol are administered exogenously, thus, disregarding the function of the corpora lutea.[51] Alternatevely, an elective cryopreservation of all embryos and transfer in a subsequent menstrual cycle presents as rational approach.

The role of GnRH-a trigger followed by luteal phase support have been explored in recent studies.

Engmann et al. (2015) reviewed the advantages and potential drawbacks of GnRH agonist triggering by performing a strengths, weaknesses, opportunities and threats (SWOT) analysis. Based on this analysis modality, the authors recommended intensive luteal support with transdermal estradiol and intramuscular progesterone alone if peak serum estradiol is 4000 or more pg/mL after GnRH-a triggering or dual triggering with GnRH agonist and hCG 1000 IU if peak serum estradiol is less than 4000 pg/mL. The recommendations of the same group based on the follicle number were as follows: administration of hCG 1500 IU 35 h after GnRH agonist trigger if there are less than 25 follicles ≥11 mm on the day of ovulation trigger, or freeze all oocytes or embryos if there are over 25 follicles.[52]

A more recent meta-analysis has compared GnRH-a trigger followed by luteal LH activity support and hCG trigger, in IVF patients undergoing fresh embryo transfer. The study demonstrated that the live birth rate was not significantly different between the GnRH-a and hCG trigger groups (OR 0.84, 95% CI 0.62, 1.14). OHSS was reported in a total of 4/413 cases in the GnRH-a group compared to 7/413 in the hCG group (OR 0.48, 95% CI 0.15, 1.60). The Authors observed a slight, but nonsignificant increase in miscarriage rate in the GnRH-a triggered group compared to the hCG group (OR 1.85; 95% CI 0.97, 3.54), and concluded that individualization of the LH activity LPS improved the luteal phase deficiency reported in the first GnRH-a trigger studies.[53]

A retrospective study to assess the cumulative probability of achieving a live birth after elective embryo cryopreservation was performed in patients that were stimulated using GnRH agonist protocol and GnRH antagonist to trigger the final oocyte maturation. All embryos were vitrified at the blastocyst stage and transferred in the subsequent menstrual cycles. Using this "conservative" approach a total of 65.9% (95% CI 57.5 to 74.3) women achieved a live birth after a maximum of six embryo transfer cycles.[54]

CONCLUSION

A long-course GnRH agonist protocol with maximum ovarian stimulation has been the standard protocol for many decades. However, it is relatively complex and expensive, requires long treatment cycles and intensive monitoring, and leads to an abnormal hormonal environment in women.

If the patient's convenience is concerned, the conventional protocols of ovarian stimulation (recombinant follicle stimulating hormone [rFSH] with gonadotropin releasing hormone agonist), have been gradually replaced by the protocols of gonadotropins with GnRH antagonist to shorten the duration of stimulation. The GnRH antagonist protocol requires a lower dose of gonadotropins without the need for a desensitization period, and yet provides remarkable outcomes with higher flexibility. With effective pituitary suppression, GnRH antagonist significantly decreases the rate of premature LH surge during stimulation to prevent early luteinization and follicular atresia.[55]

This approach meets the desire to shift to more patient-friendly mild ovarian stimulation allowing a control of risk of OHSS, and a more efficient management of patients with poor ovarian response.

In addition, GnRH antagonists protocols allow early onset of ovarian stimulation in young women with neoplastic diseases prior to the antineoplastic treatments in order to to freeze autologous oocytes for fertility preservation.

REFERENCES

1. Jianping Ou, Weilje Xing, Yubin Li, et al. Short versus long gonadotropin-releasing hormone analogue suppression protocols in IVF/ICSI in patients in various age ranges. Plos One. 2015;10(7):1-11.
2. Sistritadis CS, Gibreel A, Basios G, et al. Gonadotrophin-releasing hormone agonist protocols for pituitary suppression in assisted reproduction. Cocharane Database Syst Rev. 2015;11:1-131.
3. Loumaye E. The control of endogenous secretion of LH by gonadotrophin-releasing hormone agonists during ovarian hyperstimulation for in-vitro fertilization and embryo transfer. Hum Reprod. 1990;5:357-76.
4. Kolibianakis EM, Venetis CA, Kalogeropulou L, et al. Fixed versus flexible gonadotropin-releasing hormone antagonist administration in in vitro fertilization: a randomized controlled trial. Fertil & Steril. 2011;95(2):558-62.
5. Berin I, Stein DE, Keltz MD. A comparison of gonadotropin-releasing hormone (GnRH) antagonist and GnRH agonist flare protocols for poor responders undergoing in vitro fertilization. Fertil Steril. 2010;93:360-3.
6. Porter RN, Smith W, Craft IL, et al. Induction of ovulation for in-vitro fertilisation using buserelin and gonadotropins. Lancet. 1984;2:1284-5.
7. Caspi E, Ron-El R, Golan A, et al. Results of in vitro fertilization and embryo transfer by combined long-acting gonadotropin-releasing hormone analog D-Trip-6-luteinizing hormone releasing hormone and gonadotropins. Fertil Steril. 1989;51(1):95-9.
8. Liu HC, Lai YM, Davis O, et al. Improved pregnancy outcome with gonadotropin releasing hormone agonist (GnRH-a) stimulation is due to the improvement in oocyte quantity rather than quality. J Assist Reprod Genet. 1992;9(4):338-44.
9. Zorn JR, Boyer P, Guichard A. Never on a sunday: programming for IVF-ET and GIFT. Lancet. 1987;1(8529):385-6.
10. Tarlatzis BC, Fauser BC, Kolibianakis EM, et al. GnRH antagonists in ovarian stimulation for IVF. Hum Reprod Update. 2006;12(4):333-40.
11. Kumar P, Sharma A. Gonadotropin-releasing hormone analogs: understanding advantages and limitations. J Hum Reprod Sci. 2014;7(3):170-4.
12. Hughes EG, Fedorkow DM, Daya S, et al. The routine use of gonadotropin-releasing hormone agonists prior to in vitro fertilization and gamete intrafallopian transfer: a meta-analysis of randomized controlled trials. Fertil Steril. 1992;58:888-96.

13. Daya S. Gonadotropin releasing hormone agonist protocols for pituitary desensitization in in vitro fertilization and gamete intrafallopian transfer cycles. Cochrane Database Syst Rev. 2000;(1) CD001299.
14. Albuquerque LE, Saconato H, Maciel MC. Depot versus daily administration of gonadotropin releasing hormone agonist protocols for pituitary desensitization in assisted reproduction cycles. Cochrane database Syst Rev. 2005;(1):CD002808.
15. Lorusso F, Depalo R, Selvaggi L. Relationship between gonadotropin releasing hormone agonist dosage and in vitro fertilization outcome. Gynecol Endocrinol. 2004;18(2):69-73.
16. Olivennes F, Fanchin R, Bouchard P, et al. The single or dual administration of the gonadotropin-releasing hormone antagonists cetrorelix in an in vitro fertilization-embryo transfer program. Fertil steril. 1994;62(3):468-76.
17. Diedrich K, Diedrich C, Santos E, et al. Suppression of the endogenous luteinizing hormone surge by the gonadotropin-releasing hormone antagonist cetrorelix during ovarian stimulation. Hum Reprod. 1994;9(5):788-91.
18. Olivennes F, Alvarez S, Bouchard P, et al. The use of a GnRH antagonist (cetrorelix) in a single dose protocol in IVF-embryo transfer: a dose finding study of 3 versus 2 mg. Hum Reprod. 1998;13(9):2411-4.
19. Albano C, Smitz J, Camus M, et al. Comparison of different doses of gonadotropin-releasing hormone antagonist Cetrorelix during controlled ovarian hyperstimulation. Fertil Steril. 1997;67:917-22.
20. The Ganirelix Dose-Finding Study Group. A double-blind, randomized, dose-finding study to assess the efficacy of the gonadotropin-releasing hormone antagonist ganirelix (Org 37462) to prevent premature luteinizing hormone surges in women undergoing ovarian stimulation with recombinant follicle stimulating hormone (Puregon). Hum Reprod. 1998;13:3023-31.
21. Wilcox J, Potter D, Moore M, et al., CAP IV investigator Group. Prospective randomized trial comparing cetrorelix acetate and ganirelix acetate in a programmed, flexible protocol for premature luteinizing hormone surge prevention in assisted reproductive technologies. Fertil Steril. 2005;84(1):108-17.
22. Olivennes F, Belaisch-Allart J, Emperaire JC, et al. Prospective, randomized, controlled study of in vitro fertilization-embryo transfer with a single dose of a luteinizing hormone-releasing hormone (LH-RH) antagonist (cetrorelix) or a depot formula of an LH-RH agonist (triptorelin). Fertil Steril. 2000;73(2):314-20.
23. Al-Inany HG, Aboulghar M, Mansour R, et al. Optimizing GnRH antagonist administration: meta-analysis of fixed vs flexible protocol. Reprod Biomed Online. 2005;10:567-70.
24. Fauser BC, Van Heusden AM. Manipulation of human ovarian function: physiological concepts and clinical consequences. Endocr Rev. 1997;18(1):71-106.
25. Wikland M, Bergh C, Borg K, et al. A prospective, randomized comparison of two starting doses of recombinant FSH in combination with cetrorelix in women undergoing ovarian stimulation for IVF/ICSI. Hum Reprod. 2001;16(8):1676-81.
26. Out HJ, Rutherford A, Fleming R, et al. A randomized, double-blind, multicentre clinical trial comparing starting doses of 150 and 200 IU of recombinant FSH in women treated with the GnRH antagonist ganirelix for assisted reproduction. Hum reprod. 2004;19(1):90-5.
27. Westergaard LG, Laursen SB, Andersen CY. Increased risk of early pregnancy loss by profound suppression of luteinizing hormone during ovarian stimulation in normogonadotropic women undergoing assisted reproduction. Hum Reprod. 2000;15:1003-8.
28. Xiong Y, Bu Z, Dai WD, et al. Recombinant luteinizing hormone supplementation in women undergoing in vitro fertilization/intracytoplasmic sperm injection with gonadotropin releasing hormone antagonist protocol: a systematic review and meta-analysis. Reprod Biol and Endocrinol. 2014;12:109.
29. Schwarze JE, Crosby JA, Zegers-Hochschild F. Addition of neither recombinant nor urinary

luteinizing hormone was associated with an improvement in the outcome of autologous in vitro fertilization/intracytoplasmic sperm injection cycles under regular clinical settings: a multicenter observational analysis. Fertil Steril. 2006;106(7):1714-7.
30. Cedrin-Durnerin I, Grange-Dujardin D, Laffy A, et al. Recombinant human LH supplementation during GnRH antagonist administration in IVF/ICSI cycles: a prospective randomized study. Hum Reprod. 2004;19:1979-84.
31. Kolibianakis EM, Papanikolaou EG, Camusa M, et al. Effect of oral contraceptive pill pretreatment on ongoing pregnancy rates in patients stimulated with GnRH antagonists and recombinant FSH for IVF. A randomized controlled trial. Hum Reprod. 2006;21:352-7.
32. Kosmas IP, Zikopoulos K, Georgiou I, et al. Low-dose HCG may improve pregnancy rates and lower OHSS in antagonist cycles: a meta-analysis. Reprod Biomed Online. 2009;19(5):619-30.
33. Fauser BC, Alper MM, Ledger W, et al. Pharmacokinetics and follicular dynamics of corifollitropin alfa versus recombinant FSH during ovarian stimulation for IVF. Reprod Biomed Online. 2010;21:593-601.
34. Mahmoud Youssef MA, van Wely M, Aboulfoutouh I, et al. Is there a place for corifollitropin alfa in IVF/ICSI cycles? A systematic review and meta-analysis. Fertil Steril. 2012;97:876-85.
35. Griesinger G, Boostanfar R, Gordon K, et al. Corifollitropin alfa versus recombinant follicle stimulating hormone: an individual patient data meta-analysis. Reprod Biomed Online. 2016;33:56-60.
36. Al-Inany HG, Abou-Setta AM, Aboulghar M. Gonadotrophin-releasing hormone antagonists for assisted conception. Cochrane Database Syst Rev. 2006;19:CD001750.
37. Kolibianakis EM, Collins J, Tarlatzis BC, et al. Among patients treated for IVF with gonadotrophins and GnRH analogues, is the probability of live birth dependent on the type of analogue used? A systematic review and meta-analysis. Hum Reprod Update. 2006;12:651-71.
38. Al-Inany HG, Youssef MA, Aboulghar M, et al. Gonadotrophin-releasing hormone antagonists for assisted reproductive technology. Cochrane Database Syst Rev. 2011;11:CD001750.
39. Orvieto R, Patrizio P. GnRH agonist versus GnRH antagonist in ovarian stimulation: an ongoing debate. Reprod Biomed Online. 2013;26:4-8.
40. Jin-song Xiao, Cun-mei Su, Xian-tao Zeng. Comparisons of GnRH antagonist versus GnRH agonist protocol in supposed normal ovarian responders undergoing IVF: a systematic review and meta-analysis. PlosOne. 2014;9(9):1-10.
41. Al-Inany HG, Youssef MA, Ayleke RO, et al. Gonadotropin-releasing hormone antagonists for assisted reproductive tecnology (Review). Cochrane Database Syst Rev. 2016;4:CD001750.
42. Wang R, Shouren L, Wang Y, et al. Comparisons of GnRH antagonists protocol versus GnRH agonist long protocol in patients with normal ovarian reserve: a systematic review and meta-analysis. PlosOne. 2017;12(4):1-19.
43. Ferraretti AP, La Marca A, Fauser BC, et al. ESHRE working group on poor ovarian response definition. ESHRE consensus on the definition of "poor response" to ovarian stimulation for in vitro fertilization: the Bologna criteria. Hum Reprod. 2011;26(7):1616-24.
44. Danhua Pu, Jie Wu, Jiayin Liu. Comparisons of GnRH antagonist versus GnRH agonist protocol in poor ovarian responders undergoing IVF. Hum Reprod. 2011;26(10):2742-9.
45. Kahyaoglu S, Yilmaz B, Isik AZ. Pharmacokinetic, pharmacodynamic, and clinical aspects of ovulation induction agents; a review of the literature. J Turk Ger Gynecol Assoc. 2017;18:48-55.
46. Desouto C, Haar T, Humaidan P. Gonadotropin-releasing Hormone agonist (GnRHa) trigger- State of the art. Reprod Biol. 2017;17:1-8.
47. Humaidan P, Ejdrup Bredkjaer H, Bungum L, et al. GnRH agonist (buserelin) or hCG for ovulation induction in GnRH antagonist IVF/ICSI cycles: a prospective randomized study. Hum Reprod. 2005;20:1213-20.
48. Griesinger G, Diedrich K, Devroey P. GnRH agonist for triggering final oocyte

maturation in the GnRH antagonist ovarian hyperstimulation protocol: a systematic review and meta-analysis. Hum Reprod Update. 2006;12(2):159-68.

49. Kolibianakis EM, Schultze-Mosgau A, Schroer A, et al. A lower ongoing pregnancy rate can be expected when GnRH agonist is used for triggering final oocyte maturation instead of HCG in patients undergoing IVF with GnRH antagonists. Hum Reprod. 2005;20:2887-92.

50. Youssef MA, Van der Veen F, Al-Inany HG, et al. Gonadotropin-releasing hormone agonist versus HCG for oocyte triggering in antagonist-assisted reproductive technology. Cochrane Database Syst Rev. 2014;(10):CD008046.

51. Humaidan P, Engmann L, Benadiva C. Luteal phase supplementation after gonadotropin-releasing hormone agonist trigger in fresh embryo transfer: the American versus European approaches. Fertil Steril. 2015;103:879-85.

52. Engmann L, Benadiva C, Humaidan P. GnRH agonist trigger for the induction of oocyte maturation in GnRH antagonist IVF cycles: a SWOT analysis. Reprod Biomed Online. 2016;32:274-85.

53. Haar T, Roque M, Esteves SC, et al. GnRH agonist trigger and LH activity luteal phase support versus hCG trigger and conventional luteal phase support in fresh embryo transfer IVF/ICSI. A systematic PRISMA review and meta-analysis. Front Endocrinol. 2017;8(116):1-10.

54. Vlaisavljevic V, Kovacic B, Knez J. Cumulative live birth rate after agonist trigger and elective cryopreservation of all embryos in high responders. Reprod Biomed Online. 2017;35(1):42-8.

55. Depalo R, Jayakrishshan K, Garruti G, et al. GnRH agonist versus GnRH antagonist in in vitro fertilization and embryo transfer (IVF/ET): Reprod Biol Endocrinol. 2012; 10:26.

CHAPTER 11

Hyperprolactinemia and Infertility

Mirudhubashini Govindarajan, Ramya Jayaram

Chapter outline

- Prolactin Gene and Structure
- Prolactin Variants
- Lactotrophs
  - Extrapituitary Prolactin
- Prolactin Receptor
- Regulation of Prolactin Secretion
- Functions of Prolactin
  - Mammary Gland Development and Lactation
  - Other Reproductive Functions
  - Nonreproductive Functions
- Prolactin Secretion and Assays
- Hyperprolactinemia
- Macroprolactinemia (Big-Big Prolactin)
- Prolactin-Secreting Adenomas
- Treatment of Hyperprolactinemia
  - Prolactin-secreting Adenoma
  - Clinical Features
  - Galactorrhea
  - Hypogonadism and Menstrual Cycle Dysfunction
- Treatment Strategies
  - Observation
  - Oral Contraceptives for Hypogonadism
  - Medical Therapy
  - Time Course of Clinical Response
- Definition of Dopamine Agonist Resistance
  - Dopamine Agonist Withdrawal
  - Surgery
  - Radiotherapy
  - Management of Prolactinomas in Pregnant Women
  - Microprolactinoma Treatment in Pregnancy
  - Macroprolactinoma in Pregnancy
  - Hyperprolactinemia in Men
  - Prolactinomas in Multiple Endocrine Neoplasia
  - Giant Prolactinomas
  - Malignant Prolactinomas

INTRODUCTION

Prolactin (PRL) is an ancient hormone whose physiological function has been changing as evolution has progressed. It ensures survival of the species through its reproductive role and survival of the individuals of the species through its homeostatic role. Being an adaptive multifaceted hormone, PRL fulfills some critical, but mostly modulatory, roles in reproductive processes. The wide expression of prolactin and its receptor gene in various cells of the body speaks for its endocrine, paracrine and autocrine functions. Prolactin is a unique pituitary hormone as its release is under tonic inhibitory control exerted by the hypothalamus. The abundant pituitary lactotrophs secreting prolactin have a high basal secretory activity.

PROLACTIN GENE AND STRUCTURE

Prolactin is a polypeptide hormone that belongs to the prolactin/growth hormone/placental lactogen family. These hormones resemble each other genetically, structurally and in receptor binding. The prolactin gene in human is found on chromosome 6. It is 10 kb in size and is composed of 5 exons and 4 introns. Transcription is regulated by two independent promoter regions, responsible for its pituitary and extrapituitary expression. Mature hPRL contains 199 amino acid (aa), with a total molecular mass of 23 kDa. The prolactin molecule is arranged in a single chain of amino acids with three intramolecular disulfide bonds between six cysteine residues. According to the current three-dimensional model, prolactin contains four long α-helices arranged in antiparallel fashion.[1]

PROLACTIN VARIANTS

Prolactin variants can result from alternative splicing of the primary transcript (minority), proteolytic cleavage and other post-translational modifications of the amino acid chain (majority). Proteolytic cleavage of PRL via cathepsin D (16 and 6 kDa fragments) or via kallikrein (22 kDa fragment) result in prolactin variants. Phosphorylation of PRL constitutes 5-30% of the PRL released by the pituitary, it has been shown that it has both agonistic and antagonistic properties. The function of some other modifications of PRL (glycosylation, deamination, sulfonation and polymerization) are not well studied. Dimerization and polymerization of prolactin or aggregation with binding proteins, such as immunoglobulins, by covalent and noncovalent bonds may result in high molecular weight forms. In general, all these forms have reduced biological activity.[1]

LACTOTROPHS

Lactotrophs are cells of the anterior pituitary gland which synthesize and secrete prolactin. They comprise 20-50% of the cellular population of the anterior pituitary gland depending on the sex and physiological status of the animal. Ontogenetically, lactotrophs descend from the Pit-1-dependent lineage of pituitary cells, together with somatotrophs and thyrotrophs. The prolactin secreting cells are heterogeneous in their distribution, shape and nature of response to secretogagues. Two cell forms expressing the PRL gene include large polyhedral cells (250-800 nm granules), which are found throughout the gland, and smaller angulated or elongated cells (200-350 nm granules), which are clustered mainly in the lateral wings and median wedge. Lactotrophs from the outer zone respond greater to thyrotropin releasing hormone (TRH) while the inner zone cells are more dopamine responsive. Occasional intermediate cells called mammosomatotroph cells also secrete both PRL and GH, often stored within the same granules.[2]

Extrapituitary Prolactin

Prolactin is also secreted in other parts of the brain, the uterus, placenta, amnion, decidua, mammary gland and milk. The mammary gland is the site of formation of the important 16 kDa anti-angiogenic variant of prolactin, a possible target of breast cancer research.[1]

PROLACTIN RECEPTOR

The prolactin-R (PRL-R) is a single membrane-bound protein that belongs to class 1 of the cytokine receptor superfamily. The gene encoding human prolactin-R is located on chromosome 5p13. Numerous PRL-R isoforms exist as a result of initiation of transcription at different promoter sites as well as alternative splicing of noncoding and coding exon transcripts. Each 598 amino acid PRL-R contains an extracellular, a hydrophobic transmembrane, and intracellular domain. The different isoforms differ in the length and composition of their cytoplasmic tail and are referred to as short, intermediate, or long PRL-R with respect to their size. In addition to the membrane-anchored PRL-R, soluble isoforms have also been identified. In all cases, however, the extracellular, ligand-binding domain is identical, whatever the isoform.[1]

The activation of prolactin receptor involves the following steps.[1]

1. Prolactin induced receptor dimerization.
2. Intracellular signal transduction by Jak2 dimerization and transphosphorylation.
3. Phosphorylation of tyrosine residues of the prolactin-R itself.
4. Signal transduction pathways associated with STAT (The signal transducer and activator of transcription) proteins (STAT 5 mainly).
5. Activation of STAT DNA-binding motif in the promoter of a target GAS gene (γ-interferon activated sequence).

Other signaling pathways include Ras/Raf/MAP kinase pathway and other kinases: c-src and Fyn.

Prolactin receptors are expressed in breast, pituitary, liver, adrenal cortex, kidney, prostate, ovary, testes, intestine, epidermis, lung, myocardium, brain and lymphocytes. Estrogen induces receptor expression.[2]

REGULATION OF PROLACTIN SECRETION

Prolactin secretion is under the inhibitory control of dopamine, which is largely produced by the tuberoinfundibular (TIDA) cells and the hypothalamic tuberohypophyseal dopaminergic system and reaches the lactotrophs via the portal system.[1] The action of dopamine is through the activation of G protein coupled—D2 receptor. D2 receptor is characterized by a single polypeptide chain containing seven hydrophobic transmembrane domains. Activation of D2 receptor leads to inhibition of adenylyl cyclase activity which in turns reduces the cAMP levels and inositol phosphate production. Other inhibitory stimuli include endothelin-1, transformation growth factor β1 and calcitonin. A short loop feedback of prolactin has also been proposed. The prolactin releasing substance include TSH releasing hormone, serotonin, estrogens, endogenous opiates, and vasoactive intestinal polypeptide.[3]

FUNCTIONS OF PROLACTIN

In their classic reviews, Nicoll and Bern[4] have elaborated on 85 different biological functions of PRL subdivided into: (i) water and electrolyte balance, (ii) growth and development, (iii) endocrinology and metabolism, (iv) brain and behavior, (v) reproduction, and (vi) immunoregulation and protection. Such actions of PRL may have been lost with evolution or may only be seen in higher animals during certain stages of development. In addition, certain actions of pituitary derived.

Prolactin (endocrine) may be taken over by locally produced PRL (autocrine or paracrine).

Mammary Gland Development and Lactation

The varied effects of prolactin on the mammary gland include growth and development of the mammary gland (mammogenesis), synthesis of milk (lactogenesis), and maintenance of milk secretion (galactopoiesis). In the process of lactogenesis, prolactin stimulates uptake of some amino acids, the synthesis of the milk proteins casein and a-lactalbumin, uptake of glucose, and synthesis of the milk sugar lactose as well as milk fats.[2]

Other Reproductive Functions

Prolactin is a luteotropic hormone and enhances progesterone secretion by potentiating the steroidogenic effects of luteinizing hormone (LH) in granulosa—luteal cells and inhibiting the 20α hydroxysteroid dehydrogenase enzyme, which inactivates progesterone. In the uterus, it increases the level of progesterone and estrogen receptors, and thus promotes blastocyst implantation. The physiological role in males includes the maintenance of cellular morphology, increase in LH receptor number, steroidogenesis and androgen production in the Leydig cells and increase FSH receptor numbers in Sertoli cells. In germ cells, PRL increases the spermatocyte-spermid conversion and a reduction in the time required to achieve capacitation. All these physiological actions do not explain the gonadal dysfunction seen in hyperprolactinemia which result from attenuated gonadotropin secretion.

Nonreproductive Functions

Prolactin is lymphocyte growth factor and stimulates immune responsiveness explaining the rise in prolactin levels in autoimmune disease like SLE. Antiangiogenic activity is inherent to the 16- kDa fragment which may be exploited in the future as local inhibitors of tumorigenesis. Prolactin exerts an osmoregulatory role by controlling the transport of anion and solute across membranes. Prolactin also affects water transport across amniotic membranes.[3]

PROLACTIN SECRETION AND ASSAYS

The calculated daily production of prolactin ranges from 200-536 µg/day/m². Prolactin is rapidly cleared with the t½ ranging from 26 to 47 minutes. Prolactin secretion is pulsatile with 13-14 peaks/per/day, each lasting 67-76 minutes, occurring at intervals of 95 min. The mean pulse amplitude is about 20-30% of the upper normal value. The highest levels are achieved during REM sleep and the lowest level occur between 10 am and noon. The Prolactin is increased by meals rich in protein.

In women levels are higher at the middle and during the second half of the menstrual cycle. Prolactin levels fall with age in both men and women. So, the sample should preferably be obtained at midmorning and not after any stressful stimuli and breast examination during the early follicular phase.[2]

The prolactin radioimmunoassay is highly specific for prolactin. Improved assay efficiency, turnaround time, reproducibility and sensitivity have been achieved with immunoradiometric (IRMA) and chemiluminescent (ICMA) assays. The normal range for prolactin is 4-30 ng/mL in females and 4-23 ng/mL in males. The new unit of expression is pmol/L and for conversion, you need to multiply by 44. The normal level is less than 700 pmol/L. There are two potential pitfalls in the diagnosis of a hyperprolactinemia: the presence of macroprolactin and the so-called 'hook effect'.

Macroprolactin: The most common form of prolactin in serum is 23 kD in size. Macroprolactin is an term used to describe aggregates of prolactin and antibodies, some autoantibodies, to prolactin that range in size from approximately 150 to 170 kD. It is an IgG-PRL complex, attributing to 20% of PRL levels in hyperprolactinemic sera, resulting in pseudohyperprolactinemia and potential misdiagnosis. For confirmation of macroprolactinemia, polyethylene glycol precipitation of macroprolactin is the most practical method. Alternatively, size exclusion chromatography can be used, if so ever it is time-consuming. To avoid diagnostic and therapeutic pitfalls, it is reasonable to ascertain the presence of macroprolactin in patients with moderately elevated PRL levels (25-150 µg/L: 500-3000 mIU/L) and less typical symptoms, such as headaches or diminished libido in the presence of regular menses.

The 'hook effect': Caution should be exercised in interpreting serum prolactin concentrations between 20 and 200 ng/mL (20 to 200 µg/L SI units) in the presence of a macroadenoma because of possible artifactually low values due to the "hook effect". This effect occurs when a very high serum prolactin, e.g. 5000 ng/mL (5000 µg/L SI units), saturates both the capture and signal antibodies used in immunoradiometric and chemiluminescent assays, and interferes with antibody-antigen-antibody sandwich formation. The result is an apparent prolactin concentration that is only modestly elevated, suggesting that the macroadenoma is clinically nonfunctioning. The artifact can be avoided by repeating the assay using a 1:100 dilution of serum or alternatively should include a washout between the two steps during the assay in all new patients with large pituitary macroadenomas who have normal or mildly elevated prolactin to avoid a misdiagnosis as nonfunctioning adenoma.[5]

HYPERPROLACTINEMIA

The real frequency of hyperprolactinemia in the general population is approximately 1.2%. Transient or long-term hyperprolactinemia can develop during different physiological situations, systemic and pituitary diseases and medications. Persistent hyperprolactinemia is confirmed by a repeat properly timed sample examination.

Hyperprolactinemia in itself is simply an abnormal laboratory value that reflects the presence of an underlying pathophysiological cause. When evaluating a patient with symptoms consistent with hyperprolactinemia and persistently elevated serum PRL, secondary causes should first be ruled out by a careful clinical history, physical examination, pregnancy test, routine biochemical analysis (to evaluate kidney and liver function), and TSH determination. If the patient is taking a drug known to cause hyperprolactinemia, it is important to determine if the drug is indeed the cause by withdrawing the drug for at least 72 hours, if this can be done safely.[6] If feasible, the patient could be switched to an alternative drug that does not increase prolactin levels because hyperprolactinemia produces the adverse biological action (like osteoporosis or infertility) even when it is secondary to drug intake. It should not always be assumed that hyperprolactinemia in a patient on drugs known to elevate prolactin is in fact due to those medications. Clozapine, quetiapine and olanzapine are reported either to cause no increase in prolactin secretion at all or to increase it only transiently and mildly.[7,8] Causes of hyperprolactinemia are sown in Table 11.1.

Table 11.1: Etiology of hyperprolactinemia.

Physiologic

Stress, breast stimulation, coitus, pregnancy, lactation, corpus luteum phase, surgery, sleep, venepuncture

Pathologic

Hypothalamic-Pituitary stalk damage

Granuloma, infiltrations, Rathke's cyst, Trauma: Pituitary stalk section, suprasellar surgery

Tumors: Craniopharyngioma, dysgerminoma, hypothalamic metastases, meningioma, suprasellar mass extension.

Pituitary

Acromegaly, idiopathic, lymphocytic hypophysitis, macroadenoma, plurihormonal adenoma, prolactinoma, surgery, trauma

Contd...

Contd...

Systemic disorder
   Chest: Neurogenic chest wall trauma, surgery, herpes zoster
   Chronic renal failure, polycystic ovarian disease, pseudocyesis

Pharmacologic

Anticonvulsants: Phenytoin

Antidepressants:
   Selective serotonin reuptake inhibitor: Fluoxetine
   Tricyclic antidepressants: Amitriptyline, chlorimipramine

Antihypertensives: Labatolol, reserpine, verapamil

Dopamine receptor blocker
   Butyrophenones: Haloperidol
   Phenothiazines: Chlorpromazine, perphenazine,
   metoclopramide, thioxanthenes

Dopamine synthesis inhibitor: Alpha methyldopa

Estrogens: Oral contraceptive pills and its withdrawal

Neuroleptics:
   Butaperazine, chloropromazine, fluphenazine, haloperidol
   Molindone, perphenazine, pimozide, promazine, promethazine, thiethylperazine, thioridazine, thiothixene, trifluoperazine

Neuropeptides: Thyrotropin releasing hormone

Opiates and antagonists:
Apomorphine, heroin, methadone, morphine

MACROPROLACTINEMIA (BIG-BIG PROLACTIN)

When the serum of a hyperprolactinemic patient contains mainly big-big PRL, the condition is termed macroprolactinemia. First described by Whittaker et al. in 1981, Macroprolactinemia has been described in 31% of women with asymptomatic hyperprolactinemia. Changes in the PRL molecule may increase the antigenicity leading to the production of antiPRL autoantibodies. Macroprolactin has bioactivity *in vitro*. The absence of bioactivity *in vivo* might be a result of the high molecular mass preventing passage of PRL through the capillary endothelium to reach target receptor, delayed clearance and absence of short loop negative feedback of prolactin on its own secretion. Macroprolactinemia can be associated with PRL-secreting pituitary tumor. Because routine assays do not detect macroprolactin, most clinicians fail to consider the problem of macroprolactin and tend to treat hyperprolactinemia in both symptomatic and asymptomatic patients. The result of medical treatment of patients with macroprolactinemia could be an oversuppressed bioactive monomeric PRL leading to pharmacologically induced luteal insufficiency.[9]

An elevated circulating prolactin level without any demonstrable cause is called idiopathic hyperprolactinemia and is resistant to dopamine. The elevation in prolactin level is marginal. Mild hyperprolactinemia occurs in around 30% of patients with PCOS and 20% patients with hypothyroidism. Hypothyroidism should be ruled out in all cases with hyperprolactinemia presenting with amenorrhea or hypomenorrhea. Hyperprolactinemia occurs in 20% of women with chronic renal failure.[2]

PROLACTIN-SECRETING ADENOMAS

About 40% of all pituitary adenomas are prolactinomas. Prolactinomas are more common in women, with a peak incidence between 20- and 50-year-old, when the ratio between the sexes is estimated to be 10:1. After the fifth decade of life, the frequency of prolactinomas is similar in both sexes. In general, prolactinomas in women of childbearing age are indolent microadenomas (<10 mm in diameter) and present with symptoms of hyperprolactinemia. Most of these generally remain stable and some disappear overtime or with DA treatment while 7–14% may continue to grow (7%). In contrast, men and postmenopausal women frequently harbor a macroprolactinoma (>10 mm in diameter) with or without extrasellar extension. Prolactin secretion by adenomas is usually proportional to their size. Adenomas <1 cm in diameter are typically associated with serum prolactin values below 200 ng/mL (8.7 nmol/L), those approximately 1.0–2.0 cm in diameter with values between 200 and 1000 ng/mL (8.7–43.48 nmol/L), and those greater than 2.0 cm in diameter with values above 1000 ng/mL (43.48 nmol/L) and as high as 50,000 ng/mL (2173.91 nmol/L). There are exceptions to this generalization, however, as occasional patients have a large adenoma but only modest hyperprolactinemia. Such adenomas are generally less well differentiated and respond less well to dopamine agonists than the more typical tumors.

If prolactin levels are < 200 ng/mL in a case of macroadenoma, it indicates that the tumor is likely nonfunctional after the hook effect is ruled out. These patients require screening to rule out hyposecretion of other pituitary hormones.[2] More than 99% of prolactinoma are benign and sharply demarcated. About half invade local structure and express markers of aggressiveness namely an elevated mitotic activity, a Ki-67 labeling index >3%, and p53 immunoreactivity >3%.[10] Because acromegaly can present with elevated prolactin levels and amenorrhea, the circulating level of IGF-1 should be measured in all patients with macroadenoma.

In patients with hyperprolactinemia who desire pregnancy, a MRI should be done to rule out a prolactinoma or other pituitary or hypothalamic cause in cases with prolactin levels more than 100 ng/mL.

TREATMENT OF HYPERPROLACTINEMIA

After ruling out the secondary causes, management of hyperprolactinemia is centered on normalizing the prolactin levels with dopamine agonists.

Prolactin-Secreting Adenoma

The major objectives of treating patients with prolactinomas are:
1. To suppress excessive hormone secretion and its clinical consequences.
2. To control tumor mass in cases of macroprolactinoma.
3. To preserve or improve residual pituitary function; and
4. To prevent disease recurrence or progression.[11]

Clinical Features

Box 11.1 shows the signs and symptoms of hyperprolactinemia.

Galactorrhea

Galactorrhea is inappropriate secretion of milk-like substance from the nipple of either men or women that persist after childbirth or discontinuation of nursing for as long as 6 months. This abnormal milk secretion can be unilateral or bilateral, profuse or sparse and vary in color and thickness. Isolated galactorrhea is commonly considered indicative of hyperprolactinemia, although prolactin levels might be normal in around 50% of individual. In these cases the transient episode of hyperprolactinemia may have triggered the process or the assay would not have detected the pulsatile episodes of hyperprolactinemia. Conversly hyperprolactinemia occurs in the absence of galactorrhea (66%), which may result from inadequate estrogen and progestational priming as seen in male or adolescent patients. In patients with both galactorrhea and amenorrhea, approximately two-thirds will have hyperprolactinemia.

Box 11.1: Signs and symptoms of hyperprolactinemia.

Due to tumor mass producing effect

Blurred vision or decreased visual acuity, cranial nerve palsies, headaches

Hydrocephalus (rare), pituitary apoplexy, seizures (temporal lobe), symptoms of hypopituitarism

Unilateral exophthalmos (rare), visual field abnormality

Due to hyperprolactinemia

Amenorrhea, oligomenorrhea, primary amenorrhea, infertility, galactorrhea

Decreased libido, impotence, premature ejaculation, erectile dysfunction, oligospermia

Osteoporosis

Hypogonadism and Menstrual Cycle Dysfunction

Excluding pregnancy, hyperprolactinemia accounts for approximately 10-20% of cases of amenorrhea. The amenorrhea in hyperprolactinemia is due many factors like inhibition of pulsatile secretion of GnRH, reduction in granulosa cell number, reduced FSH receptor binding, inhibition of granulosa cell 17β estradiol level by inhibiting the aromatase activity, atresia of dominant follicle due to low estrogen levels, inadequate luteinization of corpus luteum and progesterone synthesis. Thus, hypogonadism produced reduces the mean bone mass and can lead to osteopenia and osteoporosis in a long run (Box 11.2).

The symptoms of hypogonadism due to hyperprolactinemia in premenopausal women correlate with the magnitude of the hyperprolactinemia. In most laboratories, a serum prolactin concentration above 15-20 ng/mL (15-20 μg/L SI units) is considered abnormally high in women of reproductive age.

- A serum prolactin concentration greater than 100 ng/mL (100 μg/L SI units) is typically associated with overt hypogonadism, subnormal estradiol secretion and its consequences, including amenorrhea, hot flashes, and vaginal dryness.
- Moderate degrees of hyperprolactinemia, e.g. serum prolactin values of 50-100 ng/mL (50-100 μg/L SI units), cause either amenorrhea or oligomenorrhea.
- Mild degrees of hyperprolactinemia, e.g., serum prolactin values of 20-50 ng/mL (20-50 μg/L SI units), may cause only insufficient progesterone secretion and, therefore, a short luteal phase of the menstrual cycle.

Mild hyperprolactinemia can cause infertility even when there is no abnormality of the menstrual cycle; these women account for approximately 20% of those evaluated for infertility. As prolactin levels increase

Box 11.2: Indications for therapy.

Mass effects: Hypopituitarism, visual field defects due to pressure on the optic chiasm, cranial nerve deficits, headaches.

Effects of hyperprolactinemia

      Hypogonadism: Amenorrhea or oligomenorrhea, infertility, impotence

      Osteoporosis or osteopenia

Relative indications: Bothersome hirsutism, bothersome galactorrhea

---

the women passes through phases of luteal insufficiency, intermittent anovulation and finally amenorrhea.

TREATMENT STRATEGIES

Observation

Asymptomatic patients with microprolactinomas do not have an absolute requirement for treatment examining the benign natural history of these tumors. An untreated prolactinoma should be followed closely for tumor enlargement with prolactin levels as tumor seldom grow without increase in prolactin levels in majority of cases. There is no consensus on the frequency of imaging. If PRL levels rise or symptoms of mass effects develop (such as headaches), then repeat scanning is indicated to evaluate for the possibility of significant tumor growth.

The presence of a macroadenoma raises the probability for the biological characteristics of the propensity to grow. Therefore, unless there are specific contraindications, therapy is usually advisable for these tumors.[11]

Oral Contraceptives for Hypogonadism

When fertility is not an issue in women with microprolactinomas, treatment of hypogonadal symptoms with an oral contraceptive is less expensive and has fewer side effects than treatment with a dopamine agonist. Treatment with estrogen may, however, induce or worsen pre-existing galactorrhea. Individual case reports of tumor enlargement have been documented. Because of this uncertainty, it is advisable to monitor patients who use oral contraceptives carefully with periodic measurement of prolactin levels. It is not necessary to repeat an MRI in indicated. There have been no trials examining the effect of estrogen on macroadenomas, and women with very large tumors and/or tumors with suprasellar extension should not be treated with estrogen.[11]

Medical Therapy

The compounds used in clinical practice to treat prolactinomas are all dopamine receptor agonists. Stimulation of D2 receptors by these drugs reduces adenylyl cyclase activity that consequently reduces intracellular cAMP, the key step in the inhibition of PRL release by dopamine. Dopamine agonists reduce the size of prolactinomas by inducing a reduction in cell volume (via an early inhibition of secretory mechanism, and a late inhibition of gene transcription and PRL synthesis), as well as causing perivascular fibrosis and partial cell necrosis. There may also be a true antimitotic effect of these drugs.

The adverse effects of bromocriptine may be grouped into:

Gastrointestinal (nausea, vomiting, constipation, dry mouth, dyspepsia, reflux esophagitis), cardiovascular (postural hypotension, dizziness, syncope) and neurological (headache, drowsiness, psychiatric adverse effects like auditory hallucinations, delusional ideas, paresthesia, nightmare, blurred vision and diplopia). Symptoms tend to occur after the initial dose and with dosage increases, and can be minimized by introducing the drug at a low dosage (0.625 or 1.25 mg/d) at bedtime, by taking it with food, and by very gradual dose escalation. The DA can also be administered as slow release preparation or by intravaginal route to avoid its gastrointestinal and cardiovascular side-effects. Up to 12% of patients are unable to tolerate therapeutic doses of bromocriptine.

Cerebrospinal fluid (CSF) rhinorrhea has been reported during treatment of adults with bromocriptine, in the absence of prior radiotherapy or surgical intervention due to tumor shrinkage, when the tumor previously served as a 'cork' for the tumor-induced defect in the skull base.[11]

Rarely, with very high doses of dopamine agonist, pulmonary infiltrates, valvular fibrosis and regurgitation, pleural effusions, pleural thickening, and retroperitoneal fibrosis have been described; however, these adverse effects appear to be dose-dependent and are unlikely to occur at the low doses used for treatment of prolactinomas. The abnormality is due to the ability of these drugs to stimulate serotonin 2B receptors, resulting in activation of several mitogenic pathways, ultimately causing this overgrowth valve disorder. Cabergoline and pergolide are potent serotonin 2B receptor agonists, whereas bromocriptine is only a partial agonist, and other dopamine agonists (pramipexole, lisuride, terguride, ropinirole, and roxindole) are not serotonin 2B receptor agonists.[12]

Bromocriptine (as a first generation agonist) has been largely superseded by more potent compounds with longer lasting effects and improved side effect profiles. Its long duration of action is attributable to slow elimination by the pituitary tumor cells, high affinity binding dopamine receptors and extensive enterohepatic circulation. In head-to-head randomized, prospective comparison studies, retrospective analyses, and general clinical experience, cabergoline has been shown to be more effective in lowering PRL levels to normal, reducing tumor size, and having less adverse effects in Table 11.2. Patients are less likely to

Table 11.2: Medical management of prolactinoma.

	Receptor	T1/2 (hrs)	Dosing schedule	Initiation dose	Mean dose	Maximum dose	Response
Ergot derivatives							
Bromocriptine (1.25, 2.5 mg)	D2 agonist D1 antagonist	3.3	BD, TID	1.25, 2.5 mg	7.5 mg/d (macro); 5 mg/d (micro)	30 mg/day	70% (micro) 65% (macro)
Cabergoline (0.25, 0.5 mg)	D2 agonist, D1 agonist (low affinity)	65	Once, twice weekly	0.25 mg	1 mg/wk (macro); 0.5 mg (micro)	10.5 mg/wk	80% (micro) 70% (macro)
Pergolide	D2 agonist D1 agonist	27	OD	0.025 mg	0.075 mg/d	–	80% (micro) 75% (macro)
Nonergot derivatives							
Quinagolide	D2 agonist, D1 agonist (low affinity)	22	OD	0.025 mg	0.075 mg/day	0.3–0.6 mg/d	80% (micro) 75% (macro)

be resistant to the therapeutic effects of cabergoline; furthermore, most patients found to be resistant to bromocriptine subsequently respond to cabergoline. Finally, treatment with cabergoline affords a greater chance of obtaining permanent remission and successful withdrawal of medication, compared with treatment with bromocriptine. Nevertheless, bromocriptine is still widely used to treat prolactinomas, primarily in young women desiring pregnancy. Once DA therapy is initiated, response is assessed with prolactin values after 4 to 6 weeks.[11]

Time Course of Clinical Response

The fall in serum prolactin typically occurs within the first two to three weeks of therapy with a dopamine agonist; in patients with macroadenomas, it always precedes any decrease in adenoma size. The decrease in adenoma size can, in many patients, be detected by imaging within six weeks after initiation of treatment; in some patients, however, a decrease is not apparent for six months.[18] These benefits occur even in patients who have impaired visual fields before therapy, occurring in 9 of 10 such patients in each of two reports.[13-21]

Following the decrease in serum prolactin and adenoma size in patients with macroadenomas, visual and pituitary function often return to normal. Vision usually begins to improve within days after the initiation of treatment.[20,21] There is recovery of menses and fertility in women and of testosterone secretion, sperm count, and erectile function in men.[21-25] Patients with macroadenomas who are hypothyroid and/or hypoadrenal may also have a return of these functions to normal.[21-25]

DEFINITION OF DOPAMINE AGONIST RESISTANCE

Resistance is defined as failure to normalize PRL levels, or failure to enable a 50% reduction of tumor size.[12] The major problem clinically is the patient with primary dopamine resistance. Patients who initially respond to a dopamine agonist and later become resistant are far less common; reasons include noncompliance, institution of gonadal steroid replacement which causes dopamine resistance in the lactotrophs, and the fortunately rare development of a carcinoma. Resistance is associated with a decrease in D2 receptor gene transcription, resulting in a 4-fold decrease in the number of D2 receptors on the cell membrane, a decrease in the G protein that couples the D2 receptor to adenylyl cyclase, disruptions in the autocrine growth factor signaling pathway mediated by nerve growth factor (NGF).[13]

Approximately 24%, 13%, and 11% of patients demonstrate resistance to bromocriptine, pergolide, and cabergoline, respectively. It is of clinical interest to know that the resistance is not a class effect. Approximately 80% of bromocriptine-resistant tumors respond to cabergoline. Possible explanations include the higher affinity of cabergoline for dopamine binding sites, its greater occupancy of the receptor, and slower elimination from the pituitary.[11]

Treatment approaches for resistant prolactinomas:
1. Trial of an alternative dopamine agonist
2. Escalation of the dopamine agonist beyond conventional doses (monitoring for valvular fibrosis by ECHO)
3. Surgical tumor resection
4. Radiotherapy.

Dopamine Agonist Withdrawal

The principal shortcoming of dopamine agonist treatment has been perceived to be its supposed lifelong requirement. After withdrawal of bromocriptine, remission rates vary between 0–44% in different studies. The more recent study by Colao et al.[14] reported recurrence rate of hyperprolactinemia after 5 years of cabergoline withdrawal of only 24% in patients with nontumoral hyperprolactinemia, 32.6% in patients with microprolactinomas, and 43.3% in those with macroprolactinomas. PRL levels at recurrence were significantly lower than at diagnosis in all groups. Age, basal PRL levels, nadir PRL levels, percent PRL suppression, nadir tumor diameter after cabergoline, treatment duration, cabergoline dose, small remnant tumors on MRI at treatment withdrawal, were all higher in patients developing a recurrence. Gillam et al.[11] suggested that in order to avoid unnecessary treatment, cabergoline withdrawal can be performed in patients with normoprolactinemia after at least 2 years of treatment and when the MRI demonstrates complete disappearance of the tumor. If small remnants are still visible, he recommends not withdrawing treatment. During the first year after drug withdrawal, prolactin levels and clinical symptoms should be assessed at 3-month intervals because recurrence rates are highest in the 12 months after withdrawal. Because increases in prolactin generally precede tumor growth, repeating an MRI is not necessary unless hyperprolactinemia recurs.

Surgery

Indications for surgery[6]
1. Nonresponders to dopaminergic therapy (prolactin level and tumor regression)
2. Patients with intolerable adverse effects of DA therapy
3. Patients with CSF fistulas under DA
4. Patients with rapidly progressive neurological deficits
5. Patients preference
6. Tumor with major cystic component.

Transsphenoidal surgery does not reliably lead to a long-term cure, and recurrence of hyperprolactinemia is frequent. The success rate of surgery in microadenomas is about 75%,[15] with higher rates for patients with prolactin levels lower than 200 µg/L (4000 mIU/L), small tumors, and amenorrhea of short duration. However, these results come from the most experienced neurosurgeons. The cure rate for macroprolactinomas especially those with cavernous extension are much lower with recurrence rate of 20%. Whether therapy with a dopamine agonist exerts a negative effect on surgical outcome due to perivascular and tumor fibrosis remains controversial. Complications of surgery includes cerebral carotid artery injury, diabetes insipidus, meningitis, nasal septal perforation, panhypopituitarism, CSF rhinorrhea and third nerve palsies.[11]

Radiotherapy

The role of radiotherapy in the management of prolactinomas is one of the adjunctive therapy. In most cases, radiotherapy is used after failed trans-sphenoidal surgery and medical therapy. Rarely, in a few centers, it has been administered postoperatively as a prophylactic measure to prevent growth of a remnant tumor. Several methodologies for the delivery of radiotherapy are conventional fractionated external beam radiotherapy (200 cGy 4-5 d/wk over a period of 5-6 wk up to a total dose of 4500-5000 Gy), stereotactic conformal radiotherapy, the radiation beams to conform to the shape of the tumor, thereby reducing radiation exposure to surrounding normal brain, and single dose stereotactic radiotherapy ('gamma-knife' radiotherapy). The selection of modality depends on the tumor size, its proximity to optic chiasma and cavernous sinus. In all of these settings, normalization of hyperprolactinemia was infrequent, with an overall normalization rate of 34.1%. The most frequent long-term morbidity of conventional radiotherapy is radiation-induced hypopituitarism, cerebrovascular accidents, optic nerve damage, neurological dysfunction, soft tissue reactions and risk of secondary radiation-induced intracranial malignancies.[11]

Management of Prolactinomas in Pregnant Women

Three major issues arise in the treatment of prolactinomas in pregnancy:
1. The effect of the pregnancy on the prolactinoma.
2. The effects of the dopamine agonist on early fetal development occurring before a pregnancy is diagnosed.
3. The safety and efficacy of dopamine agonists after reintroduction for symptomatic tumor growth.[2]

During pregnancy, estrogen stimulates PRL synthesis and secretion and promotes lactotroph cell hyperplasia. PRL levels in the maternal circulation rise throughout normal pregnancy, reaching a mean concentration of 150 ng/mL at term. After delivery, the gland rapidly involutes and returns to its normal size by 6 months postpartum. The potential for the enlargement of a prolactinoma during pregnancy is highly dependent upon two factors: its size and the patient's history if prior radiotherapy or surgery. The risk to tumor enlargement with microprolactinemia (2.5%) and surgically resected or irradiated pregestationally (5%) is low. There is a moderate risk of clinically significant tumor enlargement for DA treated macroprolactinomas (31%). Observational studies have shown that pregnancy has a favorable effect on the natural history of pre-existing prolactinomas. Prolactin levels are lower after delivery than before conception and complete remission of hyperprolactinemia has been reported in 17-37% of women after pregnancy. Changes in tumor vasculature resulting in pituitary necrosis, microinfarction, or hemorrhage have been suggested as potential mechanisms to explain how pregnancy might lead to normalization of prolactin.

Hyperprolactinemia associated anovulation and infertility can be corrected with placenta crossing dopamine agonists, potentially exposing the fetus to one of these drugs for at least 3 to 4 weeks of gestation, until a pregnancy can be confirmed and allow discontinuation of the medication. The use of bromocriptine, when it is taken for only the first few weeks of gestation has the largest safety database and it has not been associated with an increase in the rates of spontaneous abortions, ectopic pregnancies, trophoblastic disease, multiple pregnancies, or congenital malformations in a very large number of pregnancies. There is less data available on the effects of continuous bromocriptine (used throughout gestation) but they are largely reassuring. The database for the use of cabergoline in pregnancy is much smaller, but there is no evidence at present indicating that it exerts deleterious effects on pregnant women. For the woman who is intolerant to bromocriptine and who is doing well with cabergoline, continuation of cabergoline for facilitating pregnancy appears to be reasonable. It is recommended that patients cease cabergoline use at least 1 month prior to trying to conceive owing to the long half-life of this agent. Although the safety databases for pergolide and quinagolide are limited, the number of abortions and malformations associated with the reported pregnancies raises serious concern. Therefore, quinagolide and pergolide should not be used when fertility is desired.[11]

The optimal management approach for a woman with a prolactinoma who desires pregnancy may depend on tumor size and individual tumor characteristics.[16]

Microprolactinoma Treatment in Pregnancy

With microprolactinomas (or intrasellar macroprolactinomas), bromocriptine or cabergoline therapy with or without ovulation induction drugs are generally preferred to surgery and radiotherapy because it is safe for the fetus when discontinued early in gestation and poses only a very low risk of tumor enlargement for the mother. If substantial tumor growth is evident, immediate reinstitution of DA therapy is appropriate by specialist. Breastfeeding is not contraindicated in the presence of micro-and macroprolactinoma. If women choose to breastfeed, an MRI scan should be done to ensure that tumor size is unchanged from baseline within 4 to 6 weeks of delivery. The use of dopamine ergot derivatives can cause high blood pressure during postpartum period and is contraindicated. Management of microprolactinoma in pregnancy[16] is shown in Flowchart 11.1.

Macroprolactinoma in Pregnancy

Considering the size and the propensity of these tumors during pregnancy producing pressure symptoms, women with microprolactinoma should be advised against pregnancy until reasonable tumor size suppression. Management of macroprolactinoma during pregnancy[16] is shown in Flowchart 11.2.

Hyperprolactinemia in Men

Hyperprolactinemia causes hypogonadotropic hypogonadism in men, which is manifested by decreased libido, impotence, infertility, gynecomastia, or rarely, galactorrhea. As in women, there is a rough correlation between the presence of any of these symptoms and the degree of hyperprolactinemia. A considerably greater proportion of males with prolactinomas that come to clinical attention have macroprolactinomas, compared with women. A summary of 16 series comprising 444 men with prolactinomas indicates that 77.9% were impotent, 36.6% had visual field defects, 33.8% had partial or complete hypopituitarism, 29.1% complained of headaches, and only 10.9% had galactorrhea. Thus, about one-third of men have symptoms due to tumor size. There are some clinical and pathological data which indicate that proliferative activity and tumor aggressiveness are greater in prolactinomas from men compared with those from women.[11]

- *Hypogonadotropic hypogonadism*: Hyperprolactinemia causes decreased testosterone secretion and low serum testosterone concentrations that are not associated with an increase in LH secretion.[10] As in women, the effect of prolactin must be on the pituitary or hypothalamus. The consequences of the hypogonadism

Flowchart 11.1: Management of microprolactinoma in pregnancy.

```
                    ┌─────────────────────────────────┐
                    │ Microprolactinoma with preganancy│
                    └─────────────────┬───────────────┘
                                      ▼
┌─────────────────────────────────────────────────────────────────────────────┐
│ • Discontinue dopamine agonist on pregnancy confirmation                    │
│ • Explain the risk of tumor enlargement                                     │
│ • Prolactin levels during pregnancy do not represent tumor growth           │
│ • Remind patients to contact their physicians if symptoms of new-onset      │
│   headaches or vision changes                                               │
│                                                                             │
│ If not previously done, arrange for baseline Goldmann visual field          │
│ perimetry and repeat every 2 months during pregnancy                        │
└──────────────┬──────────────────────────────────────────┬───────────────────┘
               ▼                                          ▼
   ┌────────────────────────┐              ┌──────────────────────────────┐
   │ Symptom free           │              │ New-onset headaches, visual  │
   │ stable visual perimetry│              │ changes, or change in visual │
   │ results                │              │ perimetry results            │
   └───────────┬────────────┘              └──────────────┬───────────────┘
               ▼                                          ▼
   ┌────────────────────────┐              ┌──────────────────────────────┐
   │ No intervention        │              │ Urgent pituitary imaging     │
   │ recommended            │              │ (MRI) specialist referral    │
   └────────────────────────┘              └──────────────────────────────┘
```

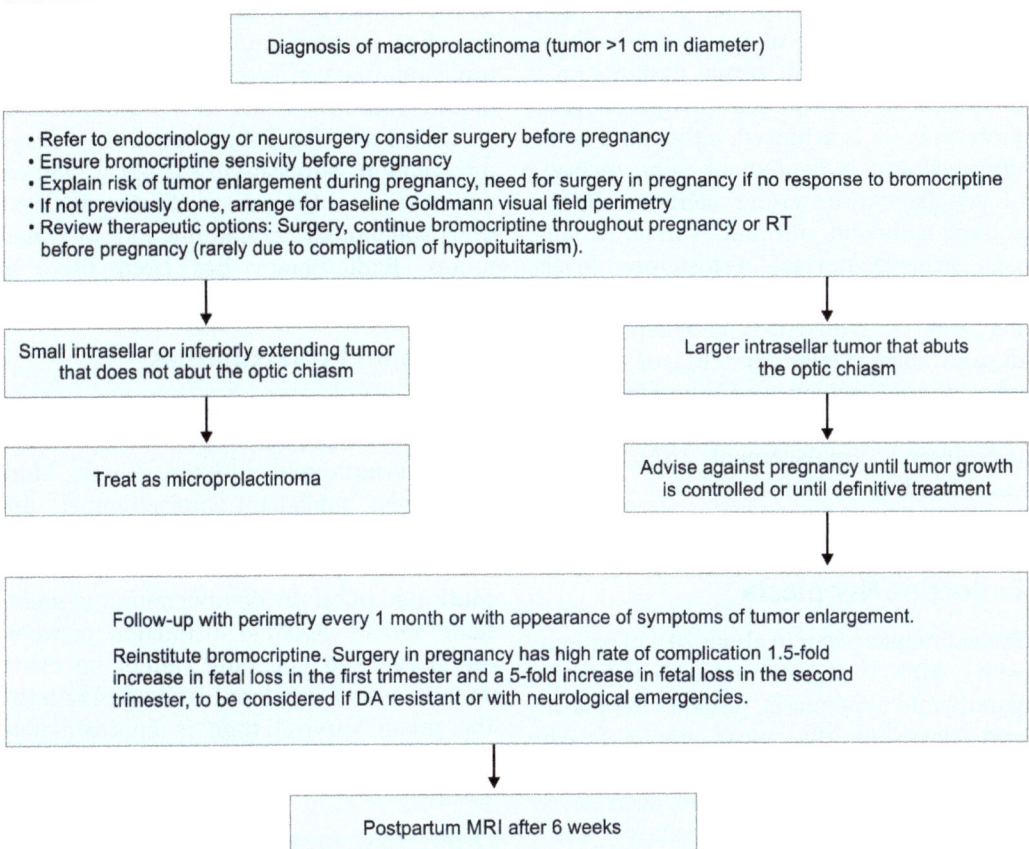

Flowchart 11.2: Management of macroprolactinoma during pregnancy.

are similar to those of hypogonadism due to other causes and include, in the short term, decreased energy and libido, and in the long term, decreased muscle mass and body hair, and osteoporosis. In one study of 20 men, for example, 16 had osteopenia in the spine and six in the hip.[12]

- *Erectile dysfunction*: Hyperprolactinemia appears to cause erectile dysfunction by a mechanism unrelated to hypogonadism because correcting the hyperprolactinemia with a dopamine agonist drug corrects the impotence. One report suggests that correcting the hypogonadism by the administration of testosterone does not correct the impotence, which corresponds to the author's anecdotal observations.[10]
- *Infertility*: Although hyperprolactinemia can cause infertility in men, probably by decreasing LH and perhaps FSH secretion, it is not a common finding among men who present for evaluation of infertility. In a study of 171 infertile men, as an example, only seven (4%) had hyperprolactinemia.[11]
- *Galactorrhea*: Men with hyperprolactinemia may develop galactorrhea. This occurs less often than in women, presumably because the glandular breast tissue in men has not been made sensitive to prolactin by preceding stimulation by estrogen and progesterone.

Data on the efficacy of medical therapy in the treatment of hyperprolactinemia in men are still limited, but similar response has been noted. Recovery from sexual dysfunction is possible with medical therapy when normoprolactinemia is achieved, although it is not universal and is dependent upon recovery of adequate testosterone secretion. Sperm volume and count normalizes in all patients who achieve normal testosterone levels, whereas sperm motility normalizes in more than 80%. For men who remain hypogonadal despite normalization of PRL, or for men who do not achieve normoprolactinemia using maximal doses of dopamine agonists, testosterone replacement should be considered.[17]

Prolactinomas in Multiple Endocrine Neoplasia

Prolactinomas occur in about 20% of patients with MEN-1 (gastrinoma, insulinoma, parathyroid hyperplasia, pituitary neoplasm) and represent the most frequent type of pituitary adenoma observed in this syndrome. They behave more aggressively than those that develop sporadically many being macroprolactinoma (84%) and invasive tumors. In general, the treatment strategy for prolactinomas in patients with MEN-1 does not differ from that for sporadic prolactinomas. The MEN-1 gene is localized to chromosome 11q13 and is a constitutive tumor suppressor gene.[11]

Giant Prolactinomas

Giant prolactinomas are defined as PRL secreting adenomas greater than 4 cm in diameter and/or those with more than 2 cm of suprasellar extension. The reported prevalences is 0.5% and 4.4% among all pituitary tumors, usually associated with very high serum PRL concentrations, in the range of 20–100,000 ng/m. Because of the excellent potential results with dopamine agonists and largely poor results of surgery in most patients, dopamine agonists is the first line of therapy. Patients with giant prolactinomas can develop pituitary apoplexy or CSF rhinorrhea due to rapid tumor size reduction with DA therapy requiring surgical intervention. Surgical cure is not a realistic attainable goal for giant prolactinomas with trans-sphenoidal, craniotomy, and combined routes. Radiotherapy has been used as adjunctive therapy.[11]

Malignant Prolactinomas

Malignant prolactinomas are rare tumors. Pituitary carcinomas represent less than 0.5% of symptomatic pituitary tumors. Most commonly, malignant prolactinomas are indistinguishable from invasive macroadenomas at presentation, the diagnosis confirmed upon the demonstration of metastatic spread. Reliable distinction between carcinoma and adenoma cannot be made on the basis of standard histological criteria. The mean survival time is approximately 10 months after metastasis. The treatment is only palliative.[11]

REFERENCES

1. Freeman ME, Kanyicska B, Lerant A, et al. Prolactin: structure, function, and regulation of secretion. Physiol Rev. 2000;80:1523-631.
2. Melmed S, Kleinberg D. Physiology and disorder of pituitary hormone axis. William's Endocrinology, 11th edition. Saunder Elsevier Publication; pp. 180-92.
3. Christine Bole-Feysot, Vincent Goffin, Marc Ederly, et al. Prolactin (PRL) and its receptor: actions, signal, transduction pathways and phenotypes observed in PRL receptor knockout mice. End Rev. 1998;19(3):225-68.
4. Nicoll CS, Bern H. On the actions of PRL among the vertebrates: is there a common denominator? In: Wolstenholme GEW, Knight J (Eds.). Lactogenic hormones. Churchill Livingstone, London. 1972; pp. 299-337.
5. Bachelot A, Binart N. Reproductive role of prolactin. Reproduction. 2007;133: 361-9.

6. Casanueva FF, Molitch ME, Schlechte JA, et al. Guidelines of the pituitary society for the diagnosis and management of prolactinomas. Clini Endo. 2006;65:265-3.
7. Wieck A, Haddad PM. Antipsychotic-induced hyperprolactinaemia in women: pathophysiology, severity and consequences. Br J Psych. 2003;182:199-204.
8. Meaney AM, Smith S, Howes OD, et al. Effects of long-term prolactin-raising antipsychotic medication on bone mineral density in patients with schizophrenia. Br J Psych. 2004; 184:503-8.
9. Nawroth F. Hyperprolactinaemia and the regular menstrual cycle in asymptomatic women: should it be treated during therapy for infertility? Reprod biomed 2005;11(5):581–88.
10. Gurlek A, Karavitaki N, Ansorge O, et al. What are the markers of aggressiveness in prolactinomas? Changes in cell biology, extracellular matrix components, angiogenesis and genetics. Euro J Endocrinol. 2007;156:143–53.
11. Gillam MP, Molitch ME, Gaetano L, et al. Advances in the treatment of prolactinomas. Endocrine Reviews. 2006;27:485–534.
12. di Sarno A, Landi ML, Cappabianca P, et al. Resistance to cabergoline as compared with bromocriptine in hyperprolactinemia: prevalence, clinical definition, and therapeutic strategy. J Clin Endocrinol Metab. 2001;86:5256-61.
13. Molitch ME. The cabergoline-resistant prolactinoma patient: new challenges. J Clin Endocrinol Metab. 2008;93(12):4643-5.
14. Colao A, Di Sarno A, Cappabianca P, et al. Withdrawal of long-term cabergoline therapy for tumoral and nontumoral hyperprolactinemia. N Engl J Med. 2003;349:2023-33.
15. Kreutzer J, Buslei R, Wallaschofski H, et al. Operative treatment of prolactinomas: indications and results in a current consecutive series of 212 patients. J Euro Endocrinol 2008;158:11-18.
16. Syed Ali Imran, Ehud Ur, Clarke DB. Managing prolactin-secreting adenomas during pregnancy. Canadian Family Physician. 2007;53:653-8.
17. Colao A, Vitale G, Cappabianca P, et al. Outcome of cabergoline treatment in men with prolactinoma: effects of a 24-month treatment on prolactin levels, tumor mass, recovery of pituitary function, and semen analysis. J Clini Endocrinol Metab. 2004;89(4):1704-11.
18. Molitch ME, Elton RL, Blackwell RE, et al. Bromocriptine as primary therapy for prolactin-secreting macroadenomas: results of a prospective multicenter study. J Clin Endocrinol Metab. 1985;60:698.
19. van der Lely AJ, Brownell J, Lamberts SW. The efficacy and tolerability of CV 205-502 (a nonergot dopaminergic drug) in macroprolactinoma patients and in prolactinoma patients intolerant to bromocriptine. J Clin Endocrinol Metab. 1991;72:1136.
20. Moster ML, Savino PJ, Schatz NJ, et al. Visual function in prolactinoma patients treated with bromocriptine. Ophthalmology. 1985; 92:1332.
21. Colao A, Di Sarno A, Landi ML, et al. Long-term and low-dose treatment with cabergoline induces macroprolactinoma shrinkage. J Clin Endocrinol Metab. 1997;82:3574.
22. De Rosa M, Colao A, Di Sarno A, et al. Cabergoline treatment rapidly improves gonadal function in hyperprolactinemic males: a comparison with bromocriptine. Eur J Endocrinol. 1998;138:286.
23. De Rosa M, Zarrilli S, Vitale G, et al. Six months of treatment with cabergoline restores sexual potency in hyperprolactinemic males: an open longitudinal study monitoring nocturnal penile tumescence. J Clin Endocrinol Metab. 2004;89:621.
24. Colao A, Vitale G, Cappabianca P, et al. Outcome of cabergoline treatment in men with prolactinoma: effects of a 24-month treatment on prolactin levels, tumor mass, recovery of pituitary function, and semen analysis. J Clin Endocrinol Metab. 2004;89:1704.
25. Warfield A, Finkel DM, Schatz NJ, et al. Bromocriptine treatment of prolactin-secreting pituitary adenomas may restore pituitary function. Ann Intern Med. 1984; 101:783.

CHAPTER 12

Poor Responder in Ovulation Induction: Management Options

Sadhana Desai, Partha Guha Roy

Chapter outline

- Cause of Decrease Ovarian Reserve
- Poor Responders: Definition
- Prediction of Ovarian Response
- Various Protocols
- Precycle Adjuvants
- Adjuvants at the Initiation of the Cycle
  - Gonadotropins
  - Corifollitropin Alpha
  - Other Approach

INTRODUCTION

In the practice of assisted reproductive technology (ART), great steps forward have been made in recent years in term of clinical knowledge and technological development especially in IVF laboratories. One of the fundamental steps to reach the success is still related to the number of eggs obtained after controlled ovarian stimulation (COS). Often the clinician comes across poor response to ovarian stimulation due to the diminished ovarian reserve which is not limited to women of advance reproductive age but occasionally also encountered in young women. The limited number of obtained eggs and thereby fewer embryos to select and transfer remains the main problem in optimizing the live birth rates in poor responders.

CAUSE OF DECREASE OVARIAN RESERVE

Physiological decline of the "Follicular Heritage" sets in every woman over time with a marked increase in the rate of follicular disappearance from age 37–38 years onwards.[1] In poor responders the mechanism of the ovarian insufficiency is prematurely determined and not fully understood. Table 12.1 enlists some causes of decrease in ovarian reserve that has been identified.[2-6]

POOR RESPONDERS: DEFINITION

Although the concept of poor ovarian response was introduced over 30 years ago, there exists a host of definition describing the poor responders. In Bologna 2011, the European Society for Human Reproductiona and Embryology (ESHRE) working group,[7] on poor ovarian response has finally given a common definition of "Poor responder" where at least two of the following three features must be present:

a. A previous episode of poor ovarian response (≤3 oocytes) with a standard dose of medication
b. An abnormal ovarian reserve with antral follicular count (ALFC) (<5–7 follicles) or anti-Müllerian harmone (AMH) (<0.5–1.1 ng/mL),

Table 12.1: Decrease in ovarian reserve.

- Ovarian surgery—Endometrioma
- Genetic defects
- Chemotherapy
- Radiotherapy
- Autoimmune disorder
- Single ovary
- Chronic smoking
- Unexplained [6,8]
- Diabetes mellitus type 1 [9]
- Transfusion dependent β-thalassemia [10]
- Uterine artery embolization for the treatment of uterine leiomyoma [11,12]

Table 12.2: Poor responders.

- Age > 40
- Basal FSH >15 IU/L
- Poor AFC < 5
- AMH < 1.0 ng/mL
- Retrieval < 3 oocytes in previous IVF cycle
- Previous IVF cycle cancellation
    - Recruitment of < 3 follicles after 8–9 days of optimum stimulation with gonadotropins
    - Estradiol <500 pg/mL on day of hCG

c. Women above 40 years of age or presenting other risk factors for poor response such as previous ovarian surgery, genetic defects, chemotherapy, radiotherapy and autoimmune disorders.

The incidence of poor response in the population undergoing ART is estimated to 9–24%. Poor responders are identified on the basis of age, previous response to stimulation, abnormal base line hormones, few antral follicles, abnormal dynamic testing and previous pelvic surgery (Table 12.2).

PREDICTION OF OVARIAN RESPONSE

Before starting controlled ovarian stimulation the prediction of ovarian response is the only way to administer an efficient and safe treatment. Age, biochemical parameters (FSH, AMH) and morphological characteristic (AFC and ovarian volume)[13] are the present markers for predicting the ovarian response to hormonal stimulation. Recently it has been demonstrated that follicle-stimulating hormone (FSH) is a good predictor only at a very high threshold levels (FSH ≥ 12 MIU/mL) which reflects a much compromised ovarian reserve.[13] AMH level has a very low inter- and intracycle variability remaining stable during menstrual cycles.[14,15] However smoking and oral contraceptive pills can affect the AMH levels.[16] A recent meta-analysis[17] has confirmed AMH as an excellent predictor of poor ovarian response to ovarian stimulation although ideal test is the response of the ovaries to hormonal stimulation itself. AMH and AFC, alone or in combination, did not improve the prediction of ongoing pregnancy rate, with the age of women being the most important factor related to live birth rate.[17] The body mass index[18,19] also plays a role in female reproduction: obese poor responder could have a lower pregnancy rate as compared to nonobese poor responders. (Table 12.3).

A word of caution when interpreting basal FSH levels in a clinical context as inconsistencies may arise from the wide inter-individual variation that exists in follicular phase FSH concentrations in the normo-ovulatory cycle. Basal FSH levels and their interpretation are depicted in Table 12.4.

Poor ovarian response to hyperstimulation is clearly associated with chronological aging. An age-related decline in response to stimulation with gonadotropins and a

Table 12.3: Predictors of ovarian response.

- Age
- FSH levels on day 3
- Anti-Müllerian hormone (AMH)
- AFC (Preferably on day 3)
- Ovarian volume
- Body mass index (BMI)

Table 12.4: Interpretation of different levels of FSH as measured on day 3.

Day 3 FSH levels	Interpretation
<10 IU/L	Normal FSH level, expect a good response
10–15 IU/L	Reduced ovarian reserve, reduced response to stimulation. Reduction in embryo quality, reduced live birth rate on average
15–20 IU/L	More marked reduction in response to stimulation. Further reduction in embryo quality. Lower live birth rates
>20 IU/L	Very poor response to stimulation. "No go at our center at this level"

Table 12.5: Outcome of IVF.[29]

Age	Live birth/cycle
30 years	17% per cycle
40 years	7% per cycle
45 years	2% per cycle

Table 12.6: Live birth rate in relation to FSH values.

FSH values	Live birth rate
• <10 IU/L	23.5%/cycle
• 10–15 IU/L	14.2%/cycle
• 15–20 IU/L	11.5%/cycle
• <20 IU/L	6.9%/cycle

reduction in the number of oocytes,[20] oocyte quality,[21] fertilization rates[22,23] and ultimately embryos[24-26] have been well documented. Many studies point to 40 years as a significant cutoff age. Although age is an important predictor of IVF outcome[27] chronological age is poorly correlated with ovarian aging (Table 12.5).[28]

Women with elevated baseline FSH levels should not be turned away from IVF treatment as reported by Thum et al. (Table 12.6).[30]

VARIOUS PROTOCOLS

Over the past 20 years for the management of the poor responder patients various protocols with different doses and types of gonadotropins have been designed but till date the clinicians are in doubt about the ideal protocol for patients defined as poor responders.

PRECYCLE ADJUVANTS

a. **Androgens:** Androgens[31] play a critical role for an adequate follicular steroidogenesis and increases FSH receptor expressions in granulosa cells amplifying the effects of FSH and thus potentially enhance responsiveness of ovaries to FSH.[31,32] Inadequate levels of androgens are associated with decreased ovarian sensitivity to FSH and low pregnancy rates after IVF.[33] Oral administration of dehydroepiandrosterone (DHEA), Transdermal application of testosterone gel before ovarian stimulation with gonadotropins could improve the response in poor responder patients. Several uncontrolled studies published in last decade showed improved clinical outcome after oral DHEA and transdermal testosterone application with a significantly higher ongoing pregnancy rate.[34] Casson et al.[35] first suggested that the oral administration of DHEA before ovarian stimulation with gonadotropin could improve the response in poor responder patients. In a few retrospective studies DHEA supplementation with 25 mg three times daily for 4 months prior to IVF, improve the number of fertilized embryos and their quality. DHEA supplementation also decreases the cancellation rate and improves the clinical pregnancy rate. DHEA supplementation for poor responders remains controversial.[36-39]

In a prospective randomized study, Kim, Howles, and Lee[40] evaluated the effects of *12.5-mg testosterone gel* pretreatment (for 21 days) prior to the start of stimulation. The testosterone gel pretreatment group and a control group both received 300 IU/day of follicle-stimulating hormone (FSH) in combination with a gonadotropin-releasing hormone antagonist for stimulation.

Women in the testosterone pretreatment group required fewer days of stimulation and fewer ampoules of gonadotropin. Cycle cancellation occurred with similar frequency. In the testosterone group, women produced more follicles and more oocytes were retrieved. The numbers of available embryos and good quality embryos also were higher. Endometrial thickness and the number of embryos transferred were the same in both groups. The implantation rate was higher in the testosterone group (14.3% vs 7.2%), and the clinical pregnancy rate per transfer was significantly higher as well (31.5% vs 15.1%). The difference in live birth rates reached borderline significance (27.3% vs 12.7%; P = 0.057). The investigators concluded that testosterone pretreatment may have a positive effect on stimulation and IVF treatment outcomes in poor responder patients.

b. **Simple cyst drainage prior to stimulation protocols**: One of the most significant side effects of pituitary down regulation with gonadotropin-releasing hormone (GnRH) agonist in COH protocols is ovarian cysts formation. Follicular cysts may be related to the endogenous gonadotropins flare in response to mid-luteal GnRH agonist. There is evidence of poor IVF performance in patients who form ovarian cysts in response to GnRH agonists in both poor responders and normal responders.

Several studies have evaluated the effect of ovarian cyst aspiration on IVF outcomes. Most of them failed to show improved outcomes with precycle aspiration.[41,42]

c. **Oral contraceptive pill (OCP) OR Antagonist suppression combined with estrogen priming**: OCP pretreatment in IVF protocols establishes an estrogenic environment and increases sex hormone-binding globulin levels while decreasing follicular androgens levels which may delay apoptosis. The progestin component of OCP suppresses luteinizing hormone thereby synchronizing follicular development, leading to a more evenly sized follicular response.

GnRH agonist flare cycles are commonly used in poor responders, and OCP pre-treatment can prevent an early rise in progesterone by eliminating the corpus luteum. OCP cause less pituitary down regulation when compared with GnRH agonist used in a long protocol.

However, numerous studies[43-45] have failed to show any difference in IVF outcomes between patients pretreated with OCP and those in whom OCP was not used. OCP significantly prolongs stimulation and increases the dose of gonadotropins.[46] Pituitary suppression with OCP may blunt a GnRH agonist or letrozole flare response in follicular phase.

d. **GnRH antagonist**: GnRH antagonists has been lately used in the late luteal phase of poor responders prior to a stimulation cycle GnRH antagonist administrated on day 25 of the menstrual cycle reduces size disparities among follicles.[47] More recent studies have resulted in similar IVF outcome when luteal E2/GnRH antagonist in GnRH antagonist protocols were compared with micro dose GnRH agonist flare protocols.[48,49]

Treatment with estrogen in the luteal phase prior to COH may promote granulosa cells FSH receptor induction and suppression of premature follicular development.[50-52] Increase number of FSH receptors and

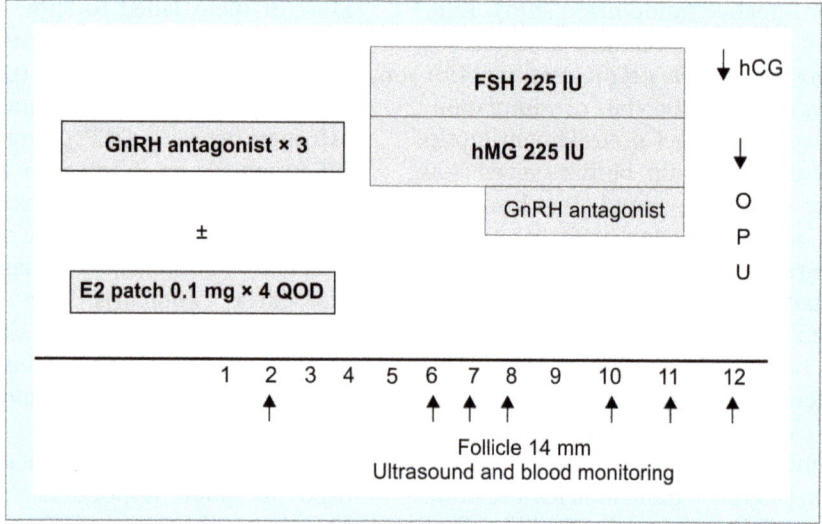

Fig. 12.1: Luteal estradiol/gonadotropins-releasing hormone antagonist protocol. (E2: estradiol; FSH: follicle stimulating hormone; hCG: human chorionic gonadotropin; hMG: human menopausal gonadotropin; IU: international unit; qod.: every other day).

improved response to FSH stimulation may promote oocyte maturation. Estrogen administered in luteal phase was shown to prevent a luteal FSH rise, decreasing luteal follicular recruitment and a premature dominant follicle.[51,52] Several studies have demonstrated decrease cancellation rate, improved number of oocyte and embryos but improved pregnancy rate have not been confirmed following luteal phase E2 patch (Fig. 12.1).[53]

ADJUVANTS AT THE INITIATION OF THE CYCLE

a. **GnRH analog flare protocol:** Use of GnRH agonist in the early follicular phase causes 24 hours long surge in endogenous FSH and LH release which is used as a strategy to improve IVF outcomes and decrease the cancellation rate in poor responders. GnRH agonists are initiated in the follicular phase of a stimulation cycle shortly before commencing the gonadotropins injection. This approach utilizes the flare response to GnRH agonist without prolonged ovarian suppression thereby reducing the required dose of gonadotropins.[53] Reported clinical pregnancy rate with flare protocol in poor responders have ranged from 12–26.3%.[54-55] In short, the success of GnRH agonist flare protocol for poor responders has led most IVF program over the last two decades to abandon long GnRH agonist protocol in the poor responder patients (Fig. 12.2).

b. **GnRh agonist's microdose flare protocol:** The desire to decrease the suppressive effects during a flare protocol has prompted the use of low-dose "micro dose" GnRH agonist flare protocol. The ideal dose should be low enough to maintain some endogens FSH and LH, yet high enough to generate a flare response early in the follicular phase and prevent an endogenous LH surge. In this protocol GnRH agonist 20–50 µg is given twice daily from the 2nd day of the cycle and is usually combined with

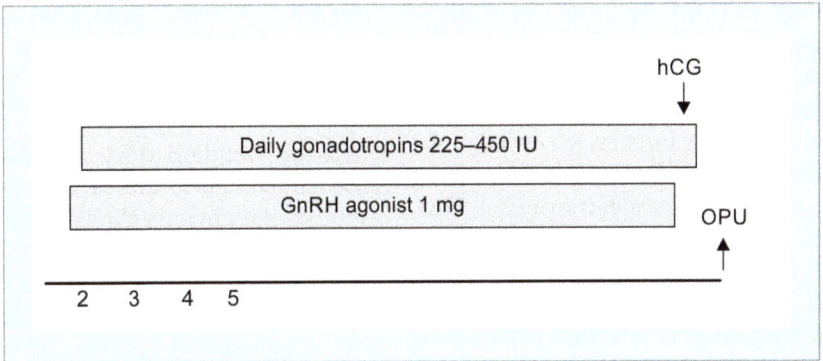

Fig. 12.2: Standard flare protocol.
(hCG: human chorionic gonadotropin ; IU: international units; OPU: ovum pickup)

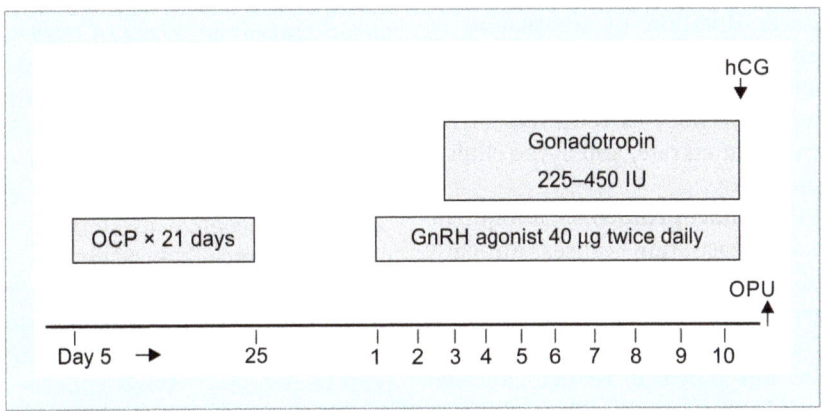

Fig. 12.3: Oral contraceptive pill/Microdose GnRH agonist protocol.
(FSH: follicle-stimulating hormone; hCG: human chorionic gonadotropin; IU: international unit; OCP: oral contraceptive pill; OPU: ovum pickup.

OCP pre-treatment in the cycle prior to COH to prevent corpus luteum rescue (Fig. 12.3).[56,57] Retrospective studies have shown that this protocol lead to improve cycle outcome with regards to the number of retrieved oocytes, percentage of patients undergoing embryo transfer, cancellation rates and pregnancy rates, when compared with traditional GnRH agonist protocols.[57]

c. **Agonist v/s Antagonist**: It is since 15 years that GnRH antagonist are available as an adjuvant to COS. It prevents a premature LH surge without early suppression of follicular development. Most protocols commence GnRH antagonists when the mean diameter of the lead follicle reaches 14 mm and continue daily until hCG administration. Multiple prospective randomized control trials compared the use of GnRH agonist flare protocols with GnRH antagonist in poor responders.[54,58,59] The result were conflicting some showing better outcomes and pregnancy rates while others showing no great significant differences.[60] A recent meta-analysis of 14 prospective randomized control trials by Pu et al.[61] documented a significant advantage of GnRH agonists over GnRH antagonist in COS for poor responders in respect to duration of stimulation. However no significant difference was found in clinical pregnancy rate, cycle cancellation rate and number of oocytes retrieved or no of mature oocytes retrieved.[54,56] The clinical issues that surround choosing an agonist flare versus an antagonist protocol include corpus luteum recovery and early rise in progesterone if a flare protocol is not pretreated with OCPs.[62]

A recent meta-analysis of 14 randomized control studies,[61] GnRH antagonist protocol resulted in a statistically significant lower duration of stimulation as compared to GnRH agonist protocols, but there was no significant difference in the number of oocytes retrieved, in the cycle cancellation rate, and in the clinical pregnancy rate.

d. **Clomiphene flare protocols**: Clomiphene citrate administration causes an early flare of endogenous gonadotropins. The endogenous LH surge can be blocked with GnRH antagonists.[63] In poor responders CC flare was shown to reduce cancellation rate, increase the number of oocyte retrieved resulting in a higher implantation rate and pregnancy rate. However the concern is about the endometrial receptivity due to its suppression. CC is commonly and successfully used both in minimal stimulation protocols and for its flare effect in high dose protocols in poor responders who are undergoing freeze all cycles.

e. **Letrozole flare protocols**: Letrozole exerts a flare effect on the pituitary by blocking estrogen synthesis and decreasing it circulating levels. Letrozoles in a dose of 2.5–5 mg daily for 5 days has been combined with gonadotropins and GnRH antagonist. It decrease the total dose of FSH used when compared with a long GnRH agonist protocol.[64] Further controlled randomized trials are needed to assess its value.

Gonadotropins

When the standard dose of gonadotropins (225–300 IU) fails to induce a proper ovarian response, the obvious clinical approach is to increase the dose. Majority of the clinicians did not report enhanced ovarian response and better pregnancy rate when the starting dose of gonadotropins was increase up to 450 IU. Increasing the FSH starting dose does not result in higher pregnancy rate and also found no difference between the starting dose of 300, 450, and 600 IU units of gonadotropins in terms of retrieved oocyte, no. of embryo obtained and pregnancy rate.[65] These patients have a reduced ovarian reserve and the recruitable follicles are fewer and the gonadotropins independently of the dosage administered can only support the cohort of follicle receptive to stimulation without manufacturing follicle de novo.

Its remains difficult to conclude based on the current literature, what the ideal starting and maintenance dose of FSH should be in poor responders.[63] What appears clear from the literature is the finding that follicular recruitment occur in the late luteal phase prior to menses and the early follicular phase therefore maximal dosing currently set at 450 IU of FSH, should be started as early in the cycle as possible. The dose may then be reduced once adequate response has been established.

hMG versus Recombinant FSH: More recent trials have suggested that hMG may have advantages for poor responders undergoing IVF, although the data are limited.[66] Mixed protocols of r-FSH and hMG have become popular to provide both a high FSH dose as well as some LH activity.

Role of LH: LH activity has been postulated to be beneficial during early follicular recruitment by increasing FSH receptors, as well as maintaining follicular development during later follicular maturation by maintaining steroid precursors LH is available as both a recombinant LH and in the standard urinary hMG, which has a 1:1 ratio of FSH and LH activity. Most reviews and meta-analysis of the role of LH, however, have been unable to confirm any benefit or detriment of LH to IVF pregnancy or live birth rates.[67] It has become clear that GnRH antagonist blunt the rise in E2 during r-FSH stimulated cycles. This decreased rise in E2 can be overcome with either hMG or r-LH, however, no advantage in IVF outcome has been established. In addition to poor responders, some authors have found a benefit to LH addition in stimulation protocols in older patients.[68]

A systematic review and meta-analysis including 603 patients by Venetis, Kolibianakis et al.[69] showed that no significant differences were present between poor responders who were treated with rLH and those who were not, regarding duration of gonadotropin stimulation, total dose of gonadotropins required for ovarian stimulation and serum E2 levels on the day of hCG. Significantly less COCs were retrieved from patients who received rLH as compared to those who did not (WMD: –0.20 COCS, 95% CI: –0.37 to –0.04). A nonsignificant increase of 6.5% in clinical pregnancy rates was present in patients who received rLH as compared to those who did not (95% CI: –0.3% to + 13.2%).

Currently, based on the best available evidence, *addition of rLH* in poor responders undergoing ovarian stimulation for IVF using rFSH and GnRH analogs does not seem to increase the probability of clinical pregnancy. However, given the magnitude of the rate difference and the confidence interval, further studies are needed for solid conclusions to be drawn.

Dosing intervals for poor responders: Despite of no documented benefit from twice daily dosing it continues to be popular, especially for mixed protocols in poor responders. Pharmacokinetics has suggested that a steady state is obtained after two days of injections, offsetting any theoretical benefits from twice daily dosing.[70]

Minimal stimulation: Role of minimal stimulation protocols though suggested for both normal and poor responder is particularly appropriate for study in poor responders, as a high dose of gonadotropins often produces no greater oocyte yield then a far less expensive cycle with oral medication or low dose of gonadotropins. Many studies have suggested natural cycle IVF or IVF with minimal stimulation as the pregnancy rates are similar as with full dose of gonadotropins.[71-74]

Natural, clomiphene or letrozole only IVF: In a natural cycle the ongoing pregnancy rate is 7.2% per cycle and 15.8% per transfer. For normal responders these ongoing pregnancy rates are unacceptably low. For poor responders one randomized trial showed higher implantation rate in natural cycle IVF but similar clinical pregnancy rate per cycle per transfer as patients treated with full dose gonadotropins.[71]

Schimberni et al.[72] evaluated the IVF outcome in large group of poor responders (500 patients) reporting very encouraging results especially in younger women (<35 years). In this group of poor responder patients the pregnancy rate was 18% per started cycle, 29% per transfer and 31% per patient. However a recent paper which analyze the natural cycles of IVF in women with poor responders, showed that the cumulative live birth per patient does not exceed 8%.

A survey of 500 consecutive cycles of natural cycle IVF by Marco S Bracia et al.[30] reported the pregnancy rate per cycle of approximately 10% and 18% per transfer. The pregnancy rate was different depending on women's age (Table 12.7). In poor responding younger women, the remaining follicle seems to be in good quality but the opposite is true of women aged 40 years or older. The efficacy

Table 12.7: Pregnancy rate in relation to the patients age.

Age	Pregnancy rate
<35 years	18%/cycle, 30%/transfer
35–39 years	11%/cycle, 20% /transfer
>40 years	6% /cycle, 10%/transfer

of natural cycle IVF is hampered by high cancellation rates mainly due to untimely LH surge. The use of GnRH antagonists in the late follicular phase, and the improvements in laboratory conditions and fertilization techniques, increase the embryo transfer rates, making this procedure more cost effective.[75]

To increase the oocyte yield by maintaining minimal cost, clomiphene citrate (CC) alone can be utilized for the IVF stimulation. As compared to natural cycle IVF CC stimulation alone in poor responders can give a pregnancy rate of 10% which is equivalent to the full dose gonadotropins. No studies are published using letrozole alone in minimal stimulation IVF. Minimal stimulation protocol with or without gonadotropins continue to be an important area of clinical investigations for poor responders.

Corifollitropin Alpha

These new gonadotropins, in hybrid molecule with prolonged half-life support the cohort of follicle receptive to stimulation for 7 days. The use of these long acting gonadotropins can exploit fully the reduced ovarian reserve by the rapid increase in serum FSH concentration which would result in a significantly higher exposure of the small antral follicles to constant high level of FSH during the early follicular phase.

Corifollitropin alpha followed by r-FSH in combination with GnRH antagonist should improve clinical results when compared to conventional stimulation protocols. Promising pregnancy rates are reported in a retrospective pilot studies (< 40 years) in poor responder patient following a combination of corifollitropin alpha with HP-hMG in a GnRH antagonist protocol.[76,77]

Other Approach

1. **Growth hormone:** Growth hormone has been added to control ovarian stimulation in poor responders to increase the probability of live birth. In fact until now there are not very recent and robust data suggesting routine use of growth hormone in ovarian stimulation protocols for poor responder patients.[78,79]
2. **Aspirin/Prednisolone:** Impaired ovarian blood flow can contribute to poor ovarian response.[80,81] Enhancing ovarian vascularization with vasoactive substances such as aspirin can improve delivery of gonadotropic hormones or other growth factors required for folliculogenesis.[82,83] However the evidence supporting the effect of a low dose of aspirin in women undergoing IVF is poor and controversial.[84] On the basis of updated evidence, a low dose of aspirin has no substantial positive effect on the likelihood of pregnancy and it should not be routinely recommended for women undergoing IVF. Prospective randomized trials demonstrated that adjuvant therapy with aspirin and prednisolone did not improve uterine blood flow, implantation and pregnancy rates.[85]
3. **Oocyte/Embryo cryopreservation:** With the advent of vitrification for cryopreservation of oocytes, treatment protocols have taken a quantum leap in the IVF program. Women with poor responders can undergo several stimulation cycles and preserve their oocytes/embryos creating a similar situation as in normal responder patients. The freeze all cycles are where oocytes are accumulated in multiple controlled ovarian stimulation cycles. The patient undergoes a FET once they have reached an optimal number of oocytes. A prospective study by Cobo

et al.[86] suggested that the cumulative life birth rate per patient was higher in the freeze all (36.4%) than the fresh group (23.7%) in a group of poor responders.

4. **IVM of human oocytes:** Oocytes are retrieved at 8–12 mm size after either priming with a few days of FSH injections followed by hCG, or during a natural cycle followed by a hCG injection. The immature retrieved oocytes are then matured *in vitro* in special media. While IVM has been proposed for patients with polycystic ovary syndrome at high risk of ovarian hyperstimulation syndrome, and cancer patients who may not undergo standard stimulation, a few case reports have described success using IVM in poor responders.

CONCLUSION

Poor ovarian responders remain one of most challenging task in ART practice. At the despite of huge publication in the last 2 decade to find the most efficient protocol for poor responders, the present systematic reviews and meta-analysis suggest the insufficient evidence exists for an optimum protocol for poor responders. Poor responders "Per se" do not represent a lower chance of successful IVF, with the age of the women being the most important predictor of live birth rate.

REFERENCES

1. Faddy MJ, Gosden RG, Gougeon A, et al. Accelerated disappearance of ovarian follicles in mid-life: implications for forecasting menopause. Hum Reprod. 1992; 7(10);1342-6.
2. de Ziegler D, Borghese B, Chapron C. Endometriosis and infertility: pathophysiology and management. The Lancet. 2010;376(9742):730-8.
3. Benaglia L, Somigliana E, Vighi V, Ragni G, Vercellini P, Fedele L. Rate of severe ovarian damage following surgery for endometriomas. Hum Reprod. 2010;25(3);678-82.
4. Streuli I, de Ziegler D, Gayet V, et al. In women with endometriosis anti-Müllerian hormone levels are decreased only in those with previous endometrioma surgery. Hum Reprod. 2012;27(11);3294-3303.
5. Raffi F, Metwally M, Amer S. The impact of excision of ovarian endometrioma on ovarian reserve: a systematic review and meta-analysis. J Clin Endocrinol Metab. 2012;97(9):3146-54.
6. De Vos M, Devroey P, Fauser BC. Primary ovarian insufficiency. Lancet. 2010;376(9744):911-21.
7. Ferraretti AP, La Marca A, Fauser BC, Tarlatzis B, Nargund G, Gianaroli L; ESHRE working group on Poor Ovarian Response Definition. ESHRE consensus on the definition of "poor response" to ovarian stimulation for in vitro fertilization: the Bologna criteria. Hum Reprod. 2011;(7):1616-24.
8. Fritz MA, Speroff L. Clinical Gynecologic Endocrinology and Infertility. Wolters Kluwer Health/Lippincott Williams & Wilkins, Philadelphia, Pa, USA, 2011.
9. Soto N, Iñiguez G, López P, et al. Anti-Müllerian hormone and inhibin B levels as markers of premature ovarian aging and transition to menopause in type 1 diabetes mellitus. Hum Reprod. 2009;24(11):2838-44.
10. Garcia-Velasco JA, Isaza V, Requena A, et al. High doses of gonadotrophins combined with stop versus non-stop protocol of GnRH analogue administration in low responder IVF patients: a prospective, randomized, controlled trial. Hum Reprod. 2000;15(11):2292-6.
11. Hehenkamp WJK, Volkers NA, Broekmans FJM, et al. Loss of ovarian reserve after uterine artery embolization: a randomized comparison with hysterectomy. Hum Reprod. 2007;22(7):1996-2005.
12. Tropeano G, Di Stasi C, Amoroso S, Gualano MR, Bonomo L, Scambia G. Long-term effects of uterine fibroid embolization on ovarian reserve: a prospective cohort study. Fertil Steril. 2010 ;94(6):2296-300.
13. Broekmans FJ, Kwee J, Hendriks DJ, et al. A systematic review of tests predicting ovarian reserve and IVF outcome. Hum Reprod Update. 2006;12(6):685-718.

14. La Marca A, Stabile G, Artenisio AC, Volpe A. Serum anti-Mullerian hormone throughout the human menstrual cycle. Hum Reprod. 2006;21(12):3103-7.
15. la Marca A, Giulini S, Tirelli A. et al. Anti-Müllerian hormone measurement on any day of the menstrual cycle strongly predicts ovarian response in assisted reproductive technology. Hum Reprod. 2007;22(3):766-71.
16. Dólleman M, Faddy MJ, van Disseldorp J, et al. The relationship between anti-müllerian hormone in women receiving fertility assessments and age at menopause in subfertile women: evidence from large population studies. J Clin Endocrinol Metab. 2013;98(5):1946-53.
17. Broer SL, Dólleman M, van Disseldorp J. et al. Prediction of an excessive response in in vitro fertilization from patient characteristics and ovarian reserve tests and comparison in subgroups: an individual patient data meta-analysis. Fertil Steril. 2013;100(2):420-9.
18. Oudendijk JF, Yarde F, Eijkemans MJC. et al. The poor responder in IVF: Is the prognosis always poor? A systematic review. Hum Reprod Update. 2012;18(1):1-11.
19. Koning AMH, Kuchenbecker WKH, Groen H. et al. Economic consequences of overweight and obesity in infertility: a framework for evaluating the costs and outcomes of fertility care. Hum Reprod Update. 2010;16(3):246-54.
20. Piette C, de Mouzon J, Bachelot A, et al. IVF: Influence of Women's Age on Pregnancy Rates. Hum Reprod. 1990;5:56-9.
21. Tucker MJ, Morton PC, Wright G, et al. Factors Affecting Success with Intracytoplasmic Sperm Injection. Reprod Fertil Dev. 1995;7:229-36.
22. Ashkenazi J, Orvieto R, Gold-Deutch R, et al. The Impact of Woman's Age and Sperm Parameters on Fertilization Rates on IVF Cycles. Eur J Obstet Gynecol Reprod Biol. 1996;66:155-9.
23. Yie SM, Collins JA, Daya S, et al. Polyploidy and fail fertilization in IVF are related to patients age and gamete quality. Hum Reprod. 1996;11:614-7.
24. Cordioro I, Calhaz-Jorge C, et al. Repercussion Da Idade de mulher, de taxa De Cliyigem e da qualidade embrionaria, na obtencao de graviez porfertilizacao in vitro. Acta Med Port. 1995;8:145-50.
25. Hull MG, Fleming CF, Hughes AO, et al. Age related decline in female fecundity: a quantitative control study of implanting capacity and survival of individual embryos after IVF. Fertil Steril. 1996;65:783-90.
26. Sharif K, Elgendy M, Lashen H, et al. Age and basal FSH as predictors of IVF outcomes. Br J Obstet Gynaecol. 1998;105:107-2.
27. Yaron Y, Botchan A, Amit A, et al. Endometrial receptivity: the age related decline in pregnancy rates and the effect of ovarian function. Fertil Steril. 1993;60:314-8.
28. Roest J, Van Heusden AM, Mous H, et al. The ovarian response as a predictor for successful IVF treatment after the age of 40 Years. Fertil Steril. 1996;66:969-73.
29. Widra EA, Botchan A, Amit A, et al. Endometrial receptivity: the age-related decline in pregnancy rates and the effect of ovarian function. Fertil Steril. 1996;65:103-8.
30. Thum MY, Abdalla H, et al. Is there any value in treating women with elevated basal FSH? Fertil Steril. 2003;80:S155 Abstract P-104.
31. Weil SJ, Vendola K, Zhou J, et al. Androgen receptor gene expression in the primate ovary: cellular localization, regulation, and functional correlations. J Clin Endocrinol Metab. 1998;83(7):2479-85.
32. Vendola KA, Zhou J, Adesanya OO, et al. Androgens stimulate early stages of follicular growth in the primate ovary. J Clin Invest. 1998;101(12):2622-9.
33. Frattarelli JL, Peterson EH. Effect of androgen levels on in vitro fertilization cycles. Fertil Steril. 2004;81(6):1713-4.
34. Sunkara SK, Coomarasamy A. Androgen pretreatment in poor responders undergoing controlled ovarian stimulation and in vitro fertilization treatment. Fertil Steril. 2011;95(8):e73-4.
35. Casson PR, Lindsay MS, Pisarska MD, et al. Dehydroepiandrosterone supplementation augments ovarian stimulation in poor responders: a case series. Hum Reprod. 2000;15(10):2129-32.
36. Barad DH, Gleicher N. Increased oocyte production after treatment with dehydroepi-androsterone. Fertil Steril. 2005;84(3):756.

37. Barad D, Gleicher N. Effect of dehydroepiandrosterone on oocyte and embryo yields, embryo grade and cell number in IVF. Hum Reprod. 2006;21(11):2845-9.
38. Barad D, Brill H, Gleicher N. Update on the use of dehydroepiandrosterone supplementation among women with diminished ovarian function. J Assist Reprod Genet. 2007;24(12):629-34.
39. Gleicher N, Ryan E, Weghofer A, et al. Miscarriage rates after dehydroepiandrosterone (DHEA) supplementation in women with diminished ovarian reserve: a case control study. Reprod Biol Endocrinol. 2009;7:108.
40. Kim CH, Howles CM, Lee HA. The effect of transdermal testosterone gel pretreatment on controlled ovarian stimulation and IVF outcome in low responders. Fertil Steril. 2011;95:679-83.
41. Qublan HS, Amarin Z, Tahat YA, et al. Ovarian cyst formation following GnRH agonist administration in IVF cycles: incidence and impact. Hum Reprod. 2006;21(3):640-4.
42. Segal S, Shifren JL, Isaacson KB, et al. Effect of a baseline ovarian cyst on the outcome of in vitro fertilization–embryo transfer. Fertil Steril. 1999;71(2):274-7.
43. Duvan CI, Berker B, Turhan NO, et al. Oral contraceptive pretreatment does not improve outcome in microdose gonadotrophin-releasing hormone agonist protocol among poor responder intracytoplasmic sperm injection patients. J Assist Reprod Genet. 2008;25(2–3):89-93.
44. Kovacs P, Barg PE, Witt BR. Hypothalamic-pituitary suppression with oral contraceptive pills does not improve outcome in poor responder patients undergoing in vitro fertilization–embryo transfer cycles. J Assist Reprod Genet. 2001;18(7):391-4.
45. Al-Mizyen E, Sabatini L, Lower AM, et al. Does pretreatment with progestogen or oral contraceptive pills in low responders followed by the GnRHa flare protocol improve the outcome of IVF–ET? J Assist Reprod Genet. 2000;17(3):140-6.
46. Lindheim SR, Barad DH, Witt B, et al. Short-term gonadotropin suppression with oral contraceptives benefits poor responders prior to controlled ovarian hyperstimulation. J Assist Reprod Genet. 1996;13(9):745-7.
47. Fanchin R, Castelo Branco A, Kadoch IJ, et al. Premenstrual administration of gonadotropin-releasing hormone antagonist coordinates early antral follicle sizes and sets up the basis for an innovative concept of controlled ovarian hyperstimulation. Fertil Steril. 2004;81(6):1554-9.
48. Ata B, Zeng X, Son WY, et al. Follicular synchronization using transdermal estradiol patch and GnRH antagonists in the luteal phase; does it increase oocyte yield in poor responders to gonadotropin stimulation for in vitro fertilization (IVF)? A comparative study with microdose flare-up protocol. Gynecol Endocrinol. 2011;27(11):876-9.
49. Weitzman VN, Engmann L, DiLuigi A, et al. Comparison of luteal estradiol patch and gonadotropin-releasing hormone antagonist suppression protocol before gonadotropin stimulation versus microdose gonadotropin-releasing hormone agonist protocol for patients with a history of poor in vitro fertilization outcomes. Fertil Steril. 2009;92(1):226-30.
50. Clark JR, Dierschke DJ, Wolf RC. Hormonal regulation of ovarian folliculogenesis in rhesus monkeys: III. Atresia of the preovulatory follicle induced by exogenous steroids and subsequent follicular development. Biol Reprod. 1981;25(2):332-41.
51. Fanchin R, Cunha-Filho JS, Schonäuer LM, et al. Coordination of early antral follicles by luteal estradiol administration provides a basis for alternative controlled ovarian hyperstimulation regimens. Fertil Steril. 2003;79(2):316-21.
52. Fanchin R, Salomon L, Castelo-Branco A, et al. Luteal estradiol pre-treatment coordinates follicular growth during controlled ovarian hyperstimulation with GnRH antagonists. Hum Reprod. 2003;18(12):2698-703.
53. Shastri SM, Barbieri E, Kligman I, et al. Stimulation of the young poor responder: comparison of the luteal estradiol/gonadotropin-releasing hormone antagonist priming protocol versus oral contraceptive microdose leuprolide. Fertil Steril. 2011;95(2):592-5.

54. Akman MA, Erden HF, Tosun SB, et al. Comparison of agonistic flare-up-protocol and antagonistic multiple dose protocol in ovarian stimulation of poor responders: results of a prospective randomized trial. Hum Reprod. 2001;16(5):868-70.
55. Fasouliotis SJ, Laufer N, Sabbagh-Ehrlich S, et al. Gonadotropin-releasing hormone (GnRH)-antagonist versus GnRH-agonist in ovarian stimulation of poor responders undergoing IVF. J Assist Reprod Genet. 2003;20(11):455-60.
56. Kahraman K, Berker B, Atabekoglu CS, et al. Microdose gonadotropin-releasing hormone agonist flare-up protocol versus multiple dose gonadotropin-releasing hormone antagonist protocol in poor responders undergoing intracytoplasmic sperm injection-embryo transfer cycle. Fertil Steril. 2009;91(6):2437-44.
57. Scott RT, Navot D. Enhancement of ovarian responsiveness with microdoses of gonadotropin-releasing hormone agonist during ovulation induction for in vitro fertilization. Fertil Steril. 1994;61(5):880-5.
58. Olivennes F, Mannaerts B, Struijs M, et al. Perinatal outcome of pregnancy after GnRH antagonist (ganirelix) treatment during ovarian stimulation for conventional IVF or ICSI: a preliminary report. Hum. Reprod. 2001;16(8):1588-91.
59. Schmidt DW, Bremner T, Orris JJ, et al. A randomized prospective study of microdose leuprolide versus ganirelix in in vitro fertilization cycles for poor responders. Fertil Steril. 2001;83(5):1568-71.
60. Lainas TG, Sfontouris IA, Papanikolaou EG, et al. Flexible GnRH antagonist versus flare-up GnRH agonist protocol in poor responders treated by IVF: a randomized controlled trial. Hum Reprod. 2008;23(6):1355-8.
61. Pu D, Wu J, Liu J. Comparisons of GnRH antagonist versus GnRH agonist protocol in poor ovarian responders undergoing IVF. Hum Reprod. 2011;26(10):2742-9.
62. Berin I, Stein DE, Keltz MD. A comparison of gonadotropin-releasing hormone (GnRH) antagonist and GnRH agonist flare protocols for poor responders undergoing in vitro fertilization. Fertil Steril. 2010;93(2):360-3.
63. Craft I, Gorgy A, Hill J, et al. Will GnRH antagonists provide new hope for patients considered "difficult responders" to GnRH agonist protocols?. Hum Reprod. 1999;14(12):2959-62.
64. Goswami SK, Das T, Chattopadhyay R, et al. A randomized single-blind controlled trial of letrozole as a low-cost IVF protocol in women with poor ovarian response: a preliminary report. Hum Reprod. 2004;19(9):2031-5.
65. Berkkanoglu M, Ozgur K. What is the optimum maximal gonadotropin dosage used in microdose flare-up cycles in poor responders? Fertil Steril. 2010;94(2):662-5.
66. Venetis CA, Kolibianakis EM, Tarlatzi TB, et al. Benefits of luteinizing hormone activity in ovarian stimulation for IVF. Reprod Biomed Online. 2009;18 (Suppl 2):31-6.
67. Kolibianakis EM, Collins J, Tarlatzis B, et al. Are endogenous LH levels during ovarian stimulation for IVF using GnRH analogues associated with the probability of ongoing pregnancy? A systematic review. Hum Reprod Update. 2006;12(1):3-12.
68. Lisi F, Rinaldi L, Fishel S, et al. Use of recombinant follicle-stimulating hormone (Gonal F) and recombinant luteinizing hormone (Luveris) for multiple follicular stimulation in patients with a suboptimal response to in vitro fertilization. Fertil Steril. 2003;79(4):1037-8.
69. Venetis CA, Kolibianakis EM, et al. Addition of recombinant LH in poor responders undergoing ovarian stimulation with recombinant FSH and GnRH analogues for in vitro fertilization: a systematic review and meta-analysis. Fertil Steril.2011;96(3):S57.
70. Seo KS, Yoon JW, Na KH, et al. Evaluation of process efficiency and bioequivalence of biosimilar recombinant human chorionic gonadotropin (rhCG). BioDrugs. 2011;25(2):115-27.
71. Morgia F, Sbracia M, Schimberni M, et al. A controlled trial of natural cycle versus microdose gonadotropin-releasing hormone analog flare cycles in poor responders undergoing in vitro fertilization. Fertil Steril. 2004;81(6):1542-7.
72. Schimberni M, Morgia F, Colabianchi J, et al. Natural-cycle in vitro fertilization in poor

responder patients: a survey of 500 consecutive cycles. Fertil Steril. 2009;92(4):1297-301.
73. Weghofer A, Margreiter M, Bassim S, et al. Minimal stimulation using recombinant follicle-stimulating hormone and a gonadotropin-releasing hormone antagonist in women of advanced age. Fertil Steril. 2004;81(4):1002-6.
74. Elizur SE, Aslan D, Shulman A, et al. Modified natural cycle using GnRH antagonist can be an optional treatment in poor responders undergoing IVF. J Assist Reprod Genet. 2005;22(2):75-9.
75. Ubaldi FM1, Rienzi L, Ferrero S, et al. Management of poor responders in IVF. Reprod Biomed Online. 2005;10(2):235-46.
76. Polyzos NP, Devos M, Humaidan P, Stoop D, Ortega-Hrepich C, Devroey P, et al. Corifollitropin alfa followed by rFSH in a GnRH antagonist protocol for poor ovarian responder patients: an observational pilot study. Fertil Steril. 2013;99(2):422-6.
77. Polyzos NP, De Vos M, Corona R, Vloeberghs V, Ortega-Hrepich C, Stoop D, et al. Addition of highly purified HMG after corifollitropin alfa in antagonist-treated poor ovarian responders: a pilot study. Hum Reprod. 2013;28(5):1254-60.
78. Dor J, Seidman DS, Amudal E, Bider D, Levran D, Mashiach S. Adjuvant growth hormone therapy in poor responders to in-vitro fertilization: a prospective randomized placebo-controlled double-blind study. Hum Reprod. 1995;10(1):40-3.
79. Eftekhar M, Aflatoonian A, Mohammadian F, et al. Adjuvant growth hormone therapy in antagonist protocol in poor responders undergoing assisted reproductive technology. Arch Gynecol Obstet. 2013;287(5):1017-21.
80. Pellicer A, Ballester MJ, Serrano MD, et al. Aetiological factors involved in the low response to gonadotrophins in infertile women with normal basal serum follicle stimulating hormone levels. Hum Reprod. 1994;9(5):806-11.
81. Battaglia C, Genazzani AD, Regnani G, et al. Perifollicular Doppler flow and follicular fluid vascular endothelial growth factor concentrations in poor responders. Fertil Steril. 2000;74(4):809-12.
82. Weiner Z, Thaler I, Levron J, et al. Assessment of ovarian and uterine blood flow by transvaginal color Doppler in ovarian-stimulated women: correlation with the number of follicles and steroid hormone levels. Fertil Steril. 1993;59(4):743-9.
83. Bassil S, Wyns C, Toussaint-Demylle D, et al. The relationship between ovarian vascularity and the duration of stimulation in in-vitro fertilization. Hum Reprod. 1997;12(6):1240-5.
84. Nardo LG, Granne I, Stewart J, et al. Medical adjuncts in IVF: evidence for clinical practice. Hum Fertil (Camb). 2009;12(1):1-13.
85. Revelli A1, Dolfin E, Gennarelli G, et al. Low-dose acetylsalicylic acid plus prednisolone as an adjuvant treatment in IVF: a prospective, randomized study. Fertil Steril. 2008;90(5):1685-91.
86. Cobo A, Garrido N, Crespo J, et al. Accumulation of oocytes: a new strategy for managing low-responder patients. Reprod Biomed Online. 2012;24(4):424-32.

CHAPTER 13

Laparoscopic Treatment of Endometriosis Focusing on Fertility Outcomes

K Jayakrishnan

Chapter outline

- Diagnosis of Endometriosis
  - Newer Classifications for Endometriosis
- Treatment
  - Preoperative and Postoperative Ovarian Suppression
  - Surgery
- Deep Infiltrating Endometriosis
- Ovarian Endometrioma and Assisted Reproduction Technique
- General Principles of Management of Endometriosis

INTRODUCTION

Infertility complaints occur in almost 60% of women with endometriosis. Mechanical interference is the most accepted phenomenon, but there is an increasing role attributed to immunological, genetic and hormonal factors, which is still under investigation and certainly contributes to the etiopathogenesis of this enigmatic disease.

Although, the etiopathogenesis of endometriosis and also its causal relationship with infertility remain unclear, the advent of assisted reproduction techniques (ARTs) allowed an important advance on infertility treatment. However, the outcomes of ART in endometriosis remain unsatisfactory, revealing impaired pregnancy and implantation rates in comparison with infertility due to tubal and male factors according to the meta-analysis of Barnhart et al. in 2002 even though other studies do not support this affirmative.

Medical treatment with gonadotropin-releasing hormone (GnRH) agonists prior to ART is associated with an increase in pregnancy rates but clinical therapy alone is considered inefficient for treating endometriosis-associated infertility. Owing to its high rates of recurrence (approximately 50% after 5 years of therapy cessation), we are frequently presented with a dilemma between performing ART or adopting a surgical approach as the first choice to achieve better results when treating infertile couples.

Undoubtedly, the best approach must be individualized to each infertile couple, combining improvement of pregnancy rates, reduction of morbidity and following good practice principles. The evaluation must be undertaken in a global manner and the essential factors to be considered are patient's age, grade and type of endometriosis (ovarian, peritoneal or deep infiltrating) and clinical symptoms of the disease.

Besides this, performing randomized, placebo-controlled studies regarding surgical treatment of endometriosis is difficult, resulting in a lack of evidence or reliable data. The aim of this review is to analyze the laparoscopic surgical procedure for infertility treatment in endometriosis in its different phenotypics presentations: peritoneal, ovarian and deep infiltrating disease.

DIAGNOSIS OF ENDOMETRIOSIS

Even before the patients presented with pain there is a delay in diagnosis of nearly nine years. Earlier diagnosis results in more focused effective care for the patients. This is the most important need for laparoscopy.

For the infertile patient, the important need to perform laparoscopy is the staging of the disease will enable the most appropriate treatment plan. This will ensure maximum pregnancy rates with greatest efficiency, safety and least cost.

Laparoscopy will enable other gynecologic problems such as ovarian cysts, myomas, adhesions tubal damage, hydrosalpinx and other conditions to be diagnosed. Diagnostic laparoscopy has been shown to identify abnormalities that could be treated in 21% of infertility patients undergoing laparoscopy after normal hysterosalpingogram (HSG) before Intrauterine insemination, with endometriosis being the most common abnormality constituting 65% of abnormalities.[1]

The prevalence of peritubal adhesions in infertile patients ranges from 10–23%. It is well recognized that it causes infertility by impairing ovum pick up, and adhesiolysis with mean pregnancy rate of 42% has been reported. For diagnosis of endometriosis visual inspection of pelvis at laparoscopy is the gold standard.[2] Figure 13.1 shows severe endometriosis with the obliteration of pouch of Douglas (POD).

Newer Classifications for Endometriosis

Endometriotic Fertility Index

Today, the most widely used staging system of endometriosis is the revised American

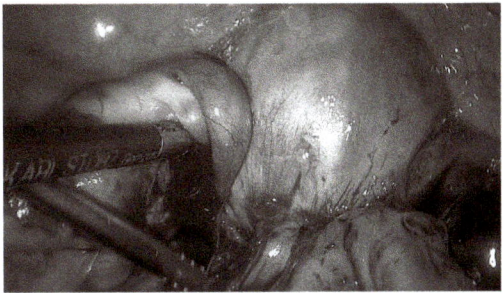

Fig. 13.1: Severe endometriosis with POD obliteration.

Fertility Society classification (r-AFS classification). The r-AFS classification is used to predict the recurrence potential of endometriosis after surgery. However, it has limited predictive ability for pregnancy after surgery. Adamson and Pasta suggested that the r-AFS classification depends mainly on morphological descriptions.[3]

The endometriosis fertility index (EFI), proposed by Adamson and Pasta in 2010, is used to predict fecundity after endometriosis surgery.

The EFI staging system is a 10-point scale system, which considers historical factors, age and length of infertility, and surgical factors, such as the least function score and the AFS score.

In addition to providing a detailed score to the appendix (fallopian tubes, fimbriae of fallopian tubes, ovaries) by calculating the least-function scores, the EFI also combines conception-related factors such as age, duration of infertility, and gravidity history. The EFI contains all of the components of the r-AFS stage score, but the r-AFS score includes only 20% of the EFI score. However, the EFI does not consider whether the patient has received *in vitro* fertilization (IVF) treatment after endometriosis surgery.

This index has been validated as clinically useful among patients with surgically confirmed endometriosis who wish to be pregnant and has been validated externally in populations of infertile patients with

Score	Description		Left	Right
4	= Normal	Fallopian tube		
3	= Mild dysfunction			
2	= Moderate dysfunction	Fimbria		
1	= Severe dysfunction			
0	= Absent or nonfunctional	Ovary		

To calculate the LF score, add together the lowest score for the left side and the lowest score for the right side. If an ovary is absent on one side, the LF score is obtained by doubling the lowest score on the side with the ovary.

Lowest score: [Left] + [Right] = [LF score]

ENDOMETRIOSIS FERTILITY INDEX (EFI)

Historical factors			Surgical factors		
Factor	Description	Points	Factor	Description	Points
Age			LF Score		
	If age is ≤ 35 years	2		If LF Score = 7 to 8 (high score)	3
	If age is 36–39 years	1		If LF Score = 4 to 6 (moderate score)	2
	If age is ≥ 40 years	0		If LF Score = 1 to 3 (low score)	0
Years infertile			AFS Endometriosis Score		
	If years infertile is ≤ 3	2		If AFS Endometriosis Lesion Score is < 16	1
	If years infertile is > 3	0		If AFS Endometriosis Lesion Score is ≥ 16	0
Prior pregnancy			AFS Total Score		
	If there is a history of a prior pregnancy	1		If AFS total score is < 71	1
	If there is no history of prior pregnancy	0		If AFS total score is ≥ 71	0
Total historical factors			**Total surgical factors**		

EFI = TOTAL HISTORICAL FACTORS + TOTAL SURGICAL FACTORS: [Historical] + [Surgical] = [EFI Score]

Fig. 13.2: Endometriosis fertility index (EFI) surgery form. (Least function (LF) score at conclusion of surgery)

endometriosis at 3 years after surgery. The higher the EFI score is, the higher their chances of spontaneous pregnancy are (Fig. 13.2).

TREATMENT

Preoperative and Postoperative Ovarian Suppression

Combined ovarian suppression prior to surgery has theoretical advantages. These include improving treatment success, facilitating surgical procedure, reducing preoperative symptoms, reducing superficial disease, reducing vascularity, reducing endometrioma size, delaying or avoiding surgery. There are potential disadvantages with preoperative therapy which include delay in diagnosis and delay in attempting pregnancy. Postoperative use of ovarian suppression, meta-analysis of published literature shows no benefit. The Cochrane database also shows an odds ratio (OR) of 0.83 for ovarian suppression versus no treatment. As an adjunct to surgery despite potential advantages, no data shows benefit of preoperative or postoperative treatment. Therefore, delay in attempting pregnancy, medication costs, side effects of ovarian suppression thir use is inappropriate for infertility patients.[3]

Surgery

Treatment of minimal/mild endometriosis by laparoscopy is superior to ovarian suppression (P = 0.01). No treatment of minimal or mild disease had similar pregnancy rates to laparoscopic treatment.

Treatment of moderate or severe disease with laparoscopy had higher pregnancy rates than treatment with laparotomy (P = 0.02).

Importantly, monthly fecundity postoperatively was 4.4% in first year, 2.9% in second year and 0.6% in the third year. Patients should be given this amount of time to conceive following surgery.

The ENDOCAN PRCT trial from Canada showed a higher pregnancy rate with surgery (37.5%) versus no treatment (22.5%). The consensus from published studies is that the treatment of minimal/mild endometriosis at time of surgery improves pregnancy rates.[4]

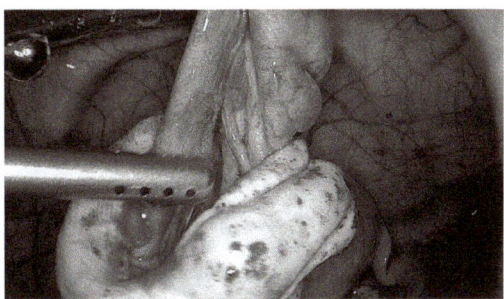

Fig. 13.3: Cystectomy in endometrioma ovary.

Moderate or severe endometriosis is usually associated with moderate or severe anatomic distortion and is associated with low pregnancy rate if untreated. Major pelvic adhesions can impair oocyte release from the ovary or inhibit ovum pick up or transport. Numerous studies have shown the benefit of surgical treatment, but in the absence PRCT it can be recommended that surgery is indicated for invasive, adhesive and cystic endometriosis.[5]

The peritoneal fluid in women with endometriosis contains an ovum capture inhibitor that prevents normal cumulus fimbriae interaction. The high pregnancy rates after surgical treatment of endometriosis suggests the reduction of endometriosis-induced tissue reaction or endometriotic derived products acting locally in the peritoneal cavity.

Laparoscopy results in fewer *de novo* adhesions and has a quick recovery time, it is generally preferred to laparotomy if surgeon has requisite expertise.[6,9]

With endometrioma, laparoscopy (Fig. 13.3) is equivalent to laparotomy with both approaches resulting in approximately 50% pregnancy rate at 2 years following surgery.[10] Pregnancy rates are not affected by size or number of endometriomas, but lower when extensive adhesions are seen in the pelvis.

A recent prospective randomized controlled trial (RCT) study demonstrated higher pregnancy rates, 59% versus 23% and lower operation rates 6% versus 23% in the group with laparoscopic ovarian cystectomy versus fenestration and coagulation.[7]

Reoperation occurs in about 8% of patients and ultrasound recurrence in 12%. It is likely that the recurrence rate of endometriomas is less than 10% with resection of the cyst wall, compared with over 20% with other techniques like drainage, wedge excision and drainage followed by GnRH-a and then repeat surgery.[8] The routine use pharmacologic agents to prevent postoperative adhesions cannot be recommended on basis of evidence.

With complete endometriotic posterior cul-de-sac obliteration the estimated life table pregnancy rates at 2 years are 29.6% for laparoscopic approach and 23.7% for laparotomy which are not different.[8,13]

There are other conditions that will enhance fertility which can be treated at time of diagnostic laparoscopy. These include treatment of myomas that may reduce pregnancy rates, polycystic ovarian disease which can be treated by drilling. Such treatments may increase the pregnancy rates and increase probability of healthy pregnancy and delivery.

Furthermore, it is easy for patients undergoing laparoscopy to have diagnostic hysteroscopy. This will enable accurate assessment of endocervical canal, uterine cavity, cervical stenosis and can be most effectively treated at time of diagnostic laparoscopy. Surgery must aim at restoration of tubo-ovarian relationship (Fig. 13.4).

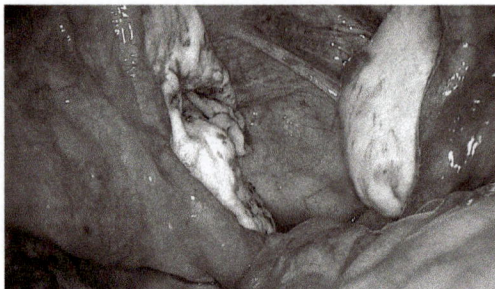

Fig. 13.4: Restoration of tubo-ovarian relationship.

DEEP INFILTRATING ENDOMETRIOSIS

Deep endometriosis of rectovaginal septum represents a separate chapter in this disease. Its characteristics are so unique that it seems inappropriate to consider it together with peritoneal and ovarian forms of the disease.

The differences of deep endometriosis begin in its lesion characteristics, histology and hormonal behavior, and also its clinical parameters, such as severity of the symptoms and therapeutic response. Deep endometriosis, in general, is defined as peritoneal invasion of over 5 mm. Its real incidence is unknown but the estimative is suggested to be one of each five endometriosis patients. In decreasing order, it affects the uterosacral ligaments, rectosigmoid colon, vagina and urinary bladder.

In spite of scores, two to eight times higher for deep endometriosis classified by revised American Society for Reproductive Medicine (ASRM) classification, pelvic pain has poor correlation with this classification. This fact is especially important when analyzing rectovaginal endometriosis, which shows an exuberant clinical presentation. New classification criteria have been proposed for this type of endometriosis.

The Adamyan classification, for example, divides rectovaginal endometriosis into three types:

1. Retrocervical endometriosis (in which the rectum is usually free of disease)
2. Rectovaginal septum
3. Bowel endometriosis (with infiltrative characteristics over the bowel thickness).

This type of classification may be more compatible with the surgical approach of this disease.

The diagnosis of rectovaginal endometriosis is also essentially surgical, but clinical and image examinations must be performed to help plan surgical strategies. At clinical examination, vaginal examination is extremely useful to reveal fibrosis or nodularity in cul-de-sac and uterosacral ligaments.

Regarding image scanning examinations, even transvaginal ultrasound can suggest rectovaginal endometriosis through visualization of a hypoecogenic lesion between rectum and vagina. In fact, it has been given particular importance to transvaginal ultrasound in the detection of rectovaginal septum endometriosis, showing high sensitivity and good correlation with laparoscopic findings. However, it is magnetic resonance imaging (MRI), in association with rectum echoendoscopy, that emerged as the best examination to identify deep endometriosis. When considering bowel endometriosis, the sensitivity is similar (90% vs 83%, respectively); however, in rectovaginal and uterosacral disease, the sensitivity is extremely different (77.7% vs 7.4% and 84.8% vs 45.6%, respectively).

There is a consensus that surgical treatment is the best option for deep endometriosis, due to high incidences of recurrence when clinical treatment is used alone.

Feasibility and advantages of laparoscopy as a surgical route for endometriosis treatment has already been proven. An important aspect may also be considered—deep endometriosis can be missed even during laparoscopy if the surgeon is not warned about it. During inspection of the peritoneal surface, the depth of invasion may not be initially noticed;

therefore, the surgeon must perform a careful palpation of any suspect lesion to check if there is infiltration of this nodule or not. The introduction of rectal and vaginal probes during the surgery also improves the exposition and excision of the lesions.

Regarding fertility outcomes, pregnancy rates after laparoscopic procedure for rectovaginal endometriosis treatment varies from 44.4% to 72%. As a matter of fact, there is no homogeneity among the studies when referring to: classification of superficial versus deep endometriosis, or (ASRM) classification; time of follow-up; if topic or ectopic pregnancy after treatment; and if spontaneous or after ART pregnancy. In spite of these differences among the studies, the pregnancy rates achieved after surgery were at least similar to pregnancy rates shown in ART.

The analysis of a prospective, randomized and placebo-controlled study for laparoscopic treatment of endometriosis, in all grades by ASRM classification, revealed spontaneous pregnancy in 12 out of 39 patients. It also showed a significant improvement of life quality after excisional surgery for grades III and IV of endometriosis in comparison with the control group. However, the relationship between fertility rates after laparoscopy and ASRM classification appears to be unsatisfactory. Chapron et al. evaluated 30 patients submitted to laparoscopy due to deep endometriosis affecting uterosacral ligaments. The spontaneous pregnancy rate was 48.5% 12 months after surgery, with only one pregnancy by IVF. There was no positive correlation between endometriosis ASRM scores and pregnancy rates.

In spite of its low incidence (5.4-12% of all endometriosis patients), bowel endometriosis is the most frequent extragenital site of endometriosis. Thus, this form of the disease must be searched preoperatively in all patients evidencing deep endometriosis approximately 9% of these patients require bowel segmental resection. The main localizations are rectum and rectosigmoid junction, responsible for 93% of all lesions. Several studies have demonstrated feasibility of laparoscopic route also for the treatment of this kind of endometriosis. Radical excision of these lesions can provide an improvement of 91-100% of the bowel endometriosis.

The impact of laparoscopic excision of colorectal endometriosis on fertility outcomes has also been studied. Hysterectomy or oophorectomy are not usually necessary in this surgery. The laparoscopic excision of bowel endometriotic lesions appears to be highly efficient in reducing pelvic pain and also restoring fertility. Darai et al. revealed pregnancy rates of 45.5% after 24 months of follow-up in 22 women who were submitted to laparoscopic resection of bowel endometriosis. Of these 22 women, 10 became pregnant (two twice), nine pregnancies were spontaneous and three occurred after one cycle of IVF. The average time for conception was 8 months after the surgery and the newborn rate was 82%. Redwine and Wright also demonstrated a fertility rate of 43% after *en bloc* resection of complete cul-de-sac obliteration due to endometriosis.[12] Other studies focusing the same goal showed pregnancy achievement in three out of seven and eight out of 15 patients. In this last study, six of these women were already submitted to IVF previously to laparoscopic procedure. Therefore, when bowel resection is necessary, the segmental colorectal resection appears to be the best option, but women must be warned about this type of surgery and mainly about its complications, once rectovaginal fistula occurs in 10% of the cases.

OVARIAN ENDOMETRIOMA AND ASSISTED REPRODUCTION TECHNIQUE

Although, we do not know the specific role of the endometriomas over the reduction of fertility potential, vascular compression is markedly observed in compromised gonads and studies have already demonstrated that 17–44% of the patients with endometriosis-related infertility present ovarian endometriotic cysts.

Therapeutic choice for infertile patients with endometriomas remains a great challenge in the assisted reproduction scenario. Once the limited efficacy of drug therapy is known laparoscopic management may be considered as a complementary approach, with satisfactory long-term fertility results whether for spontaneous pregnancies or ART, in this last one improving transvaginal accessibility and, sometimes, ovarian stimulation response. Regardless of the absence of a definitive conclusion for the ideal therapeutic management, there is a trend to indicate laparoscopy for all infertile patients presenting with endometriomas.

The surgical decision in these cases must be taken cautiously, considering factors that may influence results, such as the patient's age and ovarian reserve markers, previous pelvic surgery, presence of pain or malignancy suspicion, disease extension and the mean diameter of the lesions.

The mean diameter of the endometriotic cyst is an important issue in the decision process. Some authors have already attributed low success rates in ART cycles to large endometriomas. We believe that ART could minimize endometriosis interference over fertility in patients with superficial ovarian lesions or cysts with mean diameter of less than 4 cm and proceed cystectomy for ovarian endometriomas of over 4 cm to possibly improve the gonad response to exogenous stimulation and access to follicles, and to confirm histologically the diagnosis, as previously stated by the European Society for Human Reproduction and Embryology.

Regarding spontaneous pregnancies and recurrence of the cysts and symptoms, Hart et al. systematically reviewed the issue and concluded that laparoscopic cystectomy appears to be the best therapeutic choice if compared with drainage or coagulation. Alborzi et al. prospectively evaluated 52 patients submitted to laparoscopic cystectomy and observed spontaneous pregnancy rates of nearly 60% in the first year after surgery, which were statistically significant when compared with the 23.3% obtained after endometrioma fenestration and coagulation. Beretta et al. had already compared such techniques in 64 patients with endometriomas and shown 24-month cumulative pregnancy rates of 66.7% for exeresis versus 23.5% when the other techniques were performed.

Thus, expectant management after surgery, with the aim of achieving spontaneous pregnancy, appears to be a good choice, especially for those patients under 35 years of age. Littman et al. observed that, in a period of 8 months after endometrioma excision, almost 50% of pregnancies were obtained spontaneously or after ovulation induction with clomiphene citrate in patients previously submitted to ART. However, patients over 35 years old or presenting signs of impaired ovarian function may not be encouraged to decide on expectant management, as they usually present a lower ovarian response. In these cases, ART may be considered as the first-choice treatment, being the laparoscopic procedure dispensable, unless there is no transvaginal access to the ovarian follicles for oocytes pick-up.

Regarding ART results after endometriomas excision, Garcia-Velasco et al. retrospectively evaluated 189 women who had undergone IVF treatment following laparoscopic approach to excise lesions and observed no differences between the groups, whatever variety analyzed. They obtained 25.4% of pregnancies among operated women and 22.7% among patients with intact cysts, with no statistical significance, and concluded that no additional benefits were provided by cystectomy.

Despite the large number of studies over the theme, consequences of endometrioma excision to the remaining ovarian tissue still hinder the surgical therapeutic decision. The possibility of normal ovarian tissue resection during endometriomas excision and occurrence of vascular damage give reason to such a dilemma and, although no answer has been given, some researchers attempt to demystify this theory.

Muzii et al. confirmed that excision provides a complete treatment to the problem and, even if ovarian adjacent tissue is being excised with the cyst, there were morphologic, and supposed physiologic, changes in this adjacent tissue in more than 80% of the 70 endometriomas obtained by laparoscopic cystectomy.[11] This implicates that the permanence of such tissue should not contribute to real ovarian reserve. Even Garcia-Velasco et al. found no difference between the numbers of oocytes retrieved following endometrioma excision, advocating the surgical option.[12] As a matter of fact, controversy was created by Ragni et al. who demonstrated a significantly reduced number of dominant follicles and oocytes among operated gonads after gonadotropic stimulation in 38 patients who were previously submitted to unilateral endometrioma laparoscopic enucleation.

Several studies have already evaluated ovarian function after endometrioma excision and demonstrated that there were no significant differences between normal and cystectomized ovaries, with satisfactory pregnancy rates. Loh et al. demonstrated a 73.3% pregnancy rate in up to 42 months after surgery, a quarter of them submitted to IVF. Similarly, other studies obtained equivalent pregnancy rates, from 30.5–38% per cycle, between women submitted to laparoscopic cystectomy and tubal infertility control group, after induced ovarian cycles.

Nevertheless, individualization of each case is the prerogative for the most adequate approach. Based on the current literature, we believe that, in general terms, laparoscopic exeresis of ovarian endometriomas in infertile patients should be considered a good practice. It is important to consider the couple's opinion after clarifying the pros and cons, stimulating the patient and her partner to participate in the decision considering the distinct possible strategies. Cyst recurrences should also be criteriously evaluated and successive excisions are strongly discouraged owing to their potential risk of diminishing follicles population.

GENERAL PRINCIPLES OF MANAGEMENT OF ENDOMETRIOSIS

The estimated cumulative pregnancy rate by life tables at 2 years following laparoscopic surgery are 60% for minimal/mild disease, 50% for moderate disease, and 40% for severe disease.[13] Following ovarian suppression, the rates at 2 years are 50% for minimal/mild, 40% for moderate disease and 15% for severe disease. Therefore, not only pregnancy rates are higher following surgery but surgery allows treatment of pain, treatment of severe disease before controlled ovarian stimulation for ART.

If the surgery is well performed, it is effective in all stages of endometriosis. Endometriomas, cul-de-sac disease for symptoms of pain or infertility. If the pregnancy does not occur within 9–15 months following surgery, repeat surgery may benefit for infertility in selected patients, and for some benefit for pain. If the patient has not had a technically adequate operation with her first surgery, it is sometimes appropriate to perform the repeat surgery or go directly to IVF. Pre-ART large endometriomas surgery is usually indicated. Clinical and surgical judgment should be used to individualize the decision to operate or not.

Research need to focus on establishing a better understanding of the pathogenesis of this enigmatic disease and complex gynecological disease. More knowledge about the pathogenesis would make earlier diagnosis possible, offer new approaches for treatment, and perhaps limit the indications or extent of the surgical procedures currently performed.

REFERENCES

1. Tanahatoe SJ, Hompes PGA, Lambalk CB. Accuracy of diagnostic laparoscopy in the infertility workup before IUI. Fertil Steril. 2003;79(2):361-6.
2. Sarvelos HG, Li TC, Cooke ID. An analysis of the outcome of microsurgical and laparoscopic adhesiolysis for chronic pelvic pain. Hum Repro. 1995;10:2895-901.
3. Adamson GD, Pasta DJ. Surgical treatment of endometriosis associated infertility: meta-analysis compared with survival analysis. Am J Obste Gynecol. 1994;171:1488-504.
4. Jacobson TZ, Barlow DH, Koninckx PR. Laparoscopic surgery for subfertility associated with endometriosis. Cochrane Database Syst Rev. 2002;(4):1332-4.
5. Suginami H, Yano K. An ovum capture inhibitor in endometriosis peritoneal fluid. Fertil Steril. 1988;50;648-53.
6. Diamond MP, Daniell JF. Adhesion formation and de novo adhesion formation following reproductive pelvic surgery. Fertil Steril. 1987;47:864-6.
7. Aiborzi S, Momtahan M, Parsanezhad. A prospective study comparing laparoscopic ovarian cystectomy versus fenestration and coagulation in patients with endometriosis. Fertil Steril. 2004;82(6):1633-7.
8. Beretta P, Franchi M, Ghezzi F. Randomised clinical trial of two laparoscopic treatments of endometriosis; cystectomy versus drainage and coagulation. Fertil Steril. 1998;70:1176-80.
9. Adamson GD, Pasta DJ. Laparoscopy versus laparotomy for treatment of endometriotic post cul-de-sac obliteration abstracts. Lasers Surg Med Suppl. 1992;4:1-85.
10. The practice committee of American Society for Reproductive Medicine. Endometriosis and Infertility. Fertil Steril. 2006;86:S156-60.
11. Muzii MR. Postoperative administration of monophasic combined oral contraceptives after laparoscopic treatment of ovarian endometriomas. Am J Obstet Gynecol. 2000;183:588-92.
12. Garcia Velasco JA, Mahutte NG. Removal of endometriomas before in vitro fertilization does not improve fertility outcomes; a matched, case control study. Fertil Steril. 2004;81(5):1194-7.
13. Redwine DB, Wright JT. Laparoscopic management of complete obliteration of cul-de-sac associated with endometriosis: long-term follow-up of en bloc resection. Fertil Steril. 2001;76(2):358-65.

CHAPTER 14

Congenital Malformations of Uterus and Reproduction

Pankaj Desai, Sameer Dixit

Chapter outline

- Embryology of the Female Genital Tract
- Genetics of Müllerian Abnormalities
- Techniques to Assess the Female Genital Tract
  - History
  - Clinical Examination
  - Hysterosalpingography
  - Standard Sonography
  - Saline Infusion Sonography
  - Three Dimensional Sonography
  - Laparoscopy
- Congenital Malformations of the Uterus
  - Class I: Agenesis or Hypoplasia—Segmental or Complete
  - Class II: Unicornuate Uterus with or without Rudimentary Horn
- Class III: Didelphys Uterus
- Class IV:-Bicornuate Uterus—Complete or Partial
- Class V: Septate Uterus—Complete or Partial
- Class VI: Arcuate Uterus
- Class VII: DES Related Abnormalities
- Defects not Classified by the AFS
- Management
  - Müllerian Aplasia
  - Creation of Neovagina
  - Fertility Treatment
  - Unicornuate Uterus
  - Uterus Didelphys
  - Bicornuate Uterus
  - Septate Uterus

INTRODUCTION

Developmental abnormalities of the Müllerian system are one of the most fascinating conditions in gynecology. A wide range of abnormalities occur, ranging from mild to severe. Müllerian abnormalities are associated with renal and axial skeletal abnormalities and management also involves investigations and treatment of these conditions.

The earliest reported case of Müllerian abnormality is in 16th century.[1] The actual incidence of the Müllerian abnormalities is unknown. The true incidence may never be known as these are grossly under reported in childhood and over reported in the population undergoing infertility treatment. The incidence varies widely and depends on the type of study. Most authors report an incidence varying from 0.1-3.5%. The most accepted incidence is 4.3% for a general population and fertile women, 3.5% for infertile women and 13% in women with recurrent pregnancy loss.[2] In a study of women undergoing Müllerian assessment at the time of undergoing tubal ligation, an incidence of 3.2% was identified.[3]

The incidence also varies with the type of diagnostic test used. In a study[4] of women undergoing HSG for recurrent pregnancy loss, the incidence was 8-10%. With emergence of more sensitive diagnostic tests, standardized classification and aggressive management, a more realistic incidence of the abnormalities would emerge in future.

EMBRYOLOGY OF THE FEMALE GENITAL TRACT

The reproductive organs of a woman consist of the external genitalia, the Müllerian tubes and the gonads. All three develop from different primordial origins and in close association with the urinary system and the hind gut. In women, the Müllerian system develops over the Wolffian system. The cranial parts of the Wolffian system persist as epoophoron and the caudal parts as the Gartner's duct. The Müllerian system persists and forms the adult fallopian tubes, the uterine corpus, the cervix and part of the vagina.

At 37 weeks after fertilization, the Müllerian ducts appear on either side of the Wolffian duct as invagination of the dorsal celomic epithelium. The site of the origin remains patent as the fimbrial end of the Fallopian tubes. The paired Müllerian tubes grow caudally and medially until they meet together in the midline and become fused together. They then converge on the urogenital septum.

The solid Müllerian tubes undergo simultaneous canalization to form the tubular structures. The cranial parts which remain patent and separate evolve into the Fallopian tubes. The upper fused portions of the tubes form the uterus while the lowermost fused portion forms the cervix. The vagina is formed from both the lower end of the fused Müllerian ducts and the urogenital sinus. The mesenchyme surrounding the Müllerian ducts condenses to form the musculature of the female genital tract.

Congenital abnormalities of the female genital tract occur due to errors in this developmental process.[5] These include:
- Agenesis/Hypoplasia
- Abnormal fusion with urogenital sinus
- Abnormal lateral fusion of the paired Müllerian tubes
- Abnormal resorption of the septum of the fused Müllerian tubes.

Developing kidney and urinary system closely follows Müllerian system. So, their abnormalities are closely associated with abnormalities of Müllerian system. Disruption of developing local mesoderm and somites accounts for some axial skeletal abnormalities. Cardiac and auditory defects are occasionally associated. Ovarian morphogenesis is distinct from Müllerian organogenesis. Hence, in these conditions, the ovarian function and hormonal milieu is normal.

GENETICS OF MÜLLERIAN ABNORMALITIES

The abnormalities occur due to disruption of the morphogenesis. Various factors[6] have been implicated in this. These include:
1. Abnormal intrauterine milieu
2. Teratogens like DES and Thalidomide
3. Genetic factors

Genetic factors involved are complex. They commonly occur sporadically. If familial incidence is detected then it is usually multifactorial. Other modalities of inheritance like autosomal dominant, autosomal recessive and X-linked disorders also exist.[6] Müllerian anomalies may also represent a part of the multiple malformation syndromes.[7]

Associated anomalies are usually seen in cases of Müllerian aplasia (AFS class I). Associated urological anomalies range between 15-40% in these cases and skeletal anomalies (congenital absence or fusion of vertebrae) occur in 12-50% of these cases.[8]

An association between MRKH syndrome and Klippel-Fiel syndrome is reported. This syndrome is characterized by congenital fusion of the cervical vertebrae, a short neck, low posterior hairline and limited range of motion in cervical spine.[9] The MURCS association (Müllerian duct aplasia, Unilateral Renal aplasia, Cervicothoracic Somite dysplasia) is another variant. Infrequently auditory deficits and cardiac defects can be found. The karyotype of the females having Müllerian aplasia is 46 XX.

Müllerian agenesis has been associated with variants of galactose-1-phosphate uridyltransferase (GALT) enzyme. This finding suggests that increased exposure to galactose is responsible for abnormal Müllerian development.[10]

Other theories about genetic disorders include abnormalities in Müllerian Inhibitory Substance (MIS) gene, loss of function mutation in *WNT4* gene and abnormalities of *HOXA9-HOXA13* genes. However, none of these have been consistently associated.

TECHNIQUES TO ASSESS THE FEMALE GENITAL TRACT

History

In case of MRKH syndrome, the patient may present with primary amenorrhea. In cases of a bicornuate uterus, patient may complain of dysmenorrhea. In cases of a vertical vaginal septum, the patient may come with the complaint that a tampon is unable to stop menstrual flow. In case of an obstructive vaginal septum, the patient may complain of dyspareunia.

Clinical Examination

Per speculum examination may reveal vaginal septum or duplication of cervix. Bimanual examination may help in identifying another horn.

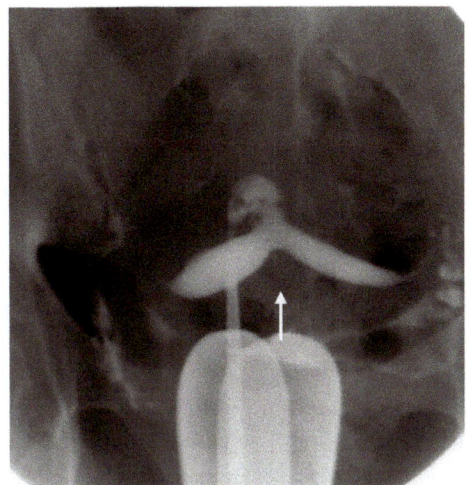

Fig. 14.1: Hysterosalpingographic image of bicornuate uterus.

Hysterosalpingography

This has been the classical tool for diagnosis of the uterine anomalies (Fig. 14.1). When the classic picture of the uterus with two fallopian tubes is seen, Müllerian abnormalities are almost ruled out.

Standard Sonography

In routine sonography, the key structure to be scrutinized is the endometrial cavity. In a normal uterus, the endometrial cavity is single. In a bicornuate uterus, two cavities are appreciated (Fig. 14.2). It must be noted that it is difficult to appreciate two cavities in a longitudinal scan. However, the clinching image is the transverse plane. The two uterine cavities in a cross section are easily identified. A TV sonography gives better diagnosis than the TA sonography. The advantages of sonography are that it is easily available; it is widely acceptable to the patients and is relatively cheap. However, the drawbacks are that the intracavitary lesions are not easily identified, a septum is not appreciated well and it does not depict the external contour of the fundus.

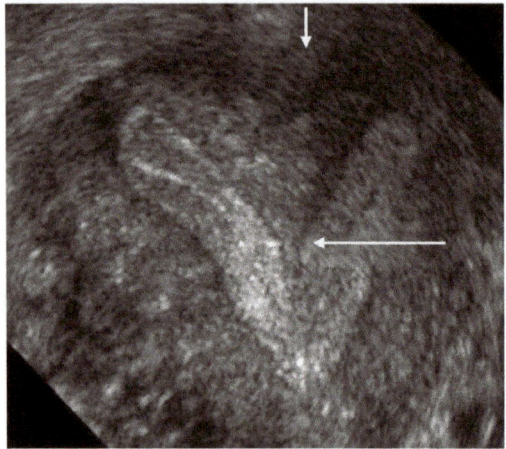

Fig. 14.2: Bicornuate uterus.

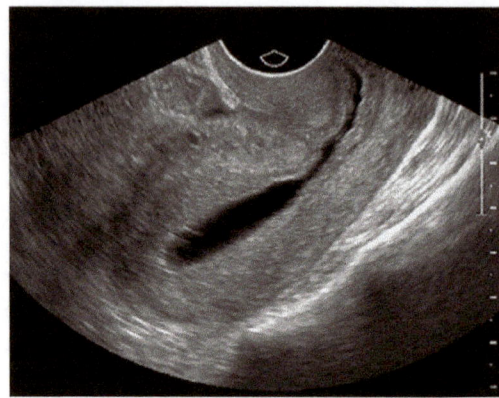

Fig. 14.3: Saline infusion sonography showing uterine cavity.

Saline Infusion Sonography (SIS)

Sline infusion sonography (SIS) combines the ultrasonography (USG) with hysterosalpingography (HSG). A catheter is placed inside the endometrial cavity and saline is instilled to achieve separation of the walls of the endometrial cavity along with continuous transvaginal ultrasound visualization. It is usually performed within first 10 days of the cycle. It is not performed after that period, firstly to avoid aborting an early pregnancy and secondly, the thick secretary endometrium may appear wrinkled to give false positive impression of endometrial pathology.

A balloon catheter like the pediatric Foley's is inserted with tip within the uterine cavity. The balloon is distended with 1 mL of water to prevent backflow of the saline. Slow instillation of 3–10 mL of prewarmed saline is done. Imaging with transvaginal sonography is done to visualize separation of the uterine walls (Fig. 14.3). Once adequate distension is confirmed, a sagittal sweep from cornu to cornu and an axial sweep from fundus to the cervix are done. The balloon is then deflated and fluid allowed to flow out. A second examination with empty uterus is performed. At the end of the examination, free fluid in the pouch of Douglas is looked for. Its presence denotes patency of at least one fallopian tube.

Potential pitfalls include blood clots or mucous plugs (created by shearing effect of the catheter) being mistaken for intrauterine pathology or overdistension of the uterus causing intrauterine pathology to be missed.

Three Dimensional Sonography

Conventional 3D sonography or 3D sonography coupled with saline infusion is better than 2D sonography (Figs. 14.4 to 14.6). It involves rapid acquisition of data volumes which are stored for subsequent analysis. Acquisition of the coronal plane improves diagnosis in almost 30.8% of the patients.[11] This includes better evaluation of the external uterine contour, detection of adhesions and identification of intrauterine pathologies.

Laparoscopy

Laparoscopy allows one to see the fundus of the uterus from outside. The differentiation between the bicornuate uterus and the septate uterus is made by the appearance of the fundus. A septate uterus shows single convex fundus while a bicornuate uterus shows two cornuae.

Congenital Malformations of Uterus and Reproduction

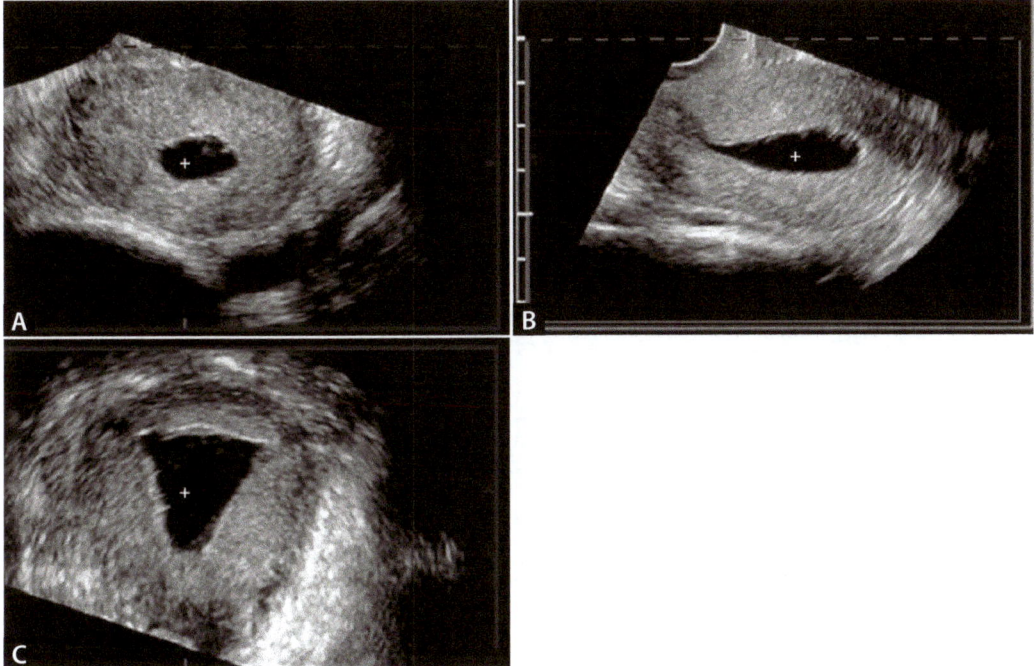

Figs. 14.4A to C: Multiplanar rendering of 3D acquisition showing all three planes.

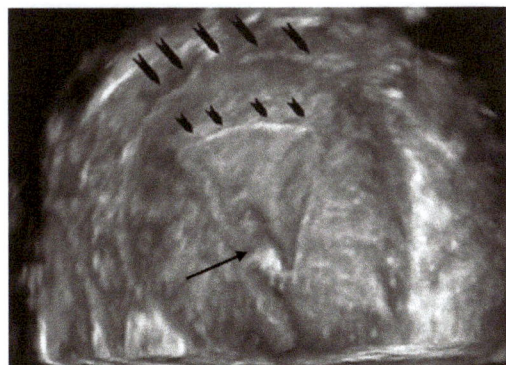

Fig. 14.5: A 3D rendered image. Outer arrows point to the fundus, inner arrows to endometrial cavity and single arrow to the catheter tip.

Figures 14.7 to 14.10 show helical CT image of normal uterus, CT image of bicornuate uterus with horse-shoe kidney, MRI image of bicornuate uterus and hysteroscopic image of subseptate uterus respectively.

ESHRE/ESGE Consensus on Diagnosis of Female Genital Anomalies[21]

Diagnostic methods

1. *Clinical examination*: An essential starting point and essential part of the evaluation. It also offers unique evaluation of vaginal and cervical abnormalities
2. *HSG*: It offers reliable information regarding uterine anatomy in the absence of cervical obstruction. It can also provide information regarding cervical cancer if it is patent. It however, does not provide any information regarding anatomy of vagina. It can not be used for diagnosing obstructive abnormalities. Its efficacy is limited by false positive and false negatives
3. *2D USG*: It is a reliable, objective and measurable tool. It is an essential part of the assessment. However, it is dynamic,

136 *Insights into Infertility Management*

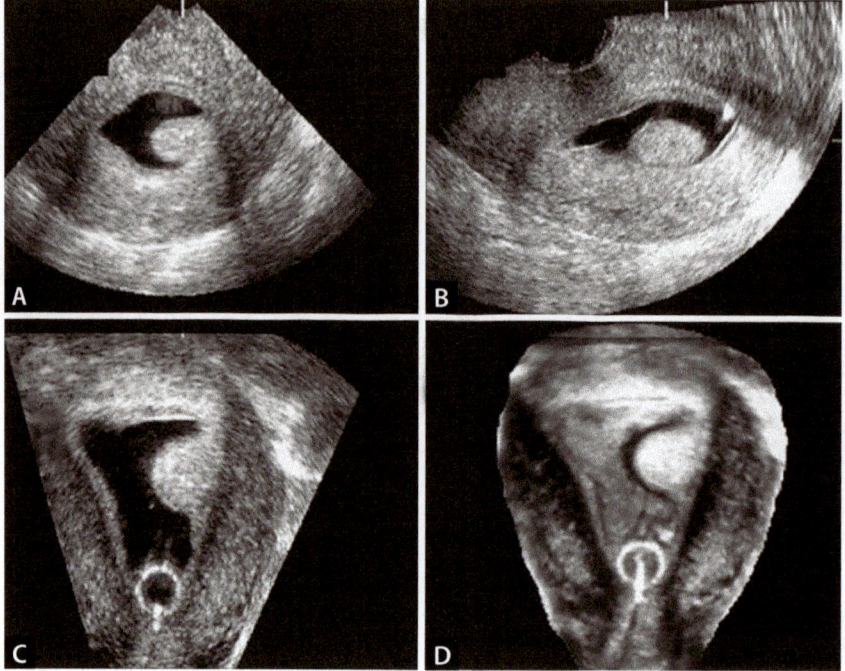

Figs. 14.6A to D: Three-dimensional Sonography.

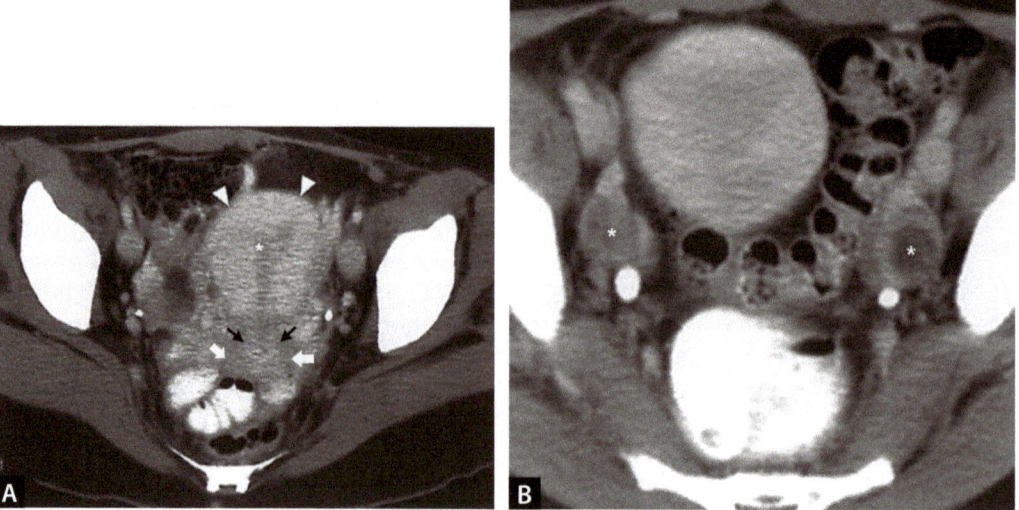

Figs. 14.7A and B: Helical CT images of normal uterus.

Congenital Malformations of Uterus and Reproduction

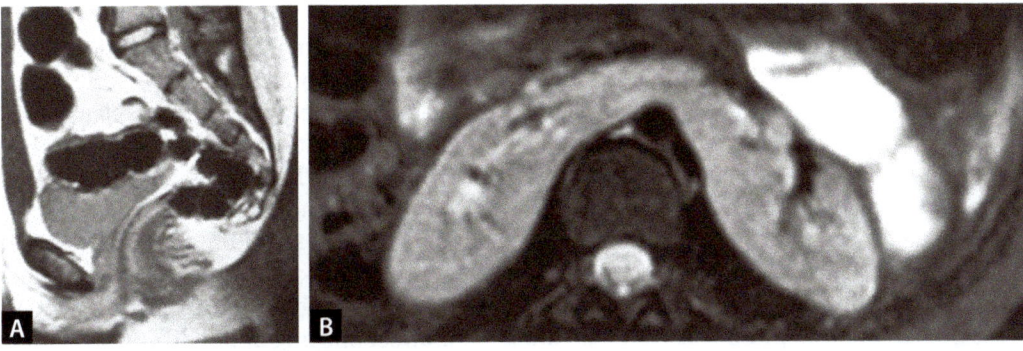

Figs. 14.8A and B: Computed tomography images of bicornuate uterus (A) with horse-shoe kidney (B).

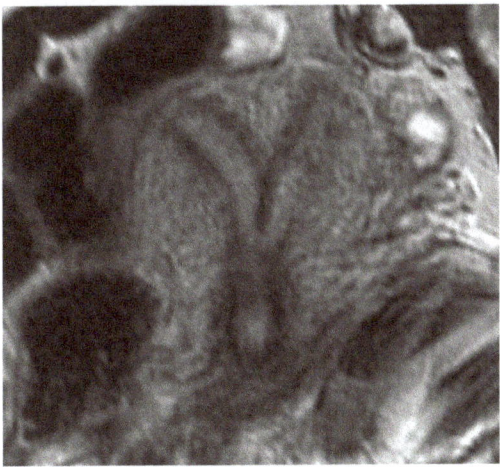

Fig. 14.9: Magnetic resonance image of bicornuate uterus.

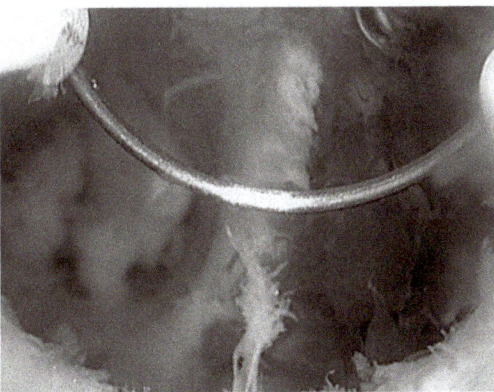

Fig. 14.10: Hysteroscopic image of subseptate uterus.

depends on experience of the clinician. It needs a systematic approach.

4. *Recommendations for proper use of 2D USG*: The endometrial line should always be visible for precise imaging of the uterus. Serial sagittal and transverse scan should be taken extending beyond the margins of the uterus.
5. *Hysterosalpingo contrast sonography*: Early follicular phase is recommended to avoid pregnancy and artefacts due to thick secretary endometrium.
6. *3D USG*: It can provide highly reliable, objective and, most importantly, measurable information for the anatomy of the cervix, uterine cavity, uterine wall, external contour of the uterus and for associated pelvic pathology; the coronal plane of the uterus does provide a clear image of the cavity and the external profile of the uterine fundus. 3D volumes give reliable and objective representation of the examined organs more independently of the examiner overcoming the limitations of obtaining coronal images with 2D sonography. It can provide, also, measurable information even for obstructed parts of the female genital tract.
7. *Recommendations for proper use of 3D USG*: This method should be started with a 2D evaluation of the uterus. Use in mid

cycle or luteal phase is encouraged as this demonstrates the endometrial wall and the outline of the cavity at its best. Contrast medium could be used for the evaluation of the cavity and the tubes; in these cases, the examination has to be performed in the early follicular phase. Save a 3D volume for off-line analysis. The reconstructed coronal plane of the uterus might show the cavity and the external uterine profile as well as the tubal angle and the junctional zone, if possible along all the endometrium and cavity. Acquisition of an isolated cervical volume, without including the uterus: from a mid-sagittal plane, an axial plane of cervix can be obtained in 80% and a coronal plane in 20% of the cases; in cases of uterine malformations, the extent of the cervix and the limits of the cervical canal may be studied better. Diagnosis of associated vaginal anomalies can be done by trans-perineal acquisition of the pelvic floor volume after filling the vagina with gel or saline; an axial plane can be obtained from a mid-sagittal plane.
8. *MRI*: It is noninvasive and it has no radiation. It gives a reliable and objective representation of the examining organs in the sagittal, transverse and coronal plane (three dimensions). It can be used for diagnosis in cases of complex and obstructing anomalies. Electronic storage of the diagnostic procedure is, nowadays, routinely done for re-evaluation.
9. *Hysteroscopy*: It is minimally invasive giving the additional opportunity of treating T-shaped, septate and bicorporeal septate uterus. Its objective includes estimation of the cervical canal and endometrial cavity (differential diagnosis of T-shaped and infantile uterus). It provides a minimal invasive evaluation of the vagina and/or cervix in case of virgo. Electronic storage of the procedure is, nowadays, routinely done for re-evaluation.
10. *Endoscopy, laparoscopy and hysteroscopy*: It provides highly reliable information for the anatomical status of the vagina (vaginoscopic approach), cervical canal, uterine cavity, tubal ostia, external contour of the uterus and the intraperitoneal structures.
11. The invasiveness of the laparoscopic approach makes it not acceptable as a first-line screening procedure; it complements indirect imaging in the diagnosis of more complex anomalies in combination with possible surgical actions. It offers supplementary information about partial or total absence of Fallopian tubes and abnormal localization of ovaries.
12. Highest degrees of overall diagnostic accuracy were in decreasing order: 3D US (97.6%), sonohysterography (SHG; 96.5%), 2D US (86.6) and hysterosalpingography (HSG; 86.9 %). MRI was shown to be able to correctly subclassifiy 85.8% of anomalies. Overall, it appears that 3D US may be more accurate than MRI in subclassifying malformations, although it should be noted that subclassification is hindered due to the subjective nature of the previous classifications adopted.

Uterine wall thickness

1. Uterine wall thickness is an important parameter and a reference point for the definitions of dysmorphic T-shaped, septate and bicorporeal uteri according to the new classification system. The adoption of an objective criterion for the definition of uterine deformity is one of the advantages of the new classification system since according to AFS classification the detection of anomalies was based only on the subjective impression of the clinician performing the test. Although myometrial thickness at the various uterine regions cannot be easily assessed with endoscopic techniques, it can be measured with ultrasound or MRI.

2. *Uterine wall thickness*: This is the distance between the line connecting the tubal ostia and the external uterine profile obtained with 3D US, MRI and, at times, with 2D US.

CONGENITAL MALFORMATIONS OF THE UTERUS

American Fertility Society has classified the malformations (Fig. 14.11, Tables 11.1 and 11.2) as:

Class I: Agenesis or Hypoplasia—Segmental or Complete

Agenesis or hypoplasia may involve the vagina, cervix, fundus, tubes or any combination of these. Mayor-Rokitansky-Kuster-Hauser (MRKH) syndrome is the most well known example of this.

Class II: Unicornuate Uterus with or without Rudimentary Horn

When an associated horn is present, this class is subdivided into communicating (continuity with main uterine cavity documented) or non-communicating. The noncommunicating variety is further subdivided on the basis of whether endometrium is present or absent in the rudimentary horn. The clinical significance of these types is that they are invariably associated with ipsilateral renal and ureteric agenesis.

Noncommunicating accessory horns that have endometrial cavity are the most common unicornuate subtype and are clinically important too. They are associated with high morbidity and mortality. When the accessory horn becomes obstructed, complication like hematometra can occur. There is also a risk of developing endometriosis.

Although normal pregnancies do occur, this type is associated with poorest obstetrical performance. This may be due to diminished uterine vasculature of deficient uterine musculature. A study[12] of 393 pregnancies revealed 54.2% had normal deliveries, 43.3% had preterm deliveries, 4.3% had ectopic pregnancies and 34.4% had spontaneous abortions. About 2% pregnancies occur in accessory horn. Hence, the noncommunicating horn should be excised prior to pregnancy.

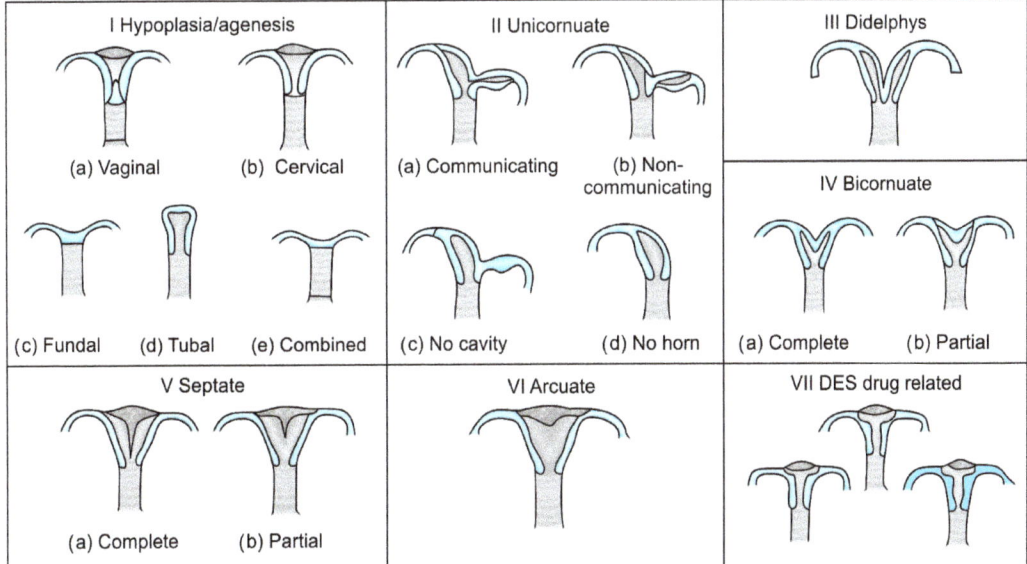

Fig. 14.11: ASRM classification of Müllerian anomalies.

Class III: Didelphys Uterus

Complete or partial duplication of vagina, cervix and uterus is a feature of this type.

About 11% of all uterine abnormalities are of this type. Complete type is characterized by two hemiuteri, two endocervical canals, with cervices fused at the lower uterine segment. Each hemiuterus is associated with a fallopian tube. Ovarian malposition may also be present. The vagina may be single or double; more commonly double (75%). Occasionally, the vaginal septum may be transverse.

This type is associated with renal abnormalities in 20% of the cases. A syndrome called is Wunderlich-Herlyn-Werner syndrome has been described.[13] This consists of obstructed unilateral vagina with uterus Didelphys with ipsilateral ureteric and renal agenesis.

Class IV: Bicornuate Uterus—Complete or Partial

Complete bicornuate uterus is characterized by a uterine septum that extends from the fundus to the cervical os. Partial type has a septum which is limited to the fundus. In both, there is a single cervix and vagina. Obstetric outcome depends on the length of the muscular septum, i.e. whether the bicornuate uterus is complete or partial. A partial bicornuate uterus has a 28% incidence of spontaneous abortion while in case of a complete bicornuate uterus; the incidence of abortion is 66%.

Class V: Septate Uterus—Complete or Partial

A single uterus has a complete or partial septum. The septum is located in the midline

Table 14.1: Classification of congenital malformations of the uterus.

	External contour	Uterine cavity	Separation of horns	Cervix
Normal	Convex, flat or, 1 cm fundal cleft	Convex or flat (Two corneal ostia)	Single triangular cavity	Single
Unicornuate	Convex or flat	Convex or flat (single corneal ostium)	Single banana shaped cavity	Single
Didelphys	Two well-formed uterine cornu, convex or flat	Two well-formed uterine cornu with convex fundal contour in each with no communication	Two horns widely divergent, at an obtuse angle	Double
Bicornuate	Fundal cleft >1 cm	Two well-formed symmetric uterine cornu with convex fundal contour in each fused caudally, communicate	Two horns widely divergent, at an obtuse angle	Single or Double
Septate	Convex, flat or <1 cm fundal cleft	Two well-formed symmetric uterine cornu, communicate	Two horns close, acute angle at the center	Single
Subseptate	Convex, flat or <1 cm fundal cleft	Two well-formed symmetric uterine cornu, communicate	Two horns close, acute angle at the center	Single
Arcuate	Convex, flat or <1 cm fundal cleft	Single cavity with a broad shallow indentation	Obtuse angle at the center	Single

fundal region. It is made up of poorly vascularized fibromuscular tissue. There are various variations of the septum. Sometimes a complete septate uterus is associated with a septate vagina. A variant septate abnormality exists which is characterized by the triad of complete septate uterus, duplicated cervix and septate vagina.[14] It is undistinguishable from uterus Didelphys except by doing laparoscopy or a 3D USG. On laparoscopy, it is identified by its convex external contour.

A rare variant of septate uterus is Robert uterus.[15] This is characterized by a complete septum and a noncommunicating hemiuteri with a blind horn.

Patients with a septate uterus have no difficulty in conceiving. Yet, they have poorest reproductive outcome of all the Müllerian anomalies.

Class VI: Arcuate Uterus

A small septate indentation is seen at the fundus.

Class VII: DES Related Abnormalities

A "T" shaped uterine cavity is seen.

Defects Not Classified by the AFS

- Transverse vaginal septum
- Vaginal atresia

Table 14.2: ESHRE/ESGE classification: Female genital tract anomalies.

ESHRE/ESGE classification
Female genital tract anomalies

	Uterine anomaly			Cervical/vaginal anomaly
Main class		**Sub-class**		**Co-existent class**
U0	Normal uterus		C0	Normal cervix
U1	Dysmorphic uterus	a. T-shaped b. Infants c. Others	C1	Septate cervix
			C2	Double 'normal' cervix
U2	Septate uterus	a. Partial b. Complete	C3	Unilateral cervical aplasia
			C4	Cervical aplasia
U3	Bicorporeal uterus	a. Partial b. Complete c. Bicorporeal septate	V0	Normal vagina
			V1	Longitudinal non-obstructing vaginal septum
U4	Hemi-uterus	a. With rudimentary cavity (communicating or not horn) b. Without rudimentary cavity (horn without cavity/no horn)	V2	Longitudinal obstructing vaginal septum
			V3	Transverse vaginal septum and/or imperforate hymen
U5	Aplastic	a. With rudimentary cavity (bi- or unilateral horn) b. Without rudimentary cavity (bi-or unilateral remnants/aplasia)	V4	Vaginal aplasia
U6	Unclassified malformations			

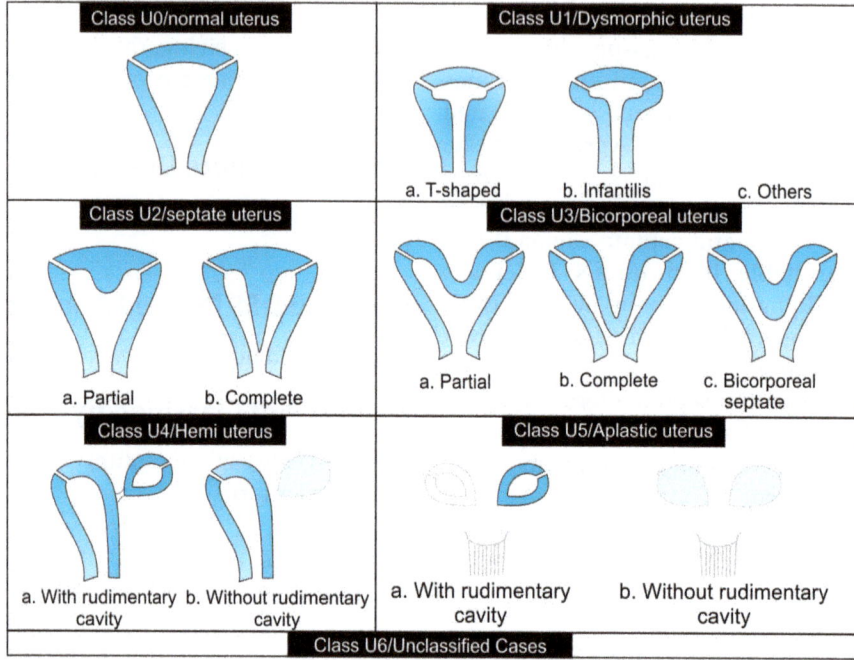

Fig. 14.12: ESHRE/ESGE classification of uterine anomalies: schematic representation (Class U2: internal indentation > 50% of the uterine wall thickness and external contour straight or with indentation <50%, Class U3: external indentation >50% of the uterine wall thickness. Class U3b: width of the fundal indentation at the midline >150% of the uterine wall thickness).

The ESHRE/ESGE Classification

It was believed that the existing AFS classification had limitations.[20] There was need to have a classification that was: Clear and accurate which correlated with patient management was simple and friendly.

MANAGEMENT

Müllerian Aplasia

This basically includes management of vaginal agenesis or MRKH syndrome. Here, the management comprises of two parts:
1. Creation of neovagina
2. Fertility treatment

Creation of Neovagina

Two methods have been described, nonsurgical and surgical. The nonsurgical method basically involves use of prosthetic moulds which deepen the existing pouch to create a satisfactory space for coitus. While surgical methods involve creation of neovagina, the strategy is to develop a space between the rectum and the bladder. Various tissues have been used to cover the newly created space. Full thickness or part thickness skin grafting is the most popular technique. However, skin grafting is associated with scar formation or contractures. Alternately, human amnion, not stripped from chorion is used as a graft material.[16]

More elaborate plastic surgical techniques include use of transposition flaps and autologous buccal mucosa. Use of artificial dermis and absorbable adhesion barrier shows promise as exogenous graft material to be used in neovagina. Interceed (Ethicon) has been used as an absorbable adhesion barrier. The neovagina epithelializes within 1 to 4 months.

Some surgeons use a bowel segment in place of skin graft. However, this is associated with troublesome leucorrhea after the surgery.

Fertility Treatment

Since, most of these women have healthy and functioning ovaries; surrogate pregnancy is a viable treatment modality.

Unicornuate Uterus

The indication for surgery is presence of endometrium in the rudimentary horn. In case the rudimentary horn does not have a functioning endometrium, then surgical intervention is not indicated.

In case surgery is contemplated, laparoscopic hemihysterectomy of the rudimentary horn is the procedure of choice. The rudimentary horn is connected to the functioning unicornuate uterus by a fibromuscular band. This band is of importance as the uterine artery courses inferior to it. The pedicle of the rudimentary horn is coagulated using bipolar cautery. Tube and the rudimentary horn are removed, leaving ipsilateral ovary which is usually healthy, *in situ*.

In the event of pregnancy in the rudimentary horn, same procedure as nonpregnant uterus is followed. However, there is a risk of increased bleeding due to pregnancy related vascularization. Methotrexate has been used to treat the pregnancy before surgical removal of the rudimentary horn.

Hysteroscopic endometrial ablation of the rudimentary horn has been reported.[17]

Uterus Didelphys

Guidelines for surgical intervention are as follows:
1. *Uterus didelphys with obstructive vaginal septum*: Full excision and marsupialization of the vaginal septum is the treatment of choice. After the septum is excised, laparoscopy may be indicated as these cases are associated with endometriosis.
2. *Uterus didelphys with nonobstructive vaginal septum*: surgery is indicated if the patient complains of dyspareunia.
3. Currently, metroplasty is not indicated in cases of nonobstructive didelphys uterus.

Bicornuate Uterus

Guidelines for surgical correction are as follows:
1. Bicornuate uterus seldom requires surgical management.[18]
2. Metroplasty should be reserved for those women with repeated pregnancy losses or rarely in those in whom no other cause for infertility is detected.

Septate Uterus

Uterine septum is associated with primary infertility, recurrent miscarriages and preterm labor. In such cases, hysteroscopic resection of the septum is indicated.[19] The decision to operate should be taken only for poor reproductive performance.

ESHRE/ESGE Consensus on workup of Female Genital Anomalies[21]

Recommended evaluation of asymptomatic women:
Clinicians should, always, be attentive for the presence of a congenital anomaly in asymptomatic women of reproductive age during their routine examination, supplementing gynecological examination with a 2D US as follows:
- *Gynecological examination*: The anatomy of the external genitalia, the vagina and the cervix should be carefully evaluated.
- *2D US*: It should be done in a predefined and systematic manner to increase its diagnostic accuracy. The shape and the dimensions of the uterine cavity, the

uterine wall (anterior, posterior, lateral and fundal width) and external uterine contour should be recorded in a systematic way in longitudinal and transverse planes.
- The absence of findings suspicious for the presence of an anomaly should not be considered as definite and the presence of one could not be excluded.
- Positive findings should be used for documentation only and counselling of the patients for further investigation given that they are asymptomatic women.

Recommended evaluation of symptomatic women
- Gynecological examination with careful evaluation and recording of the external genitalia, vaginal and cervical anatomy.
- 2D US (vaginal) in a predefined and systematic manner (to increase its diagnostic accuracy), where the shape and the dimensions of the uterine cavity, the uterine wall (anterior, posterior, lateral and fundal width) and external uterine contour should be recorded in a systematic way and predefined way in longitudinal and transverse planes. Measurements of 2D US examination should be used as a referendum for the evaluation of uterine anatomy deviations in 3D ultrasound.
- 3D US (vaginal) in a predefined and systematic manner where the shape and the deviations from normal cervical and uterine anatomy should be recorded and documented.

REFERENCES

1. Steinmetz GP. Formation of artificial vagina. West J Surg. 1940;48:169-73.
2. Grimbizis GF, Camus M, Tarlatzis BC, et al. Clinical implications of uterine malformations and hysteroscopic treatment result. Hum Reprod Update. 2001;7:161-74.
3. Frank R. The formation of an artificial vagina without operation. Am J Obstet Gynecol. 1938; 35:1053-5.
4. Stray-Pederson B, Stray-Pederson S. Etiologic factors and subsequent reproductive performance in 195 couples with a prior history of habitual abortion. Am J Obstet Gynecol. 1984;148:140-6.
5. Amesse LS, Pfaff-Amesse T. Congenital anomalies of the reproductive tract. Clinical Reproductive Medicine and Surgery. New York: Elsiever. 2000; pp. 235-9.
6. Golan A, Langer R, Bukovsky I, et al. Congenital anomalies of Müllerian system. Fertil Steril. 1989; 5:747-55.
7. Carson SA, Simpson JL, Elias S, et al. Heritable aspects of uterine anomalies. Fertil Steril. 1983;1:86-90.
8. Turunen A, Unnerus CE. Spinal changes in patients with congenital aplasia of the vagina. Acta Obstet Gynecol Scand. 1967;1:99-106.
9. Willemsen WN. Combination of Mayer-Rokitansky-Kuster and Klippel Fiel syndrome-a case report and literature review. Eur J Obstet Gynecol Reprod Biol. 1982;4: 229-35.
10. Aughton DJ. Müllerian duct abnormalities and galactosemia heterozygosity: report of a family. Clin Dysmorphol. 1993;1:55-61.
11. Erdem M, Bilgin U, Bozkurt N, et al. Comparison of transvaginal sonography and saline infusion sonohysterography in evaluating the endometrial cavity in pre and postmenopausal patients with abnormal uterine bleeding. Menopause. 2007;14: 846-52.
12. Lin P. Reproductive outcomes in women with uterine anomalies. J Womens Health (Larchmt). 2004;1:33-9.
13. Tridenti G, Bruni V, Ghirardini G. Double uterus with blind hemivagina and ipsilateral renal agenesis: clinical variants in three adolescent women. Case report and literature review. Adolesc Pediatric Gynecol. 1995;8:20.
14. Giraldo JL, Habana A, Duleba AJ, et al. Septate Uterus associated with cervical duplication and vaginal septum. J Am Assoc Gynecol Laparosc. 2000;2:277-9.
15. Robert HG. Uterus cloisonne avec cavite borgne sans hematometeri. CR Soc Fr Gynecol. 1989;767-7.
16. Nisolle M, Donnez J. Vaginoplasty using amniotic membranes in cases of vaginal

agenesis or after vaginectomy. J Gynecol Surg. 1992;1:25-30.
17. Hucke J, DeBruyne F, Campo RL, et al. Hysteroscopic treatment of congenital uterine malformations causing hemihematometra: a report of three cases. Fertil Steril. 58:823-57.
18. Jones HW. Reconstruction of congenital uterovaginal anomalies. Female Reproductive Surgery. Baltimore: Lippincott Williams and Wilkins 1992, 246.
19. Valdes C, Malini S, Malinak LR. Ultrasound evaluation of female genital tract abnormalities. Am J Obstet Gynecol. 1984;149:285-92.
20. Grimbizis GF, Gordts S, Di Spiezio Sardo A, et al. The ESHRE-ESGE consensus on the classification of female genital tract congenital anomalies. Gynecological Surgery. 2013;10(3):199-212.
21. Grimbizis GF, Di Spiezio Sardo A, Saravelos SH, et al. The Thessaloniki ESHRE/ESGE consensus on diagnosis of female genital anomalies. Gynecological Surgery. 2016;13(1):1-16.

CHAPTER 15

Medical Management of Fibroids

K Jayakrishnan, Niranjana Jayakrishnan

Chapter outline

- Oral Contraceptive Pills
- Tranexamic Acid
- Medical Management
  - Progesterone Receptor Agonists and Modulators
- Ulipristal Acetate
- Telapristone
  - Progestogen-releasing Intrauterine System
- Gonadotropin-releasing Hormone Agonist
  - Practice Guidelines: Ulipristal versus GnRHa
- Gonadotropin-releasing Hormone Antagonist
  - Promising GnRH Antagonist (Elagolix)
  - Somatostatin Analogs
- Aromatase Inhibitors
- Selective Estrogen Receptor Modulator
  - Raloxifene and Tamoxifen
  - Potential of Novel Therapies Enabled by Smart Nanocarriers
  - Halofuginone

Uterine leiomyomas are the most common gynecological tumors and are present in 30% of women in the reproductive age group. Treatment of leiomyomas must be individualized, based on symptoms, size and rate of growth of the uterus, and the woman's desire for fertility. The majority of uterine leiomyomas are asymptomatic and will not require therapy.

Medical management should be tailored to the needs of the woman presenting with uterine fibroids (UF) and geared to alleviating the symptoms. Cost and side effects of medical therapies may limit their long-term use (SOGC 111-C). The drugs used for the management of fibroids are enlisted in Table 15.1.

ORAL CONTRACEPTIVE PILLS

The influence of oral contraceptive pills (OCP) on myomata is poorly understood and data on its effect on the size of myomata are conflicting.

Mechanism of action: By inhibiting ovulation, both OCPs and pregnancy may have a protective effect against the recurrence of fibroids after myomectomy.

Review of literature: OCP appear to improve short-term menstrual irregularities through their effects on the endometrium but they do not reduce the size of myomata. In a meta-analysis, the authors reported a 17% reduction in morbidity among women who had used OCP for 5 years or more.

Side effects: Early side effects of oral contraceptives (OCs) include bloating, nausea, and breast tenderness. Although they may be bothersome enough to lead to discontinuation of the OC, these side effects usually subside in several months. Abnormal bleeding is

Medical Management of Fibroids

Table 15.1: Drugs used for management of fibroids medically.

Treatment	Contraceptic effect	Effect on pain	Effect on bleeding	Fibroid volume	Special consideration
NSAID	• No • Fertility preserved	Helpful	Reduction shown in HMB	Not evaluated	• Gastric irritation • Patients with asthma • Start at onset of bleeding • Mefenamic acid is the only NSAID with a licence for HMB but other NSAIDs may have a class effect
Tranexamic acid	• No • Fertility preserved	No effect	Reduction shown in HMB	Not evaluated	• Maximum daily dose of 4 g best given as 1 g four times daily • Start at onset of bleeding and use for up to 4 days • Available over the counter • Thromboembolic events are rare
LNG-IUS	Yes, reversed on removal	Usually helpful	Significant reduction but may take 6 months	No conclusive evidence	• Not contraindicated in nulliparous women • Clinicians who fit intrauterine devices should be appropriately trained and attend regular updates to maintain their competence • Progestogenic side effects tend to be minimal and usually settle after 6 months
CHC	Yes, reversed on stopping	Usually helpful	Reduction shown in HMB Helped by extended use (tricycling or continuous)	Not evaluated	• Commonly used in clinical practice, although oestradiol valerate/dienogest combination is only product licensed in women with HMB, with evidence of 88% reduction in menstrual blood loss • Assess risk of ATE and VTE • Refer to UKMEC
High-dose oral progestogen	No, but not recommended if trying to conceive	Usually helpful	Reduction shown in HMB if used on days 5–26 of each cycle (15 mg norethisterone or 20–30 mg/day medroxyprogesterone acetate)	Not evaluated	• Progestogenic side effects significant and limit long-term continuation • May be helpful at menopause • Avoid norethisterone if BMI >30 kg/m^2 due to risk of VTE • Use in luteal phase only (i.e. day 19–26) is not effective

Contd...

Contd...

Treatment	Contraceptive effect	Effect on pain	Effect on bleeding	Fibroid volume	Special consideration
High-dose injected progestogen	Yes, and will take up to a year before fertility returns after last injection	Usually helpful	Reduction, with high incidence of amenorrhea with continuous use	Not evaluated	• Variable weight gain • Caution in women with high risk of osteoporosis or cardiovascular disease due to hypoestrogenic effects
Ulipristal acetate (5 mg)	No. Additional non-hormonal contraception required in women at risk of pregnancy	Yes, effective within first cycle	Rapid reduction in bleeding, with many achieving amenorrhea within 7–10 days	Significant reduction of 36–42% by 3 months	• Licensed for women with fibroids suitable for surgery to relieve symptoms • 3-month course can be repeated once; second 3-month course is licensed • Benefit on fibroid volume when stopping may persist for 3–6 months
GnRH analogs	No. Additional non-hormonal contraception required in all women at risk of pregnancy	Yes, gradual reduction	Gradual reduction up to 30 days to achieve amenorrhea	Significant reduction of 53% by 3 months	• Specialist initiated; for shared care, see local guidelines • Menopausal symptoms usual • Consider add-back HRT (continuous combined or tibolone) if young • (<45 years), high osteoporotic risk, or intractable menopausal symptoms develop • Limited use because of osteoporosis risk

ATE: arterial thromboembolism; CHC: combined hormonal contraception; GnRH: gonadotropin-releasing hormone; HMB: heavy menstrual bleeding; HRT: hormone replacement therapy; LNG-IUS: levonorgestrel intrauterine system; NSAID: non-steroidal anti-inflammatory drug; VTE: venous thromboembolism. See: www.guidelines.co.uk/wpg.uterine_fibroids_2014

a common problem that often resolves. Weight gain is not a consistent finding with low-dose pills.

TRANEXAMIC ACID

Mechanism of action: This antifibrinolytic lysine derivative reduces the amount of bleeding by preventing fibrin degradation.

Dosage: The dose is usually 1–1.5 g 4 times daily; however, patients are advised to use tranexamic acid (TA) sporadically only during acute episodes of heavy bleeding.

Review of literature: FDA-approved for treatment of menorrhagia in 2009, TA decreases menstrual bleeding within 2–3 hours of administration. Low-quality evidence suggests that the drug reduces intraoperative blood loss during myomectomy.

Side effects: Include dizziness, gastrointestinal symptoms, and possible intralesional thrombosis leading to necrosis.

Long-term disadvantages: Although the evidence for risk of thromboembolic event with TA is controversial, caution should be exercised with its use in combination with hormonal treatment such as OCP.

MEDICAL MANAGEMENT

All medications currently available for fibroid treatment including gonadotropin-releasing hormone (GnRH)-agonist and sex steroids are unsuitable for long-term use because of their significant side effects. In recent years, new medications have been introduced that offer the promise of practical, long-term, medical therapy for symptomatic fibroids. To date, the most encouraging results in terms of fibroid volume reduction, symptom relief, and compliance with long-term administration have been obtained with mifepristone, a progesterone receptor antagonist, and asoprisnil, a selective progesterone receptor modulator.

Progesterone Receptor Agonists and Modulators

Mifepristone

Mechanism of action: Mifepristone has been the first available active antiprogestin. It has been shown to decrease fibroid size and blood flow to the fibroids

Dosage: Early studies of women with symptomatic fibroids reported that daily administration of mifepristone at doses ranging from 5 to 50 mg for 3 to 6 months resulted in a 26–74% reduction in fibroid volume and a decrease in the prevalence and severity of fibroid-related symptoms, including menorrhagia, dysmenorrhea and pelvic pressure (Steinauer et al., 2004).

Review of literature: More recently, in a randomized, double-blinded, placebo-controlled trial including 42 women with symptomatic fibroids, treatment with mifepristone 5 mg per day for 26 weeks led to a 47% reduction in fibroid size and a significant improvement in fibroid-related symptoms (Fiscella et al., 2006). By 12 months, 9 (41%) of 22 women randomized to mifepristone had become amenorrheic (Fiscella et al., 2006). The drug was well tolerated, and no endometrial hyperplasia was noted in any participant (Fiscella et al., 2006).

Side effects: High incidence (28%) of endometrial hyperplasia was observed in patients screened with endometrial biopsies (Steinauer et al., 2004).

Long-term benefits: Although these data are very encouraging, further studies in larger samples with longer periods of treatment are needed to reliably assess the long-term safety and efficacy of this drug.

Asoprisnil

Another promising medication for fibroid treatment is asoprisnil, a selective progesterone receptor modulator (SPRM) with mixed agonist/antagonist activity.

Mechanism of action: This drug has been shown to inhibit proliferation and induce apoptosis in uterine fibroid cells. In addition, it has an inhibitory effect on the endometrium as a result of suppressed endometrial angiogenesis and/or function of the spiral arteries (Chwalisz et al., 2004).

Dosage: Small observational studies of women with symptomatic fibroids showed that daily treatment with asoprisnil at doses ranging from 5 mg to 25 mg for 3 months reduced fibroid volume in a dose-dependent manner and suppressed both abnormal and normal uterine bleeding, with no effects on circulating estrogen levels and no breakthrough bleeding (Chwalisz et al., 2005).

Review of literature: In a recent randomized, double-blind, placebo-controlled trial involving 129 women, a 3-month treatment with asoprisnil doses of 5, 10 and 25 mg daily suppressed uterine bleeding in 28, 64 and

83% of women, respectively, and reduced fibroid volume and fibroid-related pressure symptoms (Chwalisz et al., 2007).

Side effects: Asoprisnil treatment was associated with follicular-phase estrogen concentration and minimal hypoestrogenic symptoms (Chwalisz et al., 2007).

Long-term benefits: These promising findings warrant replication through larger controlled trials over extended treatment intervals.

ULIPRISTAL ACETATE

The newest SPRM that has both agonist and antagonist selective tissue effect is ulipristal acetate.

Mechanism of action: Induces apoptosis by suppressing neovascularization and cell proliferation without proliferating healthy uterine tissue.

Dosage: At a daily dose of 5–10 mg, ulipristal acetate-induced amenorrhea in 50–70% of women in 10 days, and resulted in suppression of uterine bleeding in all patients at the end of a 13-week course.

Review of literature: A comparison of monthly injection of leuprolide acetate (3.75 mg) and daily administration 5–10 mg ulipristal for 3 months by Donnez et al. found that both drugs had the same effect on myomata. Myomata maintained a size reduction 6 months after discontinuation of ulipristal, eliminating the need for further surgical interventions.

If treatment for more than 3 months is anticipated, a patient must wait for two menstrual periods before restarting ulipristal. In the first study of long-term medical management with ulipristal, four 3-month courses led to a significant reduction in fibroid volume in 80% of cases. The volume of the largest fibroid was decreased by 72%.

Side effects: Headache, nausea, abdominal pain, dizziness, fatigue, dysmenorrhea, acne, menstrual irregularity, functional ovarian cysts, and hot flushes.

Long-term usage: Clinicians detecting endometrial thickening in women treated with UA need to be aware that administration of UA for longer than 3 months may lead to endometrial thickening. This is related to cystic glandular dilation, not endometrial hyperplasia. However, in absence of robust safety data for a period longer than 3 months or on repeat courses of treatment, treatment duration should not exceed 3 months. Clinicians should be aware of the need to investigate, as per usual clinical practice, persistence of endometrial thickening following treatment discontinuation and return of menstruation to exclude any underlying pathological conditions.

TELAPRISTONE

Mostly has progesterone antagonist activity and low antiglucocorticoid activity. It was specifically developed for use as an antiprogestin in the treatment of uterine fibroids and endometriosis. It has been shown to reduce fibroid size by up to 40% and significantly decreases vaginal bleeding. While one study reported that telapristone-induced apoptosis in fibroid cells another studies did not confirm this fact.

The US Food and Drug Administration (FDA) placed a full clinical hold on telapristone in August, 2009 because of elevated liver enzymes associated with drug treatment.

Progestogen-releasing Intrauterine System

The levonorgestrel-releasing intracauterine system (LNG-IUS) was introduced as a contraceptive device, but it was recognized as an effective treatment for non-organic abnormal uterine bleeding (AUB), decreasing its intensity and improving anemia. Its use for treating UF-related bleeding, therefore, was soon investigated. A prospective study comparing the efficacy of the LNG-IUS in improving AUB in two groups of women, with and without fibroids, has demonstrated an 86% decrease in bleeding intensity in both groups. After 4 years, there was a 99.5% decrease in both groups and also a reduction in uterine volume in the group with fibroids.

Another study, an randomized-control trial (RCT) comparing LNG-IUS with a low-dose combined oral contraceptive (COC) in women with fibroids, demonstrated that the former was more effective in reducing UF-related bleeding than the latter, although the trial suffered with high attrition rates and assessed uterine bleeding in only 22 patients. In the LNG-IUS group, there was a significant decrease in menstrual blood loss and uterine volume, while hematocrit increased. Both studies excluded women with submucous fibroids that caused distortion of the uterine cavity. Therefore, LNG-IUS is probably an effective option in selected symptomatic women with no endometrial distortion.

GONADOTROPIN-RELEASING HORMONE AGONIST

Mechanism of action: GnRHa works by desensitizing GnRH pituitary receptors. As a result, it is associated with an initial flare effect followed by a hypoestrogenic state after 2 weeks. It has been used to treat uterine myomas for more than 3 decades. The most common GnRHa used for uterine myoma is leuprolide acetate.

Dosage: Intramuscular injection of 3.75 mg monthly—or a single dose of 11.25 mg every 3 months—reduces the mean uterine volume by 36% at 12 weeks and 45% at 24 weeks. However, the effects are temporary.

Review of literature: GnRHa is useful for premenopausal women who opt for medical treatment and for preoperative treatment. It reduces the size of myomata, facilitating surgery with a minimally invasive technique and improving the patient's hematologic status. However, it may lead to degeneration of myomata, making them soft and difficult to manipulate. Occasionally, the cleavage plane between a myoma and the pseudocapsule obliterates, making myoma enucleation challenging. Whether obliteration of the surgical plane is related to the presence of adenomyosis is not entirely clear.

Side effects: GnRHa adverse effects, such as menopausal symptoms, are related to the hypoestrogenic state. When given alone, it is associated with up to 5.5% reduction in bone mass within the first 6 months of use. Due to its adverse effects, GnRHa use should be limited to 3-6 months. In order to counter adverse effects and to maintain patient compliance, add-back treatment with low-dose estrogen and progestin therapy is advisable

Practice Guidelines: Ulipristal versus GnRHa

In women with excessive uterine bleeding, the authors use ulipristal acetate 5 mg daily for 3 months. It is associated with a rapid decrease in uterine bleeding. During the first few days of treatment, when the bleeding is still excessive, supportive treatment with tranexamic acid can be given. A second course of ulipristal is administered after two menstrual cycles.

Alternatively, a single course of GnRHa for 3 months can be given. However, it may be associated with increased uterine bleeding in the first week of treatment due to initial stimulation of the endometrium. Because of GnRHa's pronounced menopausal adverse effects, add-back treatment should be considered.

Ulipristal or GnRHa can be given for 3 months preoperatively to reduce fibroid volume before myomectomy by laparoscopy or laparotomy.

For patients undergoing hysteroscopic myomectomy, the authors use GnRHa preoperatively a month before the procedure. It produces a thin endometrium, which facilitates the procedure and decreases fluid absorption. Ulipristal is associated with endometrial changes but not thin endometrium.

Side effects: Adverse effects are similar to those of GnRHa and disappear after drug discontinuation, with rapid return to the original leiomyoma size. Release of histamine by mast cells is a known adverse effect. Recent preparations are associated with less histamine release and thus better tolerated.

Long-term-benefits: Long-term therapeutic efficacy is yet to be determined.

GONADOTROPIN-RELEASING HORMONE ANTAGONIST

Mechanism of action: GnRH antagonists exert their action through the direct competitive inhibition of GnRH by occupying the pituitary GnRH receptors and therefore, blocking the access of the endogenous GnRH and exogenously administered agonists to their receptor sites. These agents may induce a deep suppression of gonadotropins and the sex steroids, while avoiding any "flare up" phenomena, which may lead to a reduction in uterine fibroids size of up to 50%. The compound has been used preoperatively to decrease myomata size before surgery. The drawbacks are absence of a long-acting preparation and cost. Daily administration may decrease patient compliance.

Review of literature: Some of the GnRH antagonists approved for clinical use by the US FDA include cetrorelix (Cetrotide; Serono) and ganirelix (Antagon; Organon International). These agents are usually used as injectables. One of the major limitations to the wide use of the GnRH antagonists in leiomyoma treatment is the short half-life of these agents and the non-availability of the Depot formulation, thus require repetitive dosing (daily for most of the antagonists).

Promising GnRH Antagonist (Elagolix)

Elagolix is a second-generation new nonpeptide (GnRH) antagonist, highly potent antagonist orally active and rapidly bioavailable after administration that is being developed by Abbott Laboratories (Abbott) in collaboration with Neurocrine Biosciences. It is finalizing the Phase III for endometriosis and finalizing Phase II for uterine leiomyoma with opportunity to be its first and only approved oral treatment for uterine leiomyoma.

This promising compound inhibits GnRH receptors in the pituitary gland leading to a dose-dependent suppression of luteirizing hormone (LH), follicle stimulating hormone (FSH), and estradiol. Consequently, suppression of E2 is more prolonged at higher doses. Pituitary suppression is maintained for only a portion of the day, and baseline gonadotropin levels return by 24 hours.

To date, Elagolix has been studied in 18 clinical trials totaling more than 1,000 subjects.

Dosage: Elagolix seems to be well tolerated for multiple doses up to 200; rapidly absorbed after oral administration, with median time of maximum plasma concentration values ranging from 0.5 h to 1 h.

The therapeutic window of E2 levels for suppression of endometriosis is attainable at a dose of 100–150 mg/day with serum estradiol remained between 20 pg/mL and 50 pg/mL. The Elagolix therapeutic dose for management of uterine fibroid is yet to be determined.

Somatostatin Analogs

Increasing evidence has demonstrated a role for growth factors, such as insulin growth factor I (IGF-I) and IGF-II, in the initiation and progression of uterine fibroids. Leiomyoma tissue expresses higher levels of IGF-I/IGF-II receptors compared to normal adjacent myometrium. Additionally, these tissues secrete their own IGF-1, probably for autocrine and paracrine use. From a clinical perspective, it has been recently reported that patients with high levels of growth hormone (acromegalic patients) have a higher prevalence of uterine fibroids than the general population.

Lanreotide, which is a long-acting somatostatin analog that has been shown to reduce growth hormone secretion, has also recently been evaluated in seven women with uterine fibroids in Italy. Interestingly, lanreotide induced a 42% mean myoma volume reduction within a 3-month period. These results show that somatostatin analogs may potentially be a new therapy for uterine fibroids.

The treatment with somatostatin analogs for diseases other than leiomyoma appears to be safe and is usually well tolerated with some reports of gallstone formation. However, the lacking of clinical trials which test the long-term use of somatostatin analogs along with the severe and adverse health implications such as decreased life expectancy due to accelerated heart disease observed in adults with growth hormone deficiency may hinder its future use for leiomyoma treatment.

AROMATASE INHIBITORS

Aromatase inhibitors (AI) work by directly blocking the conversion of androgen to estrogen, leading to a decrease in circulating estrogen levels without causing systemic adverse effects.

Letrozole: This drug is associated with a reduction in fibroid size, thinning of endometrium and cessation of bleeding. Mild side effects of hot flashes, vaginal dryness and musculoskeletal pain are reported. The LEAP (letrozole, exemestane, and anastrozole pharmacodynamics) trial was a phase I pharmacodynamic study comparing the effects of aromatase inhibitors on safety parameters such as serum markers of bone formation and resorption, in healthy postmenopausal women with normal bone mineral density. The results demonstrated that all three inhibitors administered for 24 weeks caused incremental increases in bone resorption markers such as C-telopeptide cross-links.

Anastrozole: This third-generation nonsteroidal medication does not alter cortisol or aldosterone levels. It is also not associated with androgenic, progestogenic, or estrogenic effects. At a dose of 1 mg/day for 12 weeks, anastrozole results in reduction in myoma volume of up to 32% and improves menstrual symptoms.

Fadrozole: Shozu et al. reported a case of rapid regression of myoma symptoms and a 71% reduction in their size after the use of fadrozole for 8 weeks. Today, there is still a paucity of information of the use of fadrozole for uterine myomata.

SELECTIVE ESTROGEN RECEPTOR MODULATOR

Selective estrozen receptor modulators (SERMs), like estrogen, are agents that elicit tissue-specific responses by intensely interacting with two kinds of estrogen receptors (ERs), ERα and ERβ, inhomogenenously distributed throughout the body. SERMs have complex pharmacokinetics properties due to their vaguely understood physicochemical properties and low solubility in blood (1–200 ng/mL). In addition to analytical detection limitations at such low concentrations, several of the compounds have sufficiently long half lives that impede protocol development. Since SERMs are not administered to humans intravenously, the exact bioavailability of any of these drugs has not been evaluated properly. Frequently, differences in SERM activity depend upon the target gene promoter, as well as the background of a desired cell or tissue.

The SERMs are characterized by their diverse range of agonist/antagonist actions on ER-mediated processes. SERMs belong to several different chemical classes such as benzopyran, benzothiophenes, chromane, indoles, naphthalenes, and triphenylethylenes compounds, all of which are not steroidal compounds. Many are available for clinical usage including raloxifene and tamoxifen discussed below. Novel SERMs are currently being tested in clinical trials such as LY353381 (arzoxifene), EM-652 and CP 336,156 and their structures are very similar to known SERMs.

Raloxifene and Tamoxifen

Two of the best characterized SERMs are tamoxifen and raloxifene, which are both considered to act predominantly as estrogen antagonists, blocking the effects of estrogens.

Raloxifene is a more complete uterine antagonist than tamoxifen, significantly reducing fibroid size in postmenopausal women yet is less efficacious at reducing tumor volume in premenopausal women. Clinical outcomes in premenopausal women treated with raloxifene suggest that this compound, like tamoxifen, can affect the ovaries via the hypothalamic-pituitary-ovarian (HPO) axis. Tamoxifen is associated with insidious side effects, such as thromboembolic events, vasomotor symptoms and an increased risk of developing endometrial cancer and cataracts.

Nonhormonal Agents

Vitamin D, green tea, heparin and its nonanticoagulant analogs, pioglitazone, and pirfenidone have been used to treat myomata. However, their clinical efficacy has not been proven in randomized trials.

Gestrinone

This synthetic steroid is commonly used in endometriosis and suppresses the growth of myomata by regulating the activity of multiple genes without inducing apoptosis. This drug is not available in India.

Cabergoline

Small studies reported a reduction in myomata size with cabergoline, a dopamine agonist used to treat hyperprolactinemia.

Potential of Novel Therapies Enabled by Smart Nanocarriers

The development of nanocarriers designed to deliver and protect drug therapeutics (e.g. anti-fibrotic, aromatase inhibitors, progestins, etc.) is an emerging field. Advances in guided-ultrasound technology (e.g. human *in vitro* fertilization where oocytes as small as 3–5 mm are manipulated) make it feasible to envision utilizing nanocarriers to create a drug depot inside the fibroid by local injection. Thus, skilled physicians could inject the therapy into the uterine fibroid under guided-ultrasound in an outpatient setting. This approach would impede diffusion and distribution of the drug away from the injected fibroid, prolong release, delay inactivation, and therefore reduce the need for repeat injections. Examples of the most promising thermoresponsive delivery systems are given below:

Atrigel®

Atrigel® comprises a water-insoluble biodegradable polymer. A drug is added, forming a solution or suspension. Leuprolide acetate was incorporated into Atrigel®. Clinical studies demonstrated a 22.5 mg leuprolide depot maintained an effective suppression of serum testosterone (50 ng/dL) for more than 3 months.

ReGel®

ReGel® is a ~4,000 Da triblock copolymer formed from PLGA and polyethylene glycol

(PEG) (PEG, 1000 Da or 1450 Da) in repetitions of PLGA-PEG-PLGA or PEG-PLGA-PEG. ReGel® is formulated as a 23 wt% copolymer solution in aqueous media. A drug is added to the solution and upon temperature elevation to 37°C the whole system gels. Degradation of ReGel® to final products of lactic acid, glycolic acid and PEG occurs over 1-6 weeks depending on copolymer molar composition. Chemically distinct drugs like porcine growth hormone and glucagon-like peptide-1 (GLP-1) may be incorporated, one at a time, and released from ReGel®.

LiquoGel™

Works by independent drug delivery routes—entrapment and covalent linkage: This later feature distinguishes LiquoGel from other thermoresponsive injectables, as in theory, two or more drugs can be delivered to the tumor site. *LiquoGel* is a tetrameric copolymer of thermogelling N-isopropylacrylamide; biodegrading macromer of poly(lactic acid) and 2-hydroxyethyl methacrylate; hydrophilic acrylic acid (to maintain solubility of decomposition products); and multifunctional hyperbranched polyglycerol to covalently attach drugs. *LiquoGel* is formulated as a 16.9 wt% copolymer solution in aqueous media. The solution gels at physiological conditions and degrades to release drug contents within 1-6 days.

Antifibrotics

Fibroids are characterized by altered collagen fibrils, fibrosis and tissue stiffness, as well as increased amounts of type I and V collagen.

Selective elimination of collagen producing cells or reducing their state of activation is currently limited to experimental trials. Medical strategies that interfere with collagen formation (e.g. antifibrotic drugs) should be efficacious in fibroid treatment.

A high throughput screening assay has been developed to identify drug candidates that show antifibrotic activity.

Two promising antifibrotic candidates are highlighted below, but in general this class of pharmaceuticals presents undesirable side effects when systemically administered.

Pirfenidone

Pirfenidone is an orally bioavailable antifibrotic agent that has been shown to regulate fibrosis. Pirfenidone inhibits fibroblast proliferation, diminishes the messenger ribonucteic acid (RNA) levels of collagen types I and III in a dose dependent manner, and effectively inhibits myometrial and fibroid cell proliferation *in vitro*. The drug is currently in phase III clinical trials for the treatment of pulmonary fibrosis.

Oral administration of pirfenidone in clinical trials is associated with undesirable side effects including vomiting, fever, abnormality of hepatic function, dizziness, facial paralysis, hepatoma, and skin photosensitivity.

Halofuginone

As an extract from hydrangeas, halofuginone is a small organic molecule exhibiting coccidiostat benefits in birds and more recently anti-fibrotic activity against fibroid cells. Halofuginone inhibits both fibroid and myometrial smooth muscle cell proliferation by rapidly inhibiting deoxyribonucleic acid (DNA) synthesis and later inducing apoptosis. In addition, halofuginone significantly suppressed TGFβI mRNA production.

At 3.5 mg/day, nausea, vomiting, and fatigue were reported. Several patients experienced bleeding complications on treatment with halofuginone in which a causal relationship could not be excluded. This medication is not currently used in humans and its toxicity is unknown.

Reported side effects of halofuginone when taken in patients with advanced solid tumors were nausea, vomiting and fatigue.

Purified Collagenase

Collagenase *Clostridium histolyticum* is an FDA approved drug targeting Dupuytren's contracture in adults with a palpable cord. This drug comprises a fixed-ratio mixture of two classes of purified collagenases; clostridial type I and type II collagenase. Both are metalloproteinases requiring zinc and calcium for full activity and have selective activity against collagen. These two classes of enzymes are not immunologically cross-reactive and differ from each other in domain structure substrate affinity and catalytic efficiency. When combined, they demonstrate synergistic collagenolytic activity.

In vivo, clostridial histolyticum collagenase is not effective in degrading type IV collagen. Thus in clinical studies, purified clostridial histolyticum collagenase did not degrade large blood vessel membranes or nerves.

The dose used for treatment of a Dupuytren's contracted joint is 0.58 mg per direct injection into the cord. Up to three injections may be given per affected joint. This drug is approved by FDA for the treatment of Dupuytren's contracture of the adult hand with a palpable cord present and has not yet been used in clinical trials for fibroids.

CONCLUSION

Thirty percent of women have uterine fibroids and the majority of them will not require intervention. For those women who present with symptoms, the menu of options for the treatment of uterine leiomyomas is expanding. These technologies are relatively new and although many are promising, they often lack long-term data, which interferes with our ability to present all risks and benefits with assurance. Ongoing research and data collection will help us assess the relative merit of newer options as the technology continues to expand.

BIBLIOGRAPHY

1. Chwalisz K, Demanno D, Garg R, et al. Therapeutic potential for the selective progesterone receptor modulator asoprisnil in the treatment of leiomyomata. Semin Reprod Med. 2004;22(2):113-9.
2. Chwalisz K, Larsen L, Mattia-Goldberg C, et al. A randomized, controlled trial of asoprisnil, a novel selective progesterone receptor modulator, in women with uterine leiomyomata. Fertil Steril. 2007;87(6):1399-412.
3. Donnez J, Tatarchuk TF, Bouchard P, et al; PEARL I Study Group. Ulipristal acetate versus placebo for fibroid treatment before surgery. N Engl J Med. 2012;366(5):409-20.
4. Donnez J, Vázquez F, Tomaszewski J, et al; PEARL III and PEARL III Extension Study Group. Long-term treatment of uterine fibroids with ulipristal acetate. Fertil Steril. 2014;101(6):1565-73.e1-18.
5. Fedele L, Bianchi S, Marchini M, et al. Histological impact of medical therapy-clinical implications. J Obstet Gynaecol. 1995;102 (Suppl 12):8-11.
6. Fiscella, K, Eisinger, Meldrum S, et al. Effect of mifepristone for symptomatic leiomyomata on quality of life and uterine size: a randomized controlled trial. Obstet Gynecol. 2006;108(6):1381-7.
7. Friedman AJ, Hoffman DI, Comite F, et al. Treatment of leiomyomata uteri with leuprolide acetate depot: a double-blind, placebo-controlled, multicenter study. The Leuprolide Study Group. Obstet Gynecol. 1991;77(5):720-5.
8. Grudzien MM, Low P, Mamming PC, et al. The antifibrotic drug halofuginone inhibits proliferation and collagen production by human leiomyoma and myometrial smooth muscle cells. Fertil Steril. 2010;93(4):1290-98.
9. Hilário SG, Bozzini N, Borsari R, et al. Action of aromatase inhibitor for treatment of uterine leiomyoma in perimenopausal patients. Fertil Steril. 2009;91(1):240-3.
10. Koechling W, Hjortkjaer R, Tankó LB. Degarelix, a novel GnRH antagonist, causes minimal histamine release compared with cetrorelix, abarelix and ganirelix in an ex

vivo model of human skin samples. Br J Clin Pharmacol. 2010;70(4):580587.
11. Kongnyuy EJ, Wiysonge CS. Interventions to reduce haemorrhage during myomectomy for fibroids. Cochrane Database Syst Rev. 2009:CD005355.
12. Luo X, Yin, P, Coon V JS, et al. The selective progesterone receptor modulator CDB4124 inhibits proliferation and induces apoptosis in uterine leiomyoma cells. Fertil Steril. 2010;93(8):2668-73.
13. Machado RB, de Souza IM, Beltrame A, et al. The levonorgestrel-releasing intrauterine system: its effect on the number of hysterectomies performed in perimenopausal women with uterine fibroids. Gynecol Endocrinol. 2013;29(5):492-5.
14. Macias-Barragan J, et al. The multifaceted role of pirfenidone and its novel targets. Fibrogenesis Tissue Repair. 2010;3(1):16.
15. Qin J, Yang T, Kong F, et al. Oral contraceptive use and uterine leiomyoma risk: a meta-analysis based on cohort and case-control studies. Arch Gynecol Obstet. 2013;288(1):139-48.
16. Rackow BW, Arici A. Options for medical treatment of myomas. Obstet Gynecol Clin North Am. 2006;33(1):97-113.
17. Shen Q, Hua Y, Jiang W, et al. Effects of mifepristone on uterine leiomyoma in premenopausal women: a meta-analysis. Fertil Steril. 2013;100(6):1722-6.e110.
18. Shozu M, Murakami K, Segawa T, et al. Successful treatment of a symptomatic uterine leiomyoma in a perimenopausal woman with a nonsteroidal aromatase inhibitor. Fertil Steril. 2003;79(3):628-31.
19. Spitz IM. Mifepristone: where do we come from and where are we going?: Clinical development over a quarter of a century. Contraception. 2010;82(5):442-52.
20. Steinauer J, Pritts EA, Jackson R, et al. Systematic review of mifepristone for the treatment of uterine leiomyomata. Obstet Gynecol. 2004;103(6):1331-36.
21. Tantibhedhyangkul JA, Behera M. Non-surgical treatment options for symptomatic uterine leiomyomas. Current Women's Health Reviews. 2010;6(2): 146-60.
22. Taylor DK, Leppert PC. Treatment for uterine fibroids: Searching for effective drug therapies. Drug Discov Today Their strateg. 2012; 9(1):e41-e49.
23. Wikland M, Evers H, Jacobsson, et al. A randomized controlled study comparing pain experience between a newly designed needle with a thin tip and a standard needle for oocyte aspiration. Hum Reprod. 2011;26(6):1377-83.

CHAPTER 16

Current Treatment Options and Emerging Strategies for Fibroid Management

K Jayakrishnan

Chapter outline

- Pharmacologic Treatment Options
- Hysterectomy
- Myomectomy
- Myolysis and Cryomyolysis
- MRI-guided Focused Ultrasound Surgery
- Fibroid Treatment via Uterine Artery Occlusion or Embolization
- Uterine Artery Embolization
- Laparoscopic Uterine Artery Occlusion
- Doppler-guided Uterine Artery Occlusion
- Proposed Mechanism of Action of Uterine Artery Occlusion and Embolization

INTRODUCTION

Although most uterine fibroids (leiomyomas) are asymptomatic and remain undiagnosed, these common benign tumors may cause significant gynecologic morbidity, particularly in premenopausal women.[1] Uterine fibroids may lead to abdominal pain, menorrhagia and metrorrhagia that may be associated with dysmenorrhea, reduced fertility, and increased risk for preterm labor and delivery and for cesarean delivery.[2-6]

Clearly, symptomatic uterine fibroids place a significant burden to individuals and society in terms of morbidity, medical resource utilization, and economic costs.[7-11] Recent advances in the development of minimally-invasive fibroid treatments may improve fibroid management by positively impacting patient care and reducing costs. However, a number of efficacy endpoints are used to determine the effectiveness of uterine fibroid treatment, such as reduction of fibroid size, reduction of bleeding, and quality of life (QOL) questionnaires (fibroid-related or generic),[12] and not all studies consistently report the same efficacy endpoint. Therefore, it is difficult to compare the effectiveness of the various treatment options available.

PHARMACOLOGIC TREATMENT OPTIONS

Oral contraceptives and progestins have been used to control uterine bleeding, but there is little evidence demonstrating their effectiveness in reducing the size of uterine fibroids.[13] Pharmacologic options that have some evidence of efficacy in the management of symptomatic uterine fibroids include the progesterone receptor antagonist mifepristone, the selective progesterone receptor modulator (SPRM) asoprisnil, and gonadotropin-releasing hormone (GnRH) agonists/antagonists. Small scale randomized studies showed that low-dose mifepristone reduced amenorrhea, improved anemia, and reduced uterine size, without causing endometrial hyperplasia.[14-16] A randomized placebo-controlled trial in women with evidence of uterine fibroids indicated that 24 weeks of treatment with the GnRH agonist leuprolide acetate depot was safe and caused significant, albeit temporary, reductions in uterine size and fibroid-related presenting symptoms, most prominently menorrhagia, but also bloating, pelvic pressure, and urinary frequency.[17] Long-term use of GnRH agonists is associated with loss of mineral bone. To prevent osteoporosis, estrogen/progestogen add-back therapy is used; however, the combination is not considered to be cost effective. Small studies using GnRH antagonists demonstrated rapid reduction in fibroid size, which may be explained by the lack of a flare-up of gonadotropin secretion. Treatment of leiomyoma with GnRH antagonists, by daily injections or by depot injections, resulted in shrinkage of the leiomyoma by 30–50% within 4 to 8 weeks.[18,19] Gonadotropin-releasing hormone analogs may have applications in reducing the size of uterine fibroids particularly to facilitate myomectomy or relieve compression of neighboring organs.[20]

Asoprisnil is the first SPRM to reach advanced clinical trials. The exact mechanism by which asoprisnil reduces uterine fibroid volume remains to be elucidated, but appears to involve a reduction in uterine blood flow,[21] possibly by cell-type specific inhibition of growth factor expression and activity in leiomyoma cells.[22] In a recently reported randomized, placebo-controlled trial in women with uterine fibroids, 12 weeks of asoprisnil treatment appeared to be well tolerated and significantly reduced fibroid volume, bloating, and pelvic pressure.[23] The most common adverse events associated with asoprisnil treatment were headache, abdominal pain, asthenia, pharyngitis, nausea, infection, enlarged abdomen, sinusitis, and flu syndrome. A few patients also developed asymptomatic ovarian cysts. In addition, the use of asoprisnil was associated with unique morphological changes and decreased levels of cell proliferation in fibroids.[24] Results of additional studies are forthcoming.

HYSTERECTOMY

As discussed above, uterine fibroids are the most common diagnosis associated with hysterectomy, which is performed approximately 600,000 times each year in the United States and 42,500 times each year in the United Kingdom.[7,8] Hysterectomy is the definitive treatment for women with symptomatic uterine fibroids because it removes all the fibroids without posing a risk of recurrence. This surgical procedure is usually associated with a high level of patient satisfaction. Beyond the obvious loss of fertility, other disadvantages of hysterectomy include the fact that it is a major surgery that requires prolonged recovery time and carries a risk of complications such as hemorrhage, bowel or bladder injury, infection, pain, or even death. Hysterectomy rates may be declining in favor of other less invasive procedures according to an analysis of data collected from 1997 to 2003 regarding patient members of Kaiser Permanente Northern California who had undergone hysterectomy, myomectomy, or UAE.[25] More definitive studies in different populations are needed to determine whether this is a widespread phenomenon.

MYOMECTOMY

Myomectomy via laparotomy, hysteroscopy, or laparoscopy is the surgical option of choice for the removal of uterine fibroids in symptomatic women who wish to preserve their fertility or otherwise desire to keep their uterus (Figs. 16.1 to 16.3).[13] However, these procedures should only be performed by surgeons

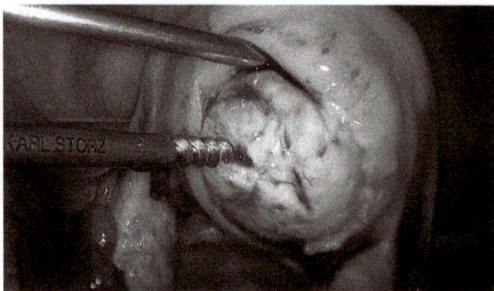

Fig. 16.1: Myoma being enucleated with myoma screw and suction irrigation cannula.

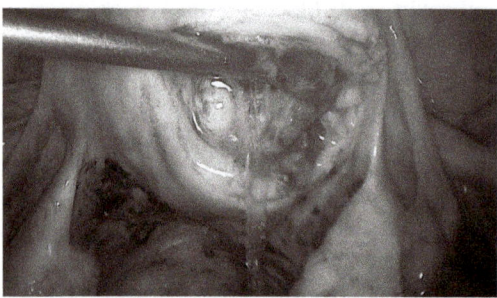

Fig. 16.2: Myoma bed after enucleation.

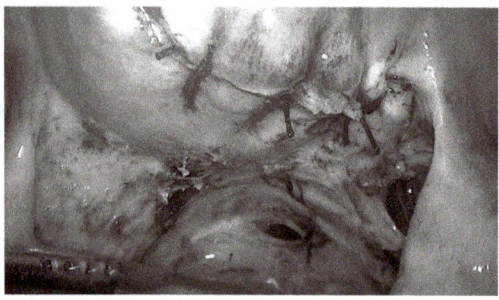

Fig. 16.3: Suturing with interrupted stitches.

with advanced training. Compared with myomectomy via laparotomy, laparoscopic myomectomy is associated with shorter hospital stays and quicker recovery time.[13] Key considerations for determining whether to proceed via laparotomy or laparoscopy are the number, location, and size of fibroids, as well as surgical considerations such as pelvic pathology and contraindications against laparoscopy, such as cardiovascular or pulmonary dysfunction.[13]

Myomectomy via both laparoscopy and laparotomy carries a significant risk of recurrence, possibly necessitating hysterectomy. Most studies reported 20% to 30% recurrence rates, but there is wide variability depending on factors such as study design, recurrence definitions, diagnostic methodology, length of observation, and patient selection.[13] For example, a study that used transvaginal ultrasonography to monitor fibroid recurrence in 149 patients who underwent myomectomy by laparotomy reported a 62% rate of fibroid recurrence and 9% rate of major surgery in 5 years with a lower risk of recurrence in women with solitary myomectomy and smaller preoperative uterine size.[26] In a case series study, Doridot and colleagues[27] reported fibroid recurrence in 45 (22.9%) of 196 women who underwent a laparoscopic myomectomy; the cumulative recurrence risk was 12.7% at 2 years and 16.7% at 5 years. These authors noted that the presence of more than one fibroid and nulliparity were risk factors for recurrence. Other potential complications of myomectomy include blood loss, infection, development of adhesions, and uterine rupture at a subsequent pregnancy.

Laparoscopic myomectomy poses a risk of necessitating conversion to laparotomy because of technical difficulties. Dubuisson and colleagues[28] observed four preoperative factors that were independent risk factors for conversion: size of largest fibroid 50 mm or more by abdominal and transvaginal ultrasonography, preoperative treatment with GnRH agonists, and intramural or anterior location of the main myoma.

MYOLYSIS AND CRYOMYOLYSIS

Myolysis, which uses laser energy or bipolar electrodes to cause coagulation necrosis in fibroids by damaging proteins and blood vessels, was originally developed as an alternative to myomectomy for women who wished to preserve their fertility.[29] Myolysis has shown some efficacy in reducing fibroid size in some patients,[30] but is associated with a risk of bowel adhesions and coagulation of the myometrium.[29] Donnez and colleagues[29] recommend that myolysis be used primarily for large, intramural, symptomatic fibroids that might be too difficult or time consuming for endoscopic myomectomy. Results from a non-randomized study suggest that, compared with endometrial ablation alone (n = 52), the combination of myolysis and endometrial ablation (n = 88) might reduce the need for subsequent surgery, including hysterectomy, in women with symptomatic fibroids and bleeding.[31] Besides the use of laser or laparoscopic bipolar needles, probes can also be placed by magnetic resonance imaging (MRI)-guided percutaneous procedures.[32]

Cryomyolysis, a refinement of the myolysis technique, entails the laparoscopic or hysteroscopic placement of a cryoprobe into the center of a fibroid and freezing to –100°C to –120°C to cause myoma coagulation.[33] Case series studies from two groups in Italy have shown that laparoscopic cryomyolysis appears to be effective in causing fibroid shrinkage (25% reduction) and symptom relief in most patients, at least up to 12 months following the procedure.[34,35]

MRI-GUIDED FOCUSED ULTRASOUND SURGERY

Magnetic resonance imaging–guided focused ultrasound surgery (MRgFUS) is a procedure approved in 2004 by the US Food and Drug Administration for the treatment of pre- or perimenopausal women with symptomatic uterine fibroids who desire to keep their uterus and have completed child bearing. Magnetic resonance imaging–guided focused ultrasound surgery combines focused high-intensity ultrasound waves to heat and destroy fibroid tissue, by induction of coagulative necrosis, and MRI to visualize anatomy, map the target fibroid tissue, and monitor the tissue temperature during treatment (Figs. 16.4 and 16.5).[36] Although the end result of this procedure is similar to myolysis and cryomyolysis, MRgFUS has the added benefit of MRI visualization of treatment effectiveness. Magnetic resonance imaging–guided focused ultrasound surgery treats one fibroid at a time, and it cannot be used to treat fibroids close to sensitive organs, such as the bowel or bladder, or those behind scar tissue. Also, the duration of the sonication portion of the procedure should be limited to 3 hours

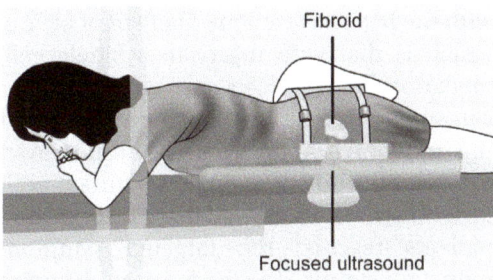

Fig. 16.4: Patient position for MRI-guided focused ultrasound surgery.

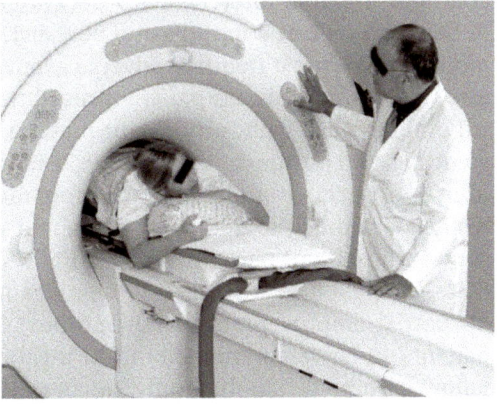

Fig. 16.5: Ex-ablate machine used for MRI-guided focused ultrasound surgery.

because prolonged immobilization may lead to increased risk of deep venous thrombosis or pulmonary embolism.[36]

The safety and efficacy of MRgFUS has been studied in single-arm prospective studies in women with clinically significant uterine fibroids. Stewart and colleagues[37] reported that among 55 enrolled patients, 76% were able to successfully complete the full treatment sessions in an outpatient setting with a small increase in pain and discomfort (as self-reported on a 4-point scale) and no major complications. In a subgroup of women who also underwent preplanned hysterectomy, pathologic examination of the uterus showed a 3-fold increase in volume of histologically confirmed necrosis compared with treatment volume ($P < 0.005$); this finding coincides with the hypothesized mechanism of action, which is that with injury to a single cell, mediators of apoptosis are generated and can spread through gap junctions to extend the area of tissue destruction. Results from the pivotal study of a single treatment with MRgFUS ($n = 109$) showed that 71% of treated patients reached the targeted symptom reduction levels (defined as a 10-point reduction in symptom severity score [SSS; 100-point scale] of the Uterine Fibroid QOL Instrument) at 6 months post-procedure and 51% at 12 months.[38] Mean decreases in SSS were 39% at 6 months and 36% at 12 months.[38] The most frequent adverse events associated with this outpatient procedure were abdominal pain, other pain, nausea/vomiting, and positional back pain.[36] Results from a prospective study in 35 symptomatic women scheduled to undergo hysterectomy showed that 1 and 6 months after MRgFUS, 61% of patients reported a significant or partial improvement of symptoms; 6 patients underwent hysterectomy during the follow-up period.[39] In this study, the uterine fibroid volume decreased 12% at 1 month and 15% at 6 months.

FIBROID TREATMENT VIA UTERINE ARTERY OCCLUSION OR EMBOLIZATION

Uterine Artery Embolization

Originally developed to manage postpartum hemorrhage,[40] UAE was later shown to reduce uterine fibroid volume and menorrhagia.[41] Performed by an interventional radiologist, UAE involves placement of a 4- or 5-French catheter into the uterine arteries via a transcutaneous femoral approach (performed under conscious sedation) and injection of trisacryl gelatin microspheres or polyvinyl alcohol particles into these arteries to cause occlusion.[33] Uterine artery embolization, which usually requires an overnight stay, normally causes a period of ischemic pain lasting 2 to 3 hours, followed by a plateau of pain, and then a gradual decrease in pain over the next 2 to 3 days.[33]

As with other procedures reviewed in this article, most of the data on UAE safety and efficacy were derived from case series rather than randomized controlled trials (RCTs). An analysis of data from 400 consecutive patients found a low rate of short-term complications, with no deaths and no major disabling injuries in women who underwent UAE at 2 institutions in Washington, DC.[42] In a study of 50 women who were asked to complete a baseline assessment and health-related QOL questionnaire, patients reported significant improvements in QOL measures and fibroid specific symptoms 3 and 6 months post-UAE.[43] Results from the voluntary, multicenter, prospective Fibroid Registry for Outcomes Data (FIBROID) showed that among 3,160 enrolled patients, 0.66% experienced a major in-hospital complication, 4.8% had a major post-discharge event within 30 days of the procedure, 2.4% had inadequate pain relief (the most common adverse event that required additional hospital treatment), and 1% required additional surgical intervention within 30 days after UAE.[44,45] A year after UAE, follow-up data from 1,701 patients showed that the mean symptom score improved from 58.6 to 18.23 (P < 0.001), but 5.3% of patients had no symptom improvement, 2.9% had a hysterectomy, and 7.3% (primarily women 45 years or older) had amenorrhea due to embolization.[46] One limitation of this study is that the 1-year data were not available for 20% of patients, which might have skewed the results if these dropouts had experienced more unfavorable outcomes than the rest of the study population.

The Dutch Uterine Artery Embolization in the Treatment of Symptomatic Uterine Fibroid Tumors (EMMY) trial compared UAE (n = 88) with hysterectomy (n = 88) for the treatment of menorrhagia caused by uterine fibroids.[47] The primary endpoint of this RCT was whether at least 75% of patients treated with UAE would avoid subsequent hysterectomy. Recently updated results showed that 2 years post-treatment, 23.5% of patients in the UAE group had undergone a hysterectomy and that there were no significant differences in improvement compared with baseline in terms of pain and bulk-related complaints.[48]

An important concern with UAE is its possible impact on menstruation and ovarian function. Chrisman and colleagues[49] reported that regular menses resumed in 56 (85%) of 66 patients (who had regular periods before the procedure) after an average of 3.5 weeks. Nine of 10 patients who failed to resume regular menstruation had laboratory results consistent with ovarian failure; also, these 9 patients were older than 45 years of age. The authors reported no difference in presenting symptoms, amount of occluding material used, or fibroid size between patients who did or did not resume regular menstruation.

Current data indicate that UAE controls menorrhagia in 85% to 95% of patients and bulk-related symptoms in 70% to 90% of patients, with a low rate of symptom recurrence.[50] In the absence of much comparative data and data with long follow-up, UAE does appear to have a lower risk of complications, shorter duration of hospitalization, and faster recovery compared with surgical alternatives such as hysterectomy and myomectomy.[50] However, the potential risk of loss of ovarian function associated with UAE is a serious consideration in women who desire to retain fertility.[51]

LAPAROSCOPIC UTERINE ARTERY OCCLUSION

Laparoscopic uterine artery occlusion uses a laparoscopic lateral retroperitoneal approach to achieve uterine artery occlusion. Unlike with UAE, patients undergoing LUAO are placed under general anesthesia, and artery occlusion is performed using ultrasonically activated sheets, clips, or electrosurgery.[52,53] Early indication of the short-term safety and efficacy of this procedure was reported by Lichtinger and colleagues[52] in a study of 8 patients who underwent LUAO for the treatment of fibroids associated with abnormal uterine bleeding, pelvic pain or pressure, or anemia. All patients in this study were discharged within 20 hours of the procedure, and all 5 patients who had abnormal bleeding at baseline reported a satisfactory decrease without developing amenorrhea. Seven of eight patients had complete disappearance of the pain or pressure they had experienced before the procedure, with the remaining patient experiencing significant relief of these symptoms. These authors cautioned that LUAO should be performed only by surgeons with advanced skills in laparoscopy.

Additional data with LUAO are available from case series and a small randomized trial. For example, a Czech study of LUAO in 68 consecutively enrolled women reported that with a median follow-up of 14.5 months, 93.2% of patients had improvement in menorrhagia or dysmenorrhea, and there was a 57.8% average reduction in volume of the dominant fibroid.[53] The mean time in surgery was 30.8 minutes (range 15–20 min), with a mean blood loss of 14.7 mL, 2.4-day mean hospital stay, and a 7.3% rate of postoperative complications. A larger retrospective analysis from the same Czech group reported that 8 (7.1%) of 114 women who underwent LUAO had complications, none had intraoperative complications or permanent injuries, and 10 (9.0%) of patients had fibroid recurrence.[54] At median follow-up at 23.6 months, the recurrence-free survival interval rate (i.e. with no clinical failure, no recurrence) was 88.3%.

An analysis of data from a Norwegian randomized controlled trial in 58 premenopausal women with symptomatic uterine fibroid showed that fewer patients treated with UAE compared with LUAO complained of heavy bleeding (4% vs 21%, P = 0.044) 6 months post-procedure.[55] However, the postoperative use of ketobemidone, an opioid analgesic, was higher after UAE compared with LUAO (46 mg vs 12 mg, P < 0.001), suggesting that LUAO caused less postoperative pain. A brief report from a prospective cohort study comparing LUAO with UAE raised concerns about increased risk for preterm birth and cesarean delivery with both procedures and higher rates of spontaneous abortion following UAE than LUAO (43.7% vs 15%).[56] Data from prospective trials with larger numbers of patients and longer follow-up are necessary to determine whether there are truly any differences in the safety and effectiveness of these procedures.

DOPPLER-GUIDED UTERINE ARTERY OCCLUSION

The positive experience with UAE and LUAO raises the question of whether temporarily occluding the uterine arteries may be just as effective as permanent occlusion or embolization in the treatment of uterine fibroids. To this end, Dickner and colleagues[57] demonstrated that a Doppler-guided nonincisional transvaginal approach could be used to successfully identify uterine arteries in 108 of 109 healthy premenopausal women despite wide variability in the position and depth of these arteries. These findings were the basis for the development of a uterine device (D-UAO) composed of a cervical tenaculum incorporating a guiding monorail and a paracervical vascular clamp with integrated Doppler ultrasound crystals, connected to a battery-powered ultrasound transceiver to generate an audible Doppler signal.

Lichtinger and colleagues[58] studied D-UAO in 10 symptomatic women with intramurally located uterine fibroids (>3 cm in average diameter by ultrasound) and found that it could be used to safely and effectively occlude the uterine arteries. After the uterine arteries were located with the audible Doppler signal, the paracervical vascular clamp was placed transvaginally and bilateral occlusion was achieved by folding the vaginal tissue around the uterine arteries to interrupt blood flow. In this pilot study, the investigators reported a 26-minute average time of clamp closure (range, 10–59 min), which resulted in the uterus remaining blanched throughout this period in all patients. Also in all patients, after the clamp was opened, the Doppler signal from the clamp returned immediately and the uterus regained a pink tonality. In addition, the ureters were never obstructed, and there was no evidence of injury in the vagina or cervix after clamp removal.

Case reports provide the initial evidence of the efficacy of D-UAO in reducing uterine volume, menorrhagia, and other fibroid-related symptoms.[59,60] Also, according to a preliminary report from a prospective study in 40 women, 6 months after D-UAO the dominant fibroid size was reduced 30% to 35%, and uterine size was reduced by an average of 20%.[61] In addition, patients with menorrhagia had a 35% to 40% reduction in menstrual blood that was associated with an average

35% reduction in Ruta Menorrhagia scores. Patients experienced few adverse events, with no reports of amenorrhea. Because 5 women experienced 6 hydronephrosis events (which spontaneously resolved in 3 patients and were effectively treated in the other 2), the procedure was successfully modified by filling the bladder to move the ureters away from the uterine arteries prior to the D-UAO, restricting excessive device movement while searching for uterine artery signal, and limiting the use of the larger clamp size to cervices larger than 4.5 cm. Since this mitigation strategy was implemented, no new cases of hydronephrosis have been reported (data on file).

Doppler-guided uterine artery occlusion is performed under anesthesia (in the form of epidural, paracervical block plus patient-controlled analgesia, or IV sedation plus patient-controlled analgesia) to prevent patient movement and potential dislodgement of the device. Deep venous thrombosis prophylaxis with pneumatic compression boots is used because the D-UAO device must stay in place for 6 hours. Anticoagulants are not recommended because they might interfere with the putative mechanism of action of this procedure. Additional clinical studies of D-UAO are ongoing.

PROPOSED MECHANISM OF ACTION OF UTERINE ARTERY OCCLUSION AND EMBOLIZATION

Burbank and Hutchins[62] proposed that uterine fibroids could be treated through the creation of transient uterine ischemia produced surgically in the case of LUAO and embolically in the case of UAE. The rationale for this hypothesis, which provides the putative mechanism of action for these procedures, is based on the fact that the uterus and, by default, uterine fibroids are mainly supplied with blood from branches of the uterine arteries. When these arteries are bilaterally occluded by surgery or injection of embolic particles, uterine blood flow is almost completely stopped, leading to blood clotting within the intrinsic arteries of the uterus and in the fibroids. The myometrial cells withstand this transient ischemia, and after approximately 6 hours, the clotted blood in the intrinsic uterine arteries lyses, reperfusing the uterus with the aid of blood flow from collateral arteries. However, fibroids are unable to lyse the clotted blood, causing eventual infarction and necrosis that results in reduced uterine volume and fibroid size.[62,63] The mechanism of action of D-UAO is thought to function in a similar way. In this case, clamp application stops uterine artery blood flow, triggering the sequence of blood clotting, uterine ischemia, and fibroid infarction and necrosis. This mechanism of fibroid death and myometrial survival following prolonged ischemia appears to use the same biological processes that cause placental death after postpartum clotting of uteroplacental arteries.[64] Some experimental evidence in support of this mechanism of action comes from monitoring of uterine pH (as a proxy for hypoxia and lactic acidosis) before, during, and 24 hours after outpatient LUAO, which showed a time course of pH drop and rise in the myometrium that appears to be consistent with the transient ischemia hypothesis.[63]

CONCLUSION

Options for the treatment of symptomatic patients with uterine fibroids have increased, particularly with the introduction of less invasive surgical procedures. Although hysterectomy remains the definitive treatment, laparoscopic myomectomy, myolysis and cryomyolysis, and MRgFUS are choices that might fulfill the needs of some women who wish to preserve their uterus or otherwise avoid major surgery. These new surgical procedures offer patients shorter hospital stays and recovery times as well as less pain and scarring, but they also pose risks such as recurrence and loss of fertility. Several studies support the safety and effectiveness of UAE and LUAO, two minimally-invasive procedures that treat fibroids via uterine artery occlusion or embolization, which produces uterine ischemia that subsequently causes fibroid infarction and necrosis. However, these procedures might affect fertility, and LUAO poses significant technical challenges. Doppler-guided Uterine Artery Occlusion is a promising new procedure currently in clinical trials in the United States and Europe that is based on the same putative mechanism of action as UAE and LUAO, without harming uterine function, at least according to initial studies. Randomized studies and prospective studies with larger numbers of patients and longer follow-up are needed to fully evaluate the safety and efficacy of all these interventions. Results from future studies should help us match the specific needs of each patient and their clinical presentation to the most appropriate treatment options

REFERENCES

1. Schwartz SM, Marshall LM, Baird DD. Epidemiologic contributions to understanding the etiology of uterine leiomyomata. Environ Health Perspect. 2000;108(suppl 5):821-7.
2. Payson M, Leppert P, Segars J. Epidemiology of myomas. Obstet Gynecol Clin North Am. 2006;33(1):1-11.
3. Ryan GL, Syrop CH, Van Voorhis BJ. Role, epidemiology, and natural history of benign uterine mass lesions. Clin Obstet Gynecol. 2005;48(2):312-24.
4. Wegienka G, Day Baird D, Hertz-Picciotto I, et al. Self-reported heavy bleeding associated with uterine leiomyomata. Obstet Gynecol. 2003;101(3):431-7.
5. Day Baird D, Dunson DB, Hill MC, et al. High cumulative incidence of uterine leiomyoma in black and white women: ultrasound evidence. Am J Obstet Gynecol 2003;188(1):100-7.
6. Keshavarz H, Hillis SD, Kieke BA, et al. Hysterectomy surveillance—United States, 1994-1999. MMWR CDC Surveill Summ. 2002;51(SS05):1-8.
7. Lepine LA, Hillis SD, Marchbanks PA, et al. Hysterectomy surveillance—United States, 1980-1993. MMWR CDC Surveill Summ. 1997;46(4):1-15.
8. Edwards RD, Moss JG, Lumsden MA, et al. Uterine-artery embolization versus surgery for symptomatic uterine fibroids. N Engl J Med. 2007;356(4):360-70.
9. Flynn M, Jamison M, Datta S, et al. Health care resource use for uterine fibroid tumors in the United States. Am J Obstet Gynecol. 2006;195(4):955-64.
10. Hartmann KE, Birnbaum H, Ben-Hamadi R, et al. Annual costs associated with diagnosis of uterine leiomyomata. Obstet Gynecol 2006;108(4):930-7.
11. Cote I, Jacobs P, Cumming D. Work loss associated with increased menstrual loss in the United States. Obstet Gynecol. 2002;100(4):683-7.
12. Spies JB, Coyne K, Guaou GN, et al. The UFS-QOL, a new disease-specific symptom and health-related quality of life questionnaire for leiomyomata. Obstet Gynecol. 2002;99(2):290-300.
13. Frishman GN, Jurema MW. Myomas and myomectomy. J Minim Invasive Gynecol. 2005;12(5):443-56.
14. Eisinger SH, Meldrum S, Fiscella K, et al. Low-dose mifepristone for uterine leiomyomata. Obstet Gynecol. 2003;101(2):243-50.
15. Eisinger SH, Bonfiglio T, Fiscella K, et al. Twelve-month safety and efficacy of low-dose mifepristone for uterine myomas. J Minim Invasive Gynecol. 2005;12(3):227-33.
16. Fiscella K, Eisinger SH, Meldrum S, et al. Effect of mifepristone for symptomatic leiomyomata on quality of life and uterine

size: a randomized controlled trial. Obstet Gynecol. 2006;108(6):1381-7.
17. Friedman AJ, Hoffman DI, Comite F, Browneller RW, Miller JD, for the Leuprolide Study Group. Treatment of leiomyomata uteri with leuprolide acetate depot: a double-blind, placebo-controlled, multicenter study. Obstet Gynecol. 1991;77(5):720-5.
18. Gonzalez-Barcena D, Alvarez RB, Ochoa EP, et al. Treatment of uterine leiomyomas with luteinizing hormone-releasing hormone antagonist Cetrorelix. Hum Reprod. 1997;12(9):2028-35.
19. Felberbaum RE, Ludwig M, Diedrich K. Medical treatment of uterine fibroids with the LHRH antagonist: Cetrorelix [in French]. Contracept Fertil Sex. 1999;27(10):701-9.
20. Chillik C, Acosta A. The role of LHRH agonists and antagonists. Reprod Biomed Online. 2001;2 (2):120-8.
21. Chwalisz K, Perez MC, Demanno D, et al. Selective progesterone receptor modulator development and use in the treatment of leiomyomata and endometriosis. Endocr Rev. 2005;26(3):423-38.
22. Wang J, Ohara N, Wang Z, et al. A novel selective progesterone receptor modulator asoprisnil (J867) down-regulates the expression of EGF, IGF-I, TGFbeta3 and their receptors in cultured uterine leiomyoma cells. Hum Reprod. 2006;21(7):1869-77.
23. Chwalisz K, Larsen L, Mattia-Goldberg C, et al. A randomized, controlled trial of asoprisnil, a novel selective progesterone receptor modulator, in women with uterine leiomyomata. Fertil Steril. 2007;87(6):1399-412.
24. Williams AR, Critchley HO, Osei J, et al. The effects of the selective progesterone receptor modulator asoprisnil on the morphology of uterine tissues after 3 months treatment in patients with symptomatic uterine leiomyomata. Hum Reprod. 2007;22(6):1696-704.
25. Jacobson GF, Shaber RE, Armstrong MA, et al. Changes in rates of hysterectomy and uterine conserving procedures for treatment of uterine leiomyoma. Am J Obstet Gynecol. 2007;196(6):601.e1-601.e6.
26. Hanafi M. Predictors of leiomyoma recurrence after myomectomy. Obstet Gynecol. 2005;105 (4):877-81.
27. Doridot V, Dubuisson JB, Chapron C, et al. Recurrence of leiomyomata after laparoscopic myomectomy. J Am Assoc Gynecol Laparosc. 2001;8(4):495-500.
28. Dubuisson JB, Fauconnier A, Fourchotte V, et al. Laparoscopic myomectomy: predicting the risk of conversion to an open procedure. Hum Reprod. 2001;16(8):1726-31.
29. Donnez J, Squifflet J, Polet R, et al. Laparoscopic myolysis. Hum Reprod Update. 2000;6(6):609-13.
30. Phillips DR, Nathanson HG, Milim SJ, et al. Laparoscopic leiomyoma coagulation. J Am Assoc Gynecol Laparosc. 1996;3(4 suppl):S39.
31. Goldfarb HA. Combining myoma coagulation with endometrial ablation/resection reduces subsequent surgery rates. JSLS. 1999;3(4):253-60.
32. Hindley JT, Law PA, Hickey M, et al. Clinical outcomes following percutaneous magnetic resonance image guided laser ablation of symptomatic uterine fibroids. Hum Reprod. 2002;17(10):2737-41.
33. Sharp HT. Assessment of new technology in the treatment of idiopathic menorrhagia and uterine leiomyomata. Obstet Gynecol. 2006;108(4):990-1003.
34. Ciavattini A, Tsiroglou D, Piccioni M, et al. Laparoscopic cryomyolysis: an alternative to myomectomy in women with symptomatic fibroids. Surg Endosc. 2004;18(12):1785-8.
35. Zupi E, Marconi D, Sbracia M, et al. Directed laparoscopic cryomyolysis for symptomatic leiomyomata: one-year follow up. J Minim Invasive Gynecol. 2005;12(4):343-6.
36. ExAblate. InSightec® ExAblate® 2000 System magnetic resonance guided focused ultrasound surgery [prescribing information]. 2004.
37. Stewart EA, Gedroyc WM, Tempany CM, et al. Focused ultrasound treatment of uterine fibroid tumors: safety and feasibility of a noninvasive thermoablative technique. Am J Obstet Gynecol. 2003;189(1):48-54.
38. Stewart EA, Rabinovici J, Tempany CM, et al. Clinical outcomes of focused ultrasound

surgery for the treatment of uterine fibroids. Fertil Steril. 2006;85(1):22-9.
39. Rabinovici J, Inbar Y, Revel A, et al. Clinical improvement and shrinkage of uterine fibroids after thermal ablation by magnetic resonance-guided focused ultrasound surgery. Ultrasound Obstet Gynecol. 2007;30(5):771-7.
40. Oliver JA J, Lance JS. Selective embolization to control massive hemorrhage following pelvic surgery. Am J Obstet Gynecol. 1979;135(3):431-2.
41. Ravina JH, Herbreteau D, Ciraru-Vigneron N, et al. Arterial embolisation to treat uterine myomata. Lancet. 1995;346(8976):671-2.
42. Spies JB, Spector A, Roth AR, et al. Complications after uterine artery embolization for leiomyomas. Obstet Gynecol. 2002;100(5 Pt 1):873-80.
43. Spies JB, Warren EH, Mathias SD, et al. Uterine fibroid embolization: measurement of health-related quality of life before and after therapy. J Vasc Interv Radiol. 1999;10(10):1293-303.
44. Myers ER, Goodwin S, Landow W, et al. Prospective data collection of a new procedure by a specialty society: the FIBROID registry. Obstet Gynecol. 2005;106(1):44-51.
45. Worthington-Kirsch R, Spies JB, Myers ER, et al. The Fibroid Registry for outcomes data (FIBROID) for uterine embolization: short-term outcomes. Obstet Gynecol. 2005;106(1):52-9.
46. Spies JB, Myers ER, Worthington-Kirsch R, et al. The FIBROID Registry: symptom and quality-of-life status 1 year after therapy. Obstet Gynecol. 2005;106(6):1309-18.
47. Hehenkamp WJ, Volkers NA, Donderwinkel PF, et al. Uterine artery embolization versus hysterectomy in the treatment of symptomatic uterine fibroids (EMMY trial): peri- and postprocedural results from a randomized controlled trial. Am J Obstet Gynecol. 2005;193(5):1618-29.
48. Volkers NA, Hehenkamp WJ, Birnie E, et al. Uterine artery embolization versus hysterectomy in the treatment of symptomatic uterine fibroids: 2 years' outcome from the randomized EMMY trial. Am J Obstet Gynecol. 2007;196(6):519.e1-519.e11.
49. Chrisman HB, Saker MB, Ryu RK, et al. The impact of uterine fibroid embolization on resumption of menses and ovarian function. J Vasc Interv Radiol. 2000;11(6):699-703.
50. Worthington-Kirsch RL. Uterine artery embolization for fibroid disease is not experimental. Cardiovasc Intervent Radiol. 2005;28(2):148-9.
51. American College of Obstetricians and Gynecologists. Uterine artery embolization. ACOG Committee Opinion No. 293. Obstet Gynecol. 2004;103:403-4.
52. Lichtinger M, Hallson L, Calvo P, et al. Laparoscopic uterine artery occlusion for symptomatic leiomyomas. J Am Assoc Gynecol Laparosc. 2002;9(2):191-8.
53. Holub Z, Jabor A, Lukac J, et al. Midterm follow-up study of laparoscopic dissection of uterine vessels for surgical treatment of symptomatic fibroids. Surg Endosc. 2004;18(9):1349-53.
54. Holub Z, Eim J, Jabor A, et al. Complications and myoma recurrence after laparoscopic uterine artery occlusion for symptomatic myomas. J Obstet Gynaecol Res. 2006;32(1):55-62.
55. Hald K, Klow NE, Qvigstad E, et al. Laparoscopic occlusion compared with embolization of uterine vessels: a randomized controlled trial. Obstet Gynecol. 2007;109(1):20-7.
56. Holub Z, Mara M, Eim J. Laparoscopic uterine artery occlusion versus uterine fibroid embolization. Int J Gynaecol Obstet. 2007;96(1):44-5.
57. Dickner SK, Cooper JM, Diaz D. A nonincisional, Doppler-guided transvaginal approach to uterine artery identification and control of uterine perfusion. J Am Assoc Gynecol Laparosc. 2004;11(1):55-8.
58. Lichtinger M, Herbert S, Memmolo A. Temporary, transvaginal occlusion of the uterine arteries: a feasibility and safety study. J Minim Invasive Gynecol. 2005;12(1):40-2.
59. Vilos GA, Vilos EC, Romano W, et al. Temporary uterine artery occlusion for treatment of menorrhagia and uterine

60. Istre O, Hald K, Qvigstad E. Multiple myomas treated with a temporary, noninvasive, Doppler-directed, transvaginal uterine artery clamp. J Am Assoc Gynecol Laparosc. 2004;11(2):273-6.
61. Vilos GA, Lichtinger M. Transvaginal Doppler-guided uterine artery occlusion for the management of leiomyomata uteri: initial pilot study results. J Minim Invasive Gynecol. 2007;14(6):S104. Abstract 286.
62. Burbank F, Hutchins FL, Jr. Uterine artery occlusion by embolization or surgery for the treatment of fibroids: a unifying hypothesis—transient uterine ischemia. J Am Assoc Gynecol Laparosc. 2000;7(suppl 4):S1-S49.
63. Lichtinger M, Burbank F, Hallson L, et al. The time course of myometrial ischemia and reperfusion after laparoscopic uterine artery occlusion—theoretical implications. J Am Assoc Gynecol Laparosc. 2003;10(4):553-66.
64. Burbank F. Childbirth and myoma treatment by uterine artery occlusion: do they share a common biology? J Am Assoc Gynecol Laparosc. 2004;11(2):138-52.

(Reference 59 continued) fibroids using an incisionless Doppler-guided transvaginal clamp: case report. Hum Reprod. 2006;21(1):269-71.

CHAPTER 17

Unexplained Infertility

Madhuri Patil

Chapter outline

- Definition
- Incidence
- Prevalence
- Standard Basic Investigations
  - RCOG Guidelines (1998) and National Guideline Clearinghouse (2000)
  - American Society of Reproductive Medicine
  - Medical History
  - Physical Examination
  - Basic Semen Analysis
- Supplementary (Advanced) Investigations
  - Laparoscopy
  - Hysteroscopy
  - Ultrasound
  - Endometrial Biopsy
  - Evaluation of Cervical Score and Postcoital Test
  - Assessment of Ovarian Reserve
  - Specialized Clinical Tests on Semen and Sperm
  - Zona-Free Hamster Oocyte Test
  - Hypo-osmotic Swelling Test
  - *In Vitro* Sperm Nuclear Chromatin Decondensation Test
- Sperm Mitochondrial Activity Index
- Hemizona Binding Assay
- Sperm DNA Fragmentation
- ESHRE Task Force on Unexplained Infertility
  - Possible Causes (Identified/Unidentified)
- Diagnosis
  - Treatment
  - Selection of Treatment Option
- Treatment Modalities
  - Antibiotic Therapy
  - Expectant Management and Lifestyle Changes
  - Clomiphene Citrate
  - Letrozole
  - Gonadotropins
  - Artificial Insemination
  - Controlled Ovarian Hyperstimulation and Artificial Insemination
  - Assisted Reproductive Technology
  - Oil Soluble HSG
  - Comparison of Different Treatments for Unexplained Infertility
- NICE Guidelines: Unexplained Infertility

DEFINITION

Diagnosis of unexplained infertility is made if the basic infertility evaluation fails to reveal an obvious cause for failure to conceive. The basic evaluation should provide evidence of adequate sperm production, ovulation and fallopian tube patency. If indicated, tests for ovarian reserve and laparoscopy should also be done.

In those patients where the results of a standard infertility evaluation are normal or whose problems do not 'explain' their infertility are assigned a diagnosis of unexplained infertility. At present, even the most sophisticated diagnostic assessment cannot reveal all of the possible abnormalities. Therefore, unexplained infertility appears to represent either the lower extreme of the normal distribution of fertility or it arises from a defect in fecundity which cannot be detected by the routine infertility evaluation. If this group of patients are followed-up without treatment 30–50% will ultimately achieve pregnancy. The success will depend on the age of the couple, the duration of their infertility and how extensive their evaluation was before being classified as 'unexplained infertility'.

INCIDENCE

Significant advances have occurred in the diagnosis and, more importantly, in the treatment of reproductive disorders over the past decade. Despite this, approximately 15–30% of couples will be diagnosed with unexplained infertility after their diagnostic workup. Defects which result in implantation failures are probably much more common than we realize and constitute another area of unexplained infertility. Assaying implantation factors like integrins may lower the incidence of unexplained infertility in our patients.

PREVALENCE

Prevalence will depend on:
- Evaluation protocol: Thoroughness of testing and use of sophisticated medical technology for evaluation
- Referral pattern
- Interpretation of diagnostic studies.

With fewer tests being performed the diagnosis is more frequent. The incidence reduces with the performance of laparoscopy. It is 10–20% without laparoscopy, the incidence reducing to < 10% after laparoscopy. It decreases further with advanced tests being performed for evaluation.[1] Literally, hundreds of molecular and biochemical events have to function properly in order to have a pregnancy develop. The standard tests for infertility barely scratch the surface and are really only looking for very obvious factors, such as blocked tubes, abnormal sperm counts and ovulation regularity. These tests do not address the molecular issues at all.

STANDARD BASIC INVESTIGATIONS

RCOG Guidelines (1998), and National Guideline Clearinghouse (2000)

Basic semen analysis (Figs. 17.1A to D) helps to identify sperm defects. Spermatogenesis takes approximately 72 days. Abnormal semen analysis results can be attributed to various unknown reasons (e.g. short period of sexual abstinence, incomplete collection, poor sexual stimulus); therefore, repeating the semen analysis at least 1 month later is important before a diagnosis is made. Explaining to the patient, the normal fluctuation that can occur between semen samples is also important.

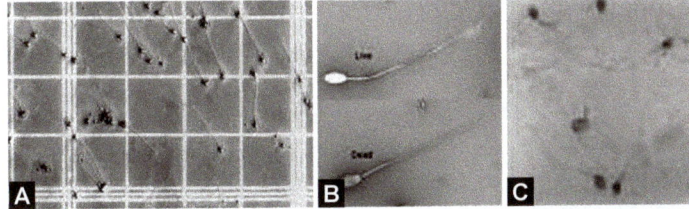
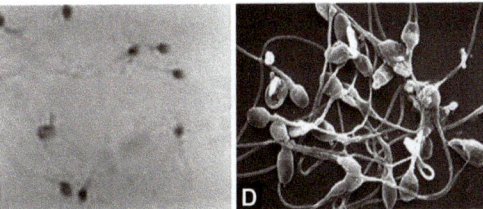

Figs. 17.1A to D: Semen analysis: (A) Count; (B) Viability; (C) Morphology; (D) Agglutination.

Normal Values for Semen Parameters

For optimum and consistent results, abstinence of at least 3 to 5 days is required prior to semen collection. The World Health Organization 2010 recommends the following as reference values:
- Volume: 1.2–5 mL
- pH: ≥ 7.2
- Sperm concentration: > 15 million/mL
- Total sperm number: > 39 million spermatozoa per ejaculate or more
- Motility: > 40% with forward progression or > 32% progressive motility (a+b)
- Vitality: > 58% live
- Morphology: > 4% with normal morphology
- White blood cells: Fewer than 1 million/mL
- Fructose (Total): >13 mol/ejaculate.

Apart from the above anti-sperm antibody testing should be done in the presence of agglutination.
- Immunobead test: Fewer than 50% motile spermatozoa with beads bound
- MAR test: Fewer than 50% motile spermatozoa with adherent particles.

Hysterosalpingography (HSG) (Fig. 17.2): Documents normal endometrial cavity and tubal patency but is of less predictive value in diagnosing pelvic pathology.

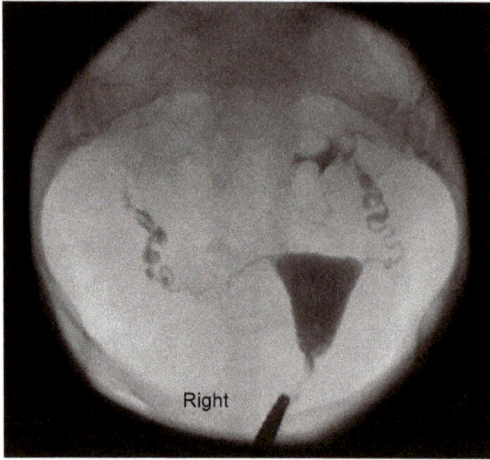

Fig. 17.2: Normal hysterosalpingography (HSG).

Mid-luteal serum progesterone: Detects ovulation.

According to these guidelines there is no value in measuring thyroid or prolactin in women with regular menstrual cycles in the absence of galactorrhea or symptoms of thyroid disease.

American Society of Reproductive Medicine

The Practice Committee of the American Society for Reproductive Medicine (ASRM) has published guidelines for a standard infertility evaluation.[2]

Evaluation of male for infertility: The full evaluation for male infertility should include a complete medical and reproductive history, a physical examination by a urologist or other specialist in male reproduction, and at least two semen analyses. Based on the results of the full evaluation, the physician may recommend other procedures and tests to elucidate the etiology of a patient's infertility. These tests may include additional semen analyses, endocrine evaluation, postejaculatory urinalysis, ultrasonography, specialized tests on semen and sperm and genetic screening.

Medical History

The patient's medical history is used to identify risk factors and behavior patterns that could have a significant impact on male infertility. The history should include the duration of infertility and prior fertility; childhood illnesses and developmental history; systemic medical illnesses (e.g. diabetes mellitus and upper respiratory diseases) and prior surgeries; a complete medical and surgical history; sexual history including history of sexually transmitted infections; coital frequency and timing; gonadal toxin exposure including heat; medications (prescription and nonprescription) and allergies; and also family reproductive history.

Physical Examination

A general physical examination is an integral part of the evaluation of male infertility. In addition to the general physical examination, particular focus should be given to the genitalia including examination of the penis, the location of the urethral meatus; palpation of the testes and measurement of their size; presence and consistency of both the vasa and epididymides; presence of a varicocele; secondary sexual characteristics including body habitus, hair distribution and breast development and digital rectal examination. The diagnosis of congenital bilateral absence of the vasa deferentia (CBAVD) is established by physical examination. Scrotal exploration is not needed to make this diagnosis.

Basic Semen Analysis (Figs. 17.3A to C)

Physicians should provide patients with standard instructions for semen collection. These instructions include a defined period of abstinence of two to three days. Semen can be collected by masturbation or by intercourse using special semen collection condoms that do not contain substances detrimental to sperm. To ensure accurate results, the laboratory should have a quality control program for semen analysis (Table 17.1).

The semen analysis provides information on semen volume as well as sperm concentration, motility and morphology. Azoospermia should not be diagnosed until the specimen is centrifuged at maximum speed (preferably 3000 g) for 15 minutes, and the pellet is examined.

Following are the references values:[3-5]

Table 17.1: Semen analysis: Reference values.

On at least two occasions	
Ejaculate volume	1.5 mL
pH	> 7.2
Sperm concentration	> 15 million/mL
Total sperm number	> 39 million/ejaculate
Percent motility	> 40%
Progressive motility (a+b)	> 32%
Sperm agglutination	< 2 (Scale 0-3)
Viscosity	< h3 (Scale 0-4)

Source: World Health Organization, 2010

HSG (Fig. 17.4): An HSG consists of radiographic evaluation of the uterine cavity and fallopian tubes after injection of a radiopaque medium through the cervical canal. Hysterosalpingography (HSG) defines the size and shape of the uterine cavity and will reveal developmental anomalies (unicornuate, septate, bicornuate uteri) or other acquired abnormalities (endometrial polyps, submucous myomas, synechiae) with potential reproductive consequences. It can document proximal and distal tubal occlusion, demonstrate salpingitis

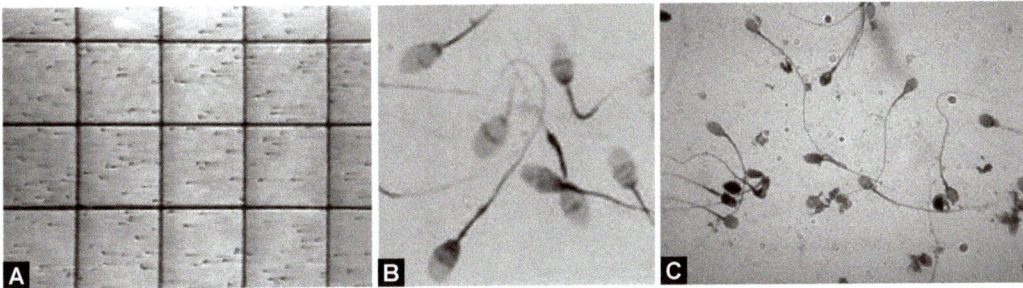

Figs. 17.3A to C: (A) Count; (B) Morphology; (C) Viability and WBCs.

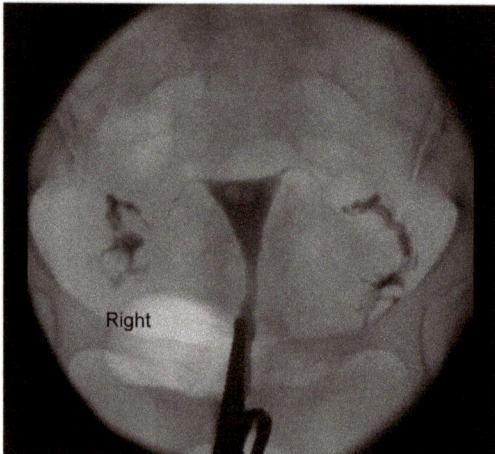

Fig. 17.4: Another image of normal hysterosalpingography.

isthmica nodosa, reveal tubal architectural detail of potential prognostic value and suggest the presence of fimbrial phimosis or peritubular adhesions when escape of contrast is delayed or becomes loculated, respectively. Findings suggesting proximal tubal obstruction require further evaluation to exclude transient occlusion resulting from tubal/myometrial contractions. However, patent fallopian tubes on HSG do not confirm that ovum pickup will occur. For example, women with severe endometriosis may have adherent ovaries in the *cul de sac* with normal fallopian tubes. When combined with laparoscopic dye chromopertubation, it can best assess tubal patency—both anatomical and physiological functioning of the tubes. The concordance of HSG with laparoscopic dye pertubation is estimated as close to 90%.[6]

Assessment of occurrence and adequacy of ovulation (Fig. 17.5): Apart from thorough menstrual history, other methods used

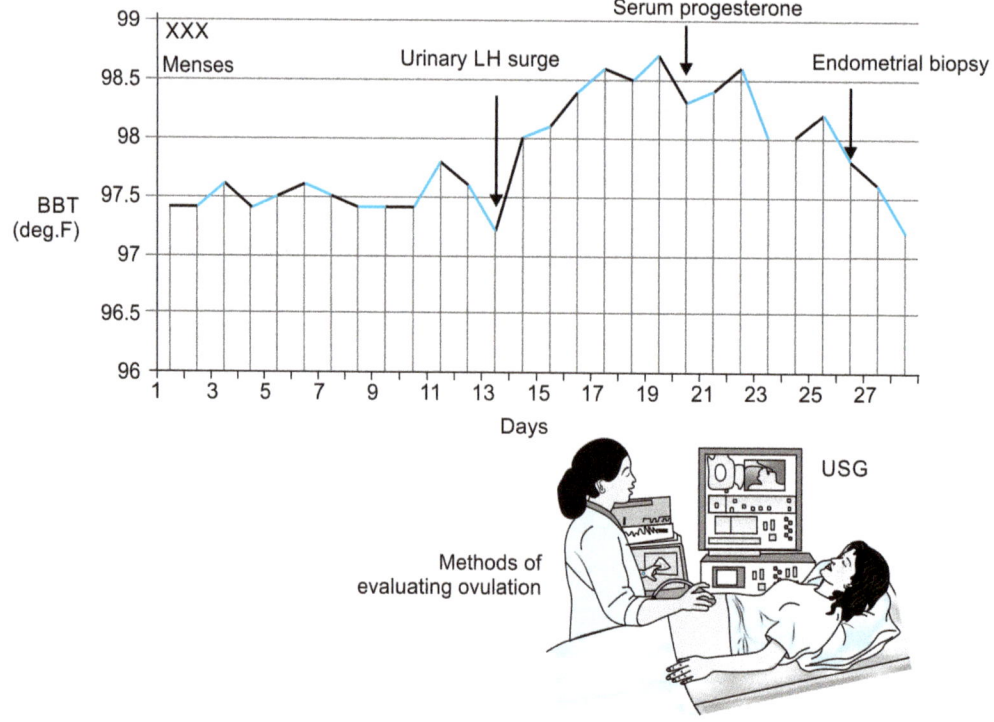

Fig. 17.5: Methods of detecting ovulation.
(BBT: basal body temperature; LH: luteinizing hormone; USG: ultrasonography)

to evaluate ovulation include basal body temperature (BBT) recordings, urinary luteinizing hormone (LH) (ovulation) predictor kits, mid luteal serum progesterone testing, and endometrial biopsy to assess for secretory endometrial development.

Basal body temperature (BBT): Recordings provide a simple and inexpensive method for evaluating ovulatory function. Whereas biphasic patterns are characteristic in ovulatory cycles, monophasic recordings or a grossly short interval of luteal phase temperature elevation (< 11 days) may identify patients with absent or poor quality ovulatory function. However, some ovulatory women may exhibit monophasic BBT patterns, and the test cannot reliably define the time of ovulation. Although BBT recordings is the least costly tool in a reliable patient, they are difficult to interpret and often frustrating for the patient.[7]

Urinary luteinizing hormone (LH) determinations using various commercial "ovulation predictor kits" can identify the midcycle LH surge, provide reliable if still indirect evidence of ovulatory function and help to define the interval in which conception is most likely (the three days ending with the day of ovulation).[8] Results generally correlate well with the peak in serum LH, particularly in evening urine specimens.[9] Urinary luteinizing hormone (LH) ovulation predictor kits are sensitive, relatively inexpensive method and pinpoint the day of ovulation, though accuracy, reliability and ease of use vary among products. Ovulation predictor kits are useful for women who do not have very long menstrual cycles and can be used by couples to appropriately time intercourse.

Serum progesterone determinations during the luteal phase also may be used to evaluate ovulatory function; values greater than 3.0 ng/mL provide presumptive evidence of ovulation.[10] Midluteal phase determinations may offer additional information regarding the quality of luteal function, although concentrations may fluctuate widely even in normal women. In spontaneous cycles, midluteal progesterone levels greater than 10.0 ng/mL correlate well with normal "in phase" endometrial histology.[11] Thus it is a less invasive way to assess luteal function, though controversy persists regarding the lower limit of normal for progesterone value. Moreover, they are often poorly timed if they are drawn on cycle day 21 in women with irregular menses. In such women, it is better to use an ovulation kit and measure the progesterone levels 7 to 8 days after the LH surge is detected.

Endometrial biopsy and histologic evaluation can demonstrate secretory endometrial development, which results from the action of progesterone and thus implies ovulation. "Dating" the endometrium using established histologic criteria[12] and demonstration of a consistent maturation delay (–2 days) is the traditional method for diagnosis of luteal phase defect (LPD). However, controversies persist regarding the accuracy of these diagnostic criteria[13,14] the prevalence of LPD,[15] and its clinical relevance as a cause of infertility. Although endometrial biopsy results are used to diagnose luteal phase defect, they do not correlate with fertility status and hence are no longer recommended (Fig. 17.6).[16]

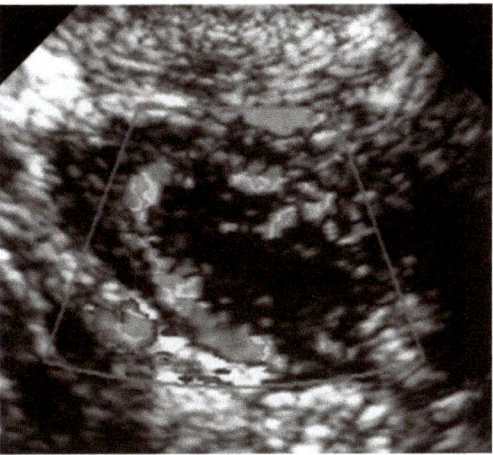

Fig. 17.6: Corpus luteum showing flare effect in color Doppler.

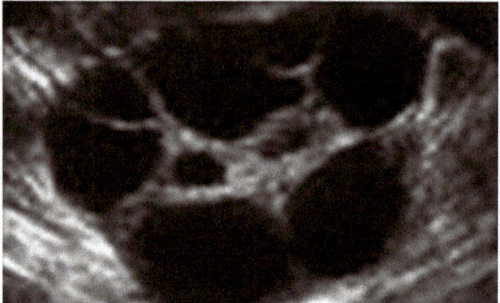

Fig. 17.7: Size and number of developing follicles.

Serial transvaginal ultrasound can reveal the size and number of developing follicles (Fig. 17.7) and provide presumptive evidence of ovulation and luteinization by demonstrating progressive follicular growth, sudden collapse of the preovulatory follicle, a loss of clearly defined follicular margins, the appearance of internal echoes and an increase in *cul de sac* fluid volume.[17] Because of the cost and logistical requirements involved, this method is generally reserved for patients in whom less complicated methods fail to provide the necessary information. Follicular monitoring today forms an important and integral part detecting ovulation (Fig. 17.8).

Serum thyroid-stimulating hormone (TSH) and prolactin determinations will identify thyroid disorders and/or hyperprolactinemia, which may require specific treatment. In amenorrheic women, a follicle-stimulating hormone (FSH) level will differentiate patients with ovarian failure from those with hypothalamic dysfunction.

If the semen analysis is abnormal, it should be repeated after at least 1 month by a laboratory that adheres to World Health Organization (WHO) guidelines, with a quality control program ensuring accurate testing.

SUPPLEMENTARY (ADVANCED) INVESTIGATIONS

The use of advanced investigations reduces the incidence of unexplained infertility. If indicated, tests for ovarian reserve and laparoscopy are included as basic tests, which otherwise are advanced tests. These tests predict the chance of conception but do not influence the outcome of treatment.

Laparoscopy (Fig. 17.9)

The role of laparoscopy in the investigation of infertility has changed over the past decade. Initially laparoscopy used to be a part of the basic infertility work-up, it is now reserved for selected cases. It allows direct visual examination of the pelvic reproductive anatomy, evaluates fallopian tubes, ovaries,

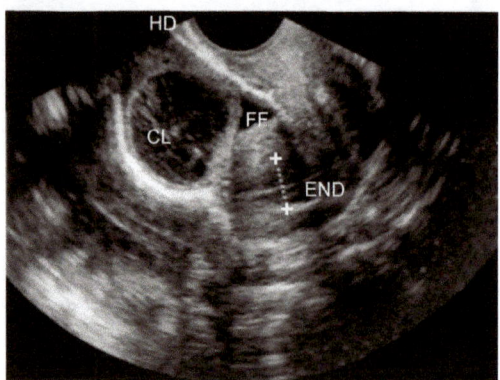

Fig. 17.8: Signs of ovulation—CL and free fluid in POD.

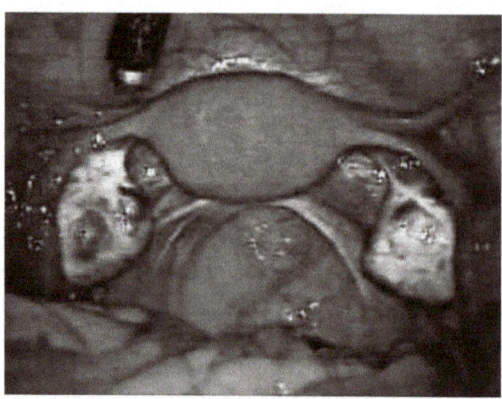

Fig. 17.9: Normal laparoscopy.

tubo-ovarian relationship, identify otherwise unrecognized peritoneal factors that influence fertility, specifically endometriosis and pelvic adhesions. It has been seen that presence of endometriosis has lower PR with OI with IUI compared to other etiologies and this could be due to defective ovarian, tubal, endometrial, sperm and coital function; macrophage invasion and sperm phagocytosis and release of chemical agents—gamete and embryo toxic. According to the guidelines of the ASRM, laparoscopy should be performed in women. It is generally indicated in women with unexplained infertility or signs and symptoms of endometriosis and in those whose history, physical examination, and/or HSG demonstrates or suggests tubal disease that may be amenable to repair.[6]

Laparoscopy may be considered early in an infertile couple if:
- Age of female partner is >35 years
- Married > 3 years
- Presence of an abnormal HSG
- History or symptoms suggestive of pelvic disease
- Elevated chlamydia IgG titers
- Presence of dyspareunia, dysmenorrhea
- History of previous pelvic surgery.

Hysteroscopy (Figs. 17.10A to E)

It is the definitive method for evaluation of the uterine cavity and diagnosis of associated abnormalities. It is indicated in the presence of an abnormal HSG or in the presence of history and symptoms suggestive of endometrial or uterine pathology. It is highly sensitive method for diagnosis of uterine anomalies, polyps, submucous myomas, and synechiae.

Ultrasound

Evaluation in the follicular phase is used to identify a normal endometrial cavity (Fig. 17.11), uterine fibroids, polyps (Figs. 17.12A and B), intrauterine adhesions (Figs. 17.13A and B) and congenital anomalies such as a bicornuate uterus (Figs. 17.14A and B) or septate uterus (Figs. 17.15A to C). At the same

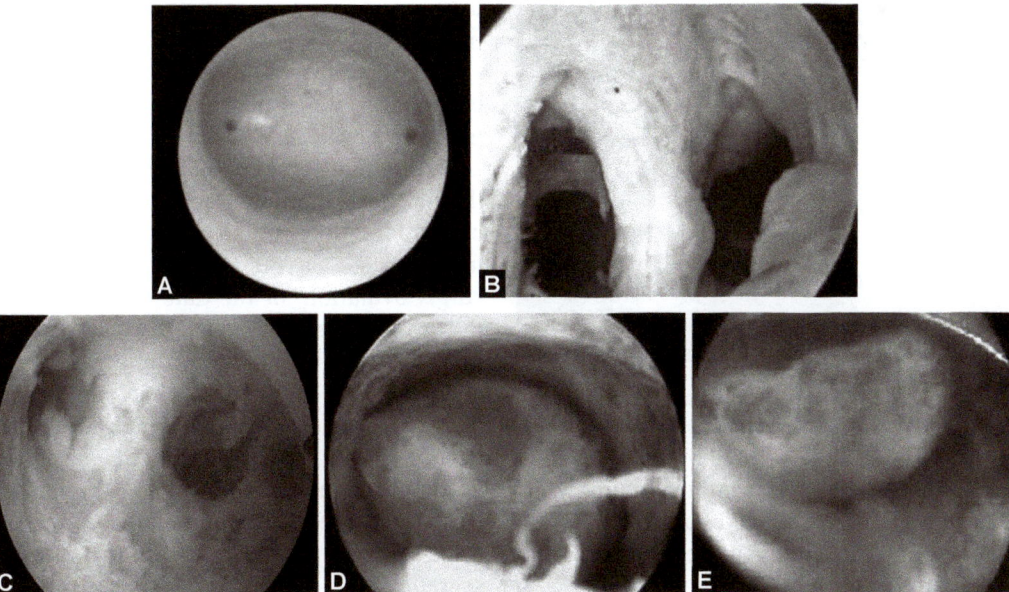

Figs. 17.10A to E: Normal and abnormal hysteroscopy pictures: (A) Normal; (B) Septum; (C) Septum and adhesions; (D) Submucous myoma; (E) Polyp.

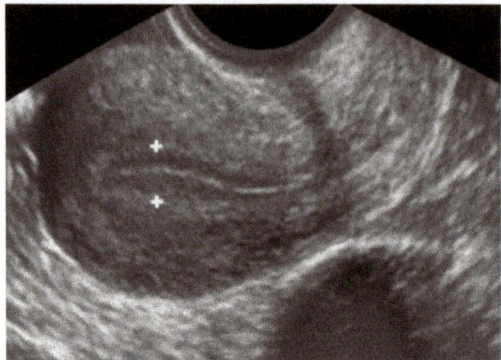

Fig. 17.11: Normal endometrial cavity.

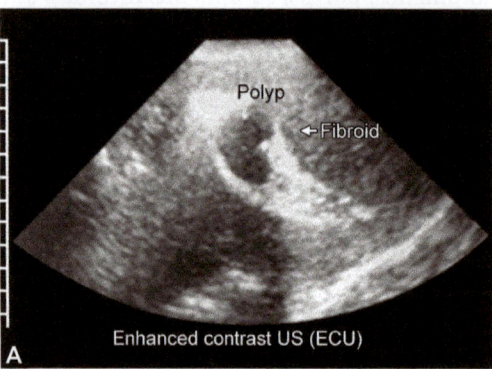

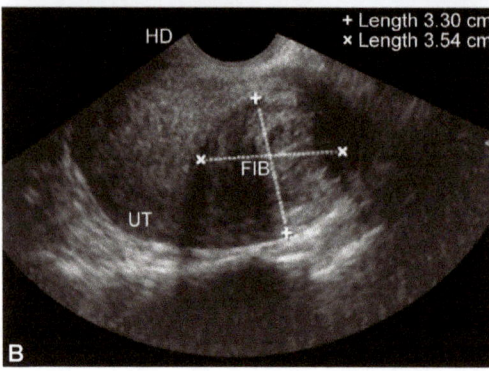

Figs. 17.12A and B: (A) Polyp and submucous myoma; (B) Intramural myoma.

time, information on ovarian volume (Fig. 17.16) and antral follicle counts (Fig. 17.17) can be obtained, making pelvic ultrasound part of the initial work-up for infertility.

A complete cavitary assessment, however, necessitates either sonohysterography for conditions such as uterine polyps, submucus leiomyomas, or Asherman's syndrome (uterine synechiae).[18] Sonohysterography, an office procedure, involves assessing the uterine cavity with ultrasound with concurrent instillation of sterile water. Some practitioners prefer diagnostic office hysteroscopy as it allows direct visualization of the uterine cavity.

Endometrial Biopsy

During the menstrual cycle, the sequential action of estrogen (E) derived from the developing follicle(s) followed by the combined action of E and P on the endometrium after ovulation causes morphological and molecular changes in endometrial cells rendering them receptive to the adhesive and migratory properties of the trophoblast cells of the implanting embryo. Thus, it has long been advocated that the clinical evaluation of the infertile couple includes an evaluation of the quality of the luteal phase. During the luteal phase, the morphological changes observed in the endometrium occur in a predictable pattern.[12]

Traditionally, the endometrium is considered 'out-of-phase' if the standardized menstrual cycle date based on morphological criteria assigned by a pathologist lags by more than 2 days than the 'actual' standardized cycle date determined by a physiological marker such as the urinary or serum LH surge, ovulation, or the date of the onset of the next menstrual cycle. The endometrial biopsy, with evaluation of morphological changes, has been considered superior to alternatives such as serum P measurements, because of the pulsatile nature of P secretion and a belief that these morphological changes better represent the cumulative effect of cycle-specific patterns of ovarian hormone secretion.[19]

The endometrial biopsy has been used for decades in the screening evaluation of the

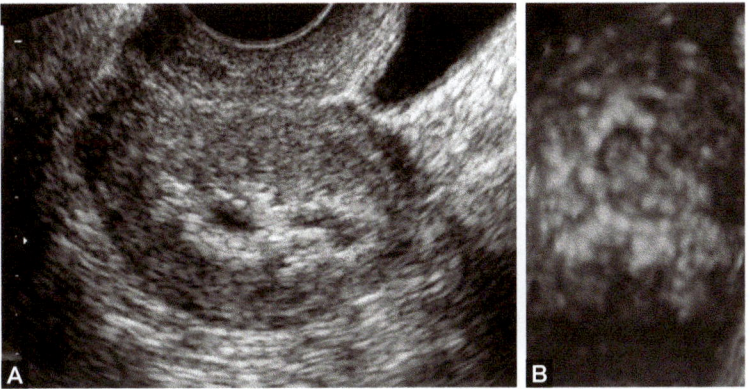

Figs. 17.13A and B: Intrauterine adhesions: (A) 2D image; (B) 3D image.

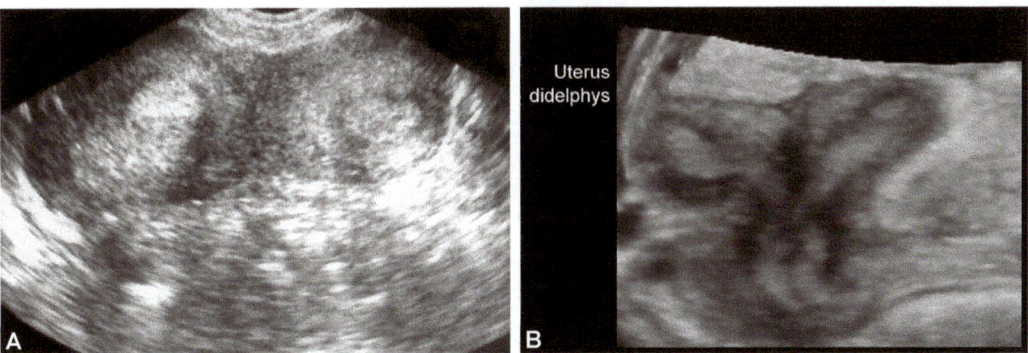

Figs. 17.14A and B: Bicornuate uterus: (A) 2D image; (B) 3D image.

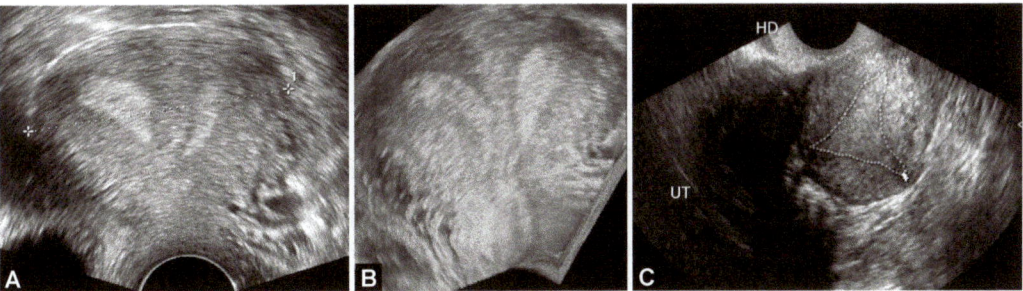

Figs. 17.15A to C: Septate uterus: (A) 2D image; (B) 3D image; (C) Triradiate appearance of endometrium.

infertile couple to confirm ovulation and to also evaluate the histological maturation of the endometrium.

Nevertheless, the surprising fact is that the ability of the histological evaluation of the endometrium to distinguish between women of fertile and infertile couples has not been rigorously ascertained and thus, prescription of treatment based on histological evaluation of the endometrium may be inappropriate.

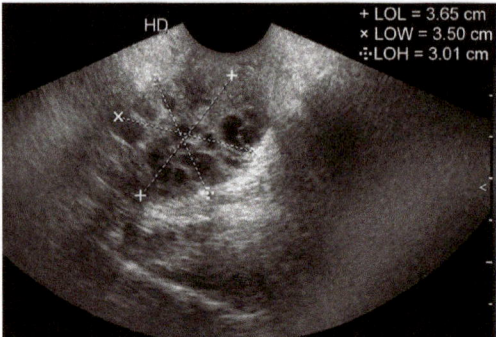

Fig. 17.16: Ovarian volume.

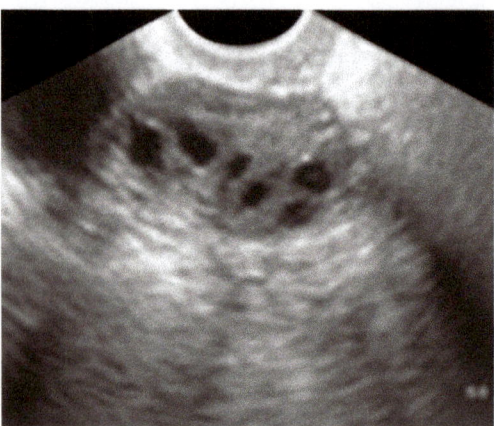

Fig. 17.17: Antral follicle count.

Moreover, the prevalence of 'out-of-phase' biopsies in the fertile population has been reported to range between <5% to as high as 50%, thus making this test difficult to interpret.[20-22]

This high variability of results casts doubt on the validity of the histological dating of the endometrium as a clinical tool for the evaluation of the luteal phase in women of infertile couples. Furthermore, even among those who advocate the routine use of the endometrial biopsy, there is controversy over the optimal timing of the procedure. Today it is indicated only when we suspect genital tuberculosis. Genital TB is always difficult to diagnose, because of the fact that it is a silent invader of the genital tract. The only reliable way of making a diagnosis is by actually culturing the tubercle bacillus from tissue sampled from the genital tract.

Evaluation of Cervical Score and Postcoital Test

It can identify abnormalities of cervical mucus production or sperm/mucus interaction. Examination of cervical mucus may reveal gross evidence of chronic cervicitis that deserves treatment. Previously, the postcoital test (PCT) assessing the sperm motility in a sample of postcoital cervical mucus was considered an integral part of the basic infertility evaluation. However, past investigations revealed a poor correlation between postcoital sperm motility and pregnancy outcome.[23] This is because results are subjective and exhibit high intra- and interobserver variation. In 1995 a blinded, prospective study demonstrated poor reproducibility of the test among trained observers, further questioning the validity of the PCT as a diagnostic tool.[24] Although its utility and predictive value have been seriously questioned,[25] some still consider it a useful diagnostic test.[26] Today, the PCT has been largely abandoned and is reserved for patients in whom results will clearly influence treatment strategy.[2]

Assessment of Ovarian Reserve

Women with advanced age or history of prior ovarian surgery are at risk for diminished ovarian function or reserve. Given the relatively noninvasive nature of the testing, several practitioners are including the evaluation of ovarian reserve as first-line work-up for infertility. The testing includes a cycle day 3 serum follicle-stimulating hormone (FSH) and estradiol level, clomiphene citrate challenge test, and/or an ultrasonographic ovarian antral follicle count.[2] The results of these tests are not absolute indicators of infertility but abnormal levels correlate with decreased response to ovulation induction medications and lowered live birth rates after IVF.

Values for Normal Ovarian Reserve

1. Day 2/3: FSH < 10 mIU/mL
2. Day 2/3: E2 < 75 pg/mL
3. Basal FSH:LH ratio < 1.5
4. Absent intercycle variability in basal FSH
5. P4: Day 10 of COH < 1.1 ng/mL
6. Day 3: Inhibin – B > 45 pg/mL
7. AMH: > 0.35 ng/mL
8. AFC > 4 at baseline scan
9. Ovarian volume > 3 cm^3
10. CC challenge test: Normal values after administration of CC 100 mg Day 5–9
    - Cycle Day 2 or 3 E2 < 65–70 FSH < 10
    - Cycle Day 10 LH < 10 FSH < 12
11. GnRH agonist stimulation test – (GAST): Increase in the E2 levels after administration of GnRh agonist on Day 2
12. Exogenous FSH ovarian reserve test (EFORT): Increment of inhibin B and E2 24 hours after administration of 300 IU of FSH on day 3 of the menstrual cycle.

Specialized Clinical Tests on Semen and Sperm

These tests are not required for routine diagnosis of male infertility. In some cases, semen analyses have failed to accurately predict a man's fertility. Therefore, there has been a search for other tests to improve the evaluation of the infertile male. They may be useful for identifying a male factor contributing to unexplained infertility or for selecting therapy.

Quantitation of leukocytes in semen: An elevated number of white blood cells in the semen has been associated with deficiencies in sperm function and motility. Patients with true pyospermia (greater than 1 million leukocytes per mL) should be evaluated for a genital tract infection or inflammation.

Tests for antisperm antibodies: Pregnancy rates may be reduced by antisperm antibodies (ASA) in the semen.[27]

Antisperm antibodies testing should be considered when there is isolated asthenospermia with normal sperm concentration, sperm agglutination or an abnormal postcoital test or in couples with unexplained infertility.

Many physicians recommend ASA testing for couples with unexplained infertility. ASA found on the surface of sperm by direct testing are more significant than ASA found in the serum or seminal plasma by indirect testing. ASA testing is not needed if sperm are to be used for ICSI.

Testing for antibody-coating of spermatozoa is done for both IgA and IgG. IgA is of greater clinical importance and the screening is performed on fresh semen samples by either:

i. Immunobead test
ii. Mixed antiglobulin reaction (MAR) test

For validity, at least 200 motile sperms must be available for counting. The diagnosis of immunological infertility is possible when 50% or more of motile sperms have adherent particles.

Computer-aided sperm analysis: Computer-aided sperm analysis (CASA) requires sophisticated instruments for quantitative assessment of sperm from a microscopic image or from videotape. CASA can be used to objectively measure sperm numbers, motility and morphology. CASA instruments are most useful clinically for assessing sperm motility and motion parameters, such as velocity or speed and head movement.

Zona-free Hamster Oocyte Test

Removal of the zona pellucida from hamster oocytes allows human sperms to fuse with hamster ova. This test is often termed as a sperm penetration assay (SPA). For penetration to occur, sperm must undergo capacitation, acrosome reaction, fusion with the oolemma, and incorporation into the ooplasm. This test should also be reserved for patients in whom results will influence treatment strategy. False negative results have frequently been recorded. The value of the test results depends, in part, on the experience of the laboratory performing the assay.

Hypo-osmotic Swelling (HOS) Test

These assays determine whether nonmotile sperm are viable by identifying which sperm have intact cell membranes. Nonmotile but viable sperm, as determined by the HOS test, may be used successfully for ICSI.
- Interpretation of HOS
- Normal > 60%—patients may benefit with IUI
- Borderline-50% and 60%: These patients are in the gray zone and may be subjected to IVF if the post wash count is at least 10 million/mL
- Abnormal <50% benefit by ICSI

Surface toxin factor, which immobilizes the sperm is present in HOS negative sperms. In patients with good count and motility but <50% HOS positive sperms, results in fertilization and cleavage, but the surface toxin factor is transferred to the zona pellucida, which prevents implantation and so ICSI is preferred.

Acrosome reaction of human sperm can be detected using specialized staining techniques. Rates of spontaneous acrosome reactions and acrosome reactions induced by agents such as calcium ionophore and progesterone have been measured. Samples from infertile men tend to demonstrate higher spontaneous acrosome reaction levels and lower levels in the presence of inducers.[28]

Test for acrosome intactness: This test is based on the principle that the acrosomal enzyme dissolves protein (e.g. gelatin). This consists of counting at least 200 spermatozoa in different optical fields and determining the incidence of those having halos measuring > 120 um and expressing data as a percentage.

A fertile sample will have > 60% spermatozoa with halos having a diameter of >120 um.

An incidence of < 60% is indicative of acrosomal inadequacy and therefore, the sample is likely to be subfertile.

In Vitro Sperm Nuclear Chromatin Decondensation Test

One of the early events of fertilization following the sperm penetration into the egg is the decondensation of the sperm nuclear chromatin. The test is designed to pick out semen samples containing spermatozoa which are capable of decondensing following penetration of an egg.

A normal, fertile sample will show > 70% spermatozoa whose nuclear chromatin has decondensed.

Sperm Mitochondrial Activity Index (SMAI)

This test estimates the incidence of spermatozoa having a full complement of mitochondria containing respiratory enzymes which are essential for providing energy for the spermatozoa motility. Lack of mitochondrial enzymes impair sperm motility and may thus contribute to subfertility.

SMAI of >50 is characteristic of a fertile semen sample.

SMAI of <50 is characteristic of an infertile semen sample.

Hemizona Binding Assay

The hemizona assay (HZA) measures the binding of capacitated sperm to isolated human zona pellucida. Human oocytes are bisected by micromanipulation, thus, allowing for an internally controlled comparison of sperm binding (from patient versus a fertile control) to match hemizonae surfaces. The two matched hemizona of the human oocytes have the advantage of providing functionally equal surfaces allowing a controlled comparison of sperm binding and therefore, limiting the amounts of oocytes used. The tightly bound spermatozoa on the outer surface of the hemizona are counted. The number of spermatozoa bound to ZP has been shown to correlate with the fertilization rate.[29]

The HZA has been found to be predictive of IVF outcome with positive and negative predictive values of 83% and 95% respectively. The major problem with this assay is the limited availability of human oocytes.

Sperm DNA Fragmentation (SDFA)

The SDFA accurately assesses the level of fragmentation, providing additional clinically significant diagnostic information on the potential of a patient's sperm to achieve pregnancy and eventually produce a live birth. It serves as a tool for measuring important properties of sperm chromatin integrity. TUNEL and Comet assays analyze directly the number of DNA breaks; the sperm chromatin structure assay (SCSA) measures the susceptibility of sperm DNA to breakage after acid treatment using flow cytometry to determine the proportions of spermatozoa having single-strand (abnormal) and double-strand (normal) DNA.

Comet Assay (Figs. 17.18A and B)

Examines DNA structure independent of chromatin folding Healthy DNA in male sperm nuclei resembles bright stars, while defective DNA looks more diffuse and appears to trail comet like tails.

TUNEL Assay (Figs. 17.19A to C)

TUNEL-positive nuclei (with double-strand nuclear DNA fragmentation) of spermatozoa as represented by the intense (A) and dull (B) Texas red fluorescence in the nuclear region.

Healthy nuclei (without DNA fragmentation) are stained blue with DAPI (C) used as counter stain.

Halosperm (Fig. 17.20)

Ready to use kit to determine DNA fragmentation.

DNA Fragmentation Index (DFI) helps in further assessment of fertility in the male despite a normal count.

0–15%	High fertility potential
> 15% and < 30%	Good to fair fertility potential
30% and higher	Low to poor fertility potential

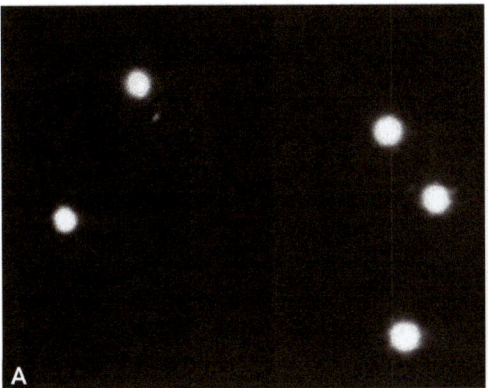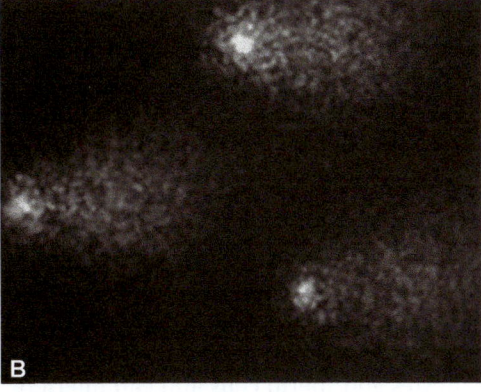

Figs. 17.18A and B: Comet assay.

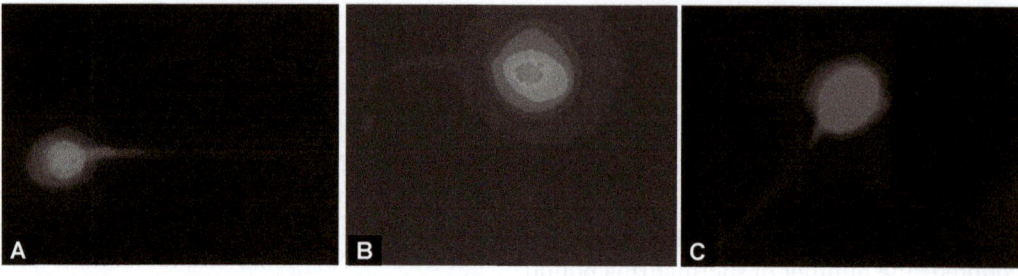

Figs. 17.19A to C: TUNEL assay.

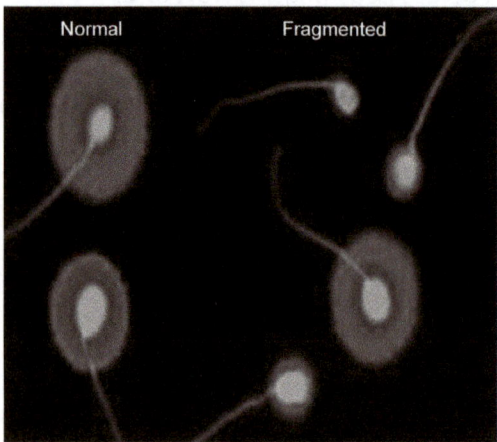

Fig. 17.20: Halosperm.

Summarizing the cut off values for sperm function test is given below:

Test	Fertile
i. HOS test	>60%
ii. Acrosome intactness	>60%
iii. Decondensation test	>70%
iv. Sperm mitochondrial activity index	>50%
v. Hemizona binding assay	
vi. Sperm DNA fragmentation	< 15%

Values for subfertile samples lesser than those shown for the fertile sample.

Biochemical tests of sperm function: These include measurements of sperm creatine kinase[30] and reactive oxygen species (ROS). ROS appear to be generated by both seminal leukocytes and sperm cells and can interfere with sperm function by peroxidation of sperm lipid membranes and creation of toxic fatty acid peroxides.[31]

Thus, these specialized tests on semen are important investigative tools, but are not necessary for the routine evaluation of men with infertility.

But today IVF serves as a best diagnostic test to assess egg quality, sperm-egg interaction, embryo development and quality of embryo.

ESHRE TASK FORCE ON UNEXPLAINED INFERTILITY

According to ESHRE infertility testing should be classified into three groups depending on correlation with pregnancy rates.

I. Tests that have an established association with pregnancy (Figs. 17.21A and B):
   - Conventional semen analysis
   - Tubal patency tests
   - Tests of ovulation.
II. Tests that are not consistently associated with pregnancy (Figs. 17.22A to C):
   - Postcoital test
   - Antisperm antibody tests
   - Zona-free hamster egg penetration test.
III. Tests that have no association with pregnancy (Figs. 17.23A and B):
   - Endometrial biopsy
   - Varicocele assessment
   - Chlamydia testing.

Though we cannot really tell why this group of patients has not conceived, it is possible to draw long-list of subtle causes of

Unexplained Infertility

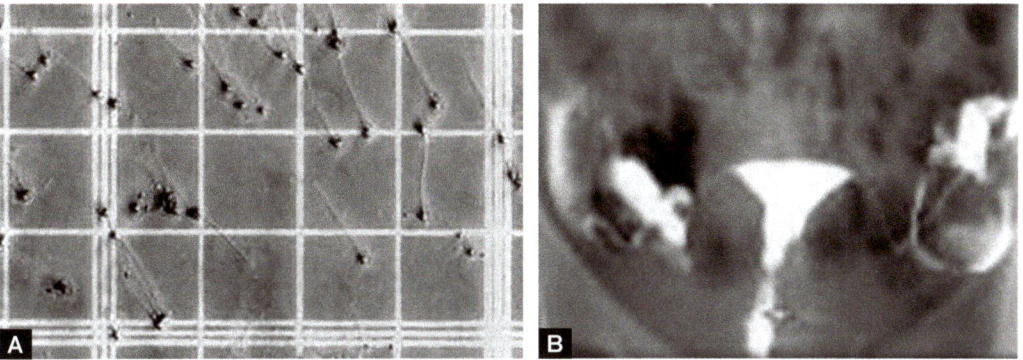

Figs. 17.21A and B: Tests that have an established association with pregnancy.

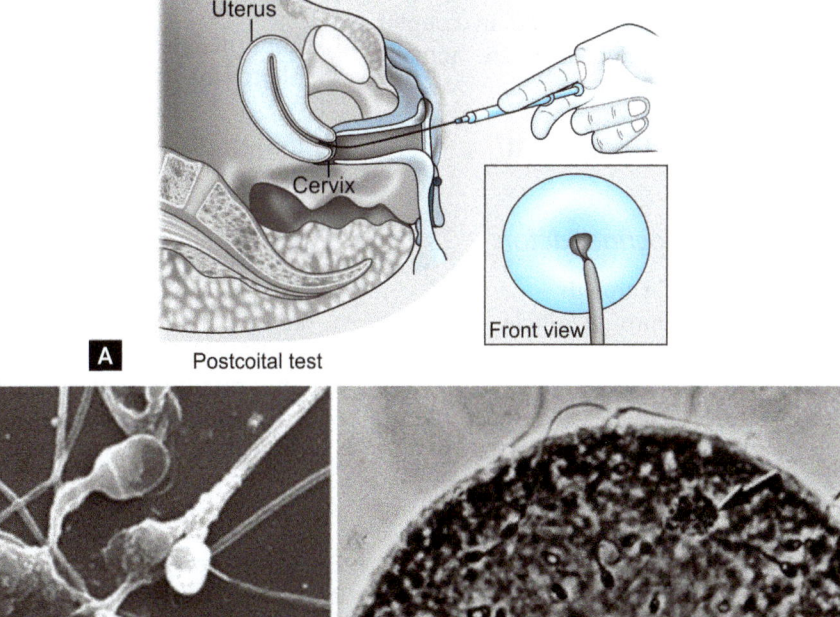

Figs. 17.22A to C: Tests that are not consistently associated with pregnancy.

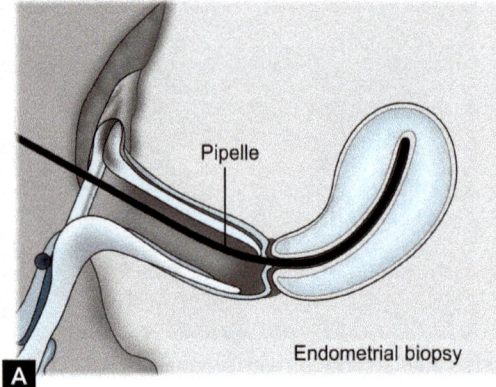
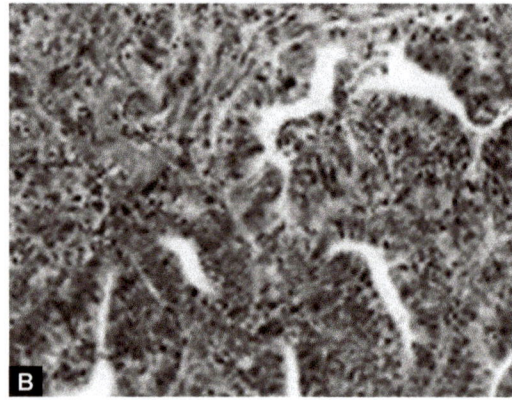

Figs. 17.23A and B: Tests that have no association with pregnancy.

infertility. But many cannot be proven with certainty and have been found in couples of normal fertility. Only few are actually treatable (Balen,1997).

Possible Causes (Identified/Unidentified)

Ovarian and Endocrine Factors

1. Abnormal follicle growth
2. Luteinized unruptured follicle
3. Hypersecretion of LH
4. Hypersecretion of prolactin in the presence of ovulation
5. Reduced growth hormone secretion/sensitivity
6. Cytologic abnormalities in oocytes
7. Genetic abnormalities in oocytes
8. Antibodies to zona pellucida.

Peritoneal Factors

1. Altered macrophage and immune activities
2. Mild endometriosis
3. Antichlamydial antibodies.

Tubal Factors

1. Abnormal peristalsis or cilial activity
2. Altered macrophage and immune activity.

Endometrial Factors

1. Abnormal secretion of endometrial proteins
2. Abnormal integrin/adhesion molecule
3. Abnormal T cell and natural killer cell activity
4. Secretion of embryotoxic factors
5. Abnormalities in uterine perfusion
6. Poor estrogen receptors in endometrial cells.

Cervical Factors

1. Altered cervical mucus
2. Increased cell-mediated immunity.

Embryological Factors

1. Poor quality embryo
2. Reduced progression to blastocyst
3. Abnormal chromosomal complement.

Male Factors

1. Reduction in sperm motility, acrosome reaction, oocyte binding and zona penetration
2. Ultrastructural abnormalities of head, neck.

Psychological

Hormonal cycle with its delicate adjustments, is controlled by brain and emotional disturbances have significant effect on fertility.

Inherited Thrombophilia

It is a risk factor for cardiovascular disease, including deep venous thrombosis,[32] as well as reproductive disorders, including recurrent pregnancy loss[33-35] (and recurrent implantation failure (RIF).[36] Women with a history of RIF after *in vitro* fertilization and embryo transfer displayed a higher prevalence of total gene mutations as well as of the plasminogen activator inhibitor (PAI)-1 4G/4G specific mutation than control women (P¼.007).

Genes that encode for proteins labeled as thrombogenic have been shown to be involved not only in coagulation and fibrinolysis but also in fertilization, embryonic development and tissue remodelling,[37] as well as recurrent implantation failure, recurrent pregnancy loss and congenital abnormalities.[38] Although the mechanisms by which thrombophilic gene mutations impact the frequency of recurrent miscarriage are thought to be related to clotting of placental vessels,[39] and the methods involved in recurrent implantation failure appear to involve the effects of hypofibrinolysis on trophoblast migration,[40,41] the influence on unexplained infertility seems to entail folic acid metabolism.

DIAGNOSIS

Unexplained infertility is a diagnosis of exclusion. To establish the diagnosis of UI, the clinician should consider the following:

1. Was the infertility evaluation complete in terms of modern standard?
2. Were the studies performed correctly?
3. Were the results interpreted appropriately?

Treatment

The treatment for unexplained infertility is therefore, by definition, empiric because it does not address a specific defect or functional impairment.[2] The principal treatment for unexplained infertility include antibiotic treatment, expectant observation with timed intercourse and lifestyle changes, ovulation induction with timed intercourse, clomiphene citrate/aromatase inhibitors and intrauterine insemination (IUI), controlled ovarian hyperstimulation (COH) with IUI and IVF.

The treatment helps to increase the chances of conception and also allows it to happen more quickly. Once obvious causes of infertility have been excluded, the treatment of couples with unexplained infertility is the same.

Aim of the treatment is to increase the monthly pregnancy rate above the natural rate of 1.5–3% by improving gamete quality, increasing gamete numbers and facilitating gamete interaction.

Selection of Treatment Option

- Duration of infertility
- Woman's age
- How extensive was the evaluation?
- Estimated chance of success
- Cost involved
- Risk and side effects of each method
- Couples own preference.

But generally the treatment should follow an orderly progression of intensity and expense. It has been seen that 75% of couples with unexplained infertility will conceive after this treatment. One could offer expectant therapy for 6 to 12 months if the women is < 35 years and is trying to conceive for about 2 years. Aggressive therapy is indicated if the women is > 35 years or is trying to conceive for >2 years (Soules, 2000).

TREATMENT MODALITIES

In the absence of a correctable abnormality, the therapy for unexplained infertility is, by default, empiric. Proposed treatment regimens include intrauterine insemination (IUI), ovulation induction with oral or injectable medications, combination of IUI with ovulation induction and assisted reproductive technologies (ARTs).

Antibiotic Therapy

A course of doxycycline for both partners is effective for most cases of pyospermia, cervicitis and/or endometritis.

Expectant Management and Lifestyle Changes

Epidemiological studies indicate cigarette smoking, abnormal body mass index (BMI), and excessive caffeine and alcohol consumption reduce fertility in the female partner. The female partner should be counseled to achieve a normal BMI, reduce caffeine intake to no more than 250 mg daily (2 cups of coffee), and reduce alcohol intake to no more than 4 standardized drinks per week.[42]

The likelihood of pregnancy without treatment among couples with unexplained infertility is less than that of fertile couples but greater than zero. It is possible that unexplained infertility represents the lower extreme of the normal distribution of fertility with no defect present. However, the routine infertility evaluation misses subtle defects because of imperfect or incomplete testing methods. Studies of couples with unexplained infertility who are followed without any treatment report, a broad variation in cumulative pregnancy rates. A retrospective review of 45 studies by Guzick and colleagues found an average cycle fecundity of 1.3-4.1% in the untreated groups, which was lower than most treatment interventions.[43]

The currently available evidence suggests that methods prospectively identifying the window of fertility are likely to be more effective for optimally timing intercourse than calendar calculations or BBT. Although expectant management is associated with the lowest cost, it results in the lowest cycle fecundity rates, and is therefore inferior to the commonly available reproductive techniques. It may provide an option for a couple with unexplained infertility in whom the female partner is young and the problem of oocyte depletion is not an immediate concern.

The spontaneous monthly fecundity rate in unexplained infertility is 1.3%. It was also observed that 60% will conceive spontaneously after 3 years (Gordon & Sperof, 2002) and 80% will conceive after 5 years (Randolph, 2000).

The duration of infertility is important. The longer the infertility, the less likely the couple is to conceive on their own. After 5 years of infertility, a couple with unexplained infertility has less than a 10% chance for success on their own.

One study showed that for couples with unexplained infertility and over 3 years of trying on their own, the cumulative pregnancy rate after 24 months of attempting conception without any treatment was 28%. This number was found to be reduced by 10% for each year that the female is over 31.[44]

Unfortunately, it is not yet possible to predict which couples will conceive spontaneously or in what time frame and so active management will help in hastening the occurrence of pregnancy.

Ovulation Induction

The underlying principle for superovulation in women with unexplained infertility, who by definition have regular ovulatory menstrual cycles, is to augment the probability of pregnancy by increasing the number of oocytes on hand for fertilization. The goal is to prevail over a possible flaw in ovulatory function that is not uncovered by conformist testing. When used in conjunction with IUI to increase the density of motile sperm available to these oocytes, the likelihood of pregnancy may be further increased.

Clomiphene Citrate

It can be given for a maximum of six cycles. Three to six months of treatment with clomiphene citrate might improve fertility by as much as 2 times as compared to no treatment. This is a very low level infertility treatment. Clomiphene citrate corrects subtle defect in ovarian function which includes both follicular development and luteal phase defect. It also increases the number of follicles that develop and consequently oocytes that are released improving the pregnancy rate. Although there is a small increase in fecundity, the low cost and ease of administration makes Clomiphene citrate a sensible first choice treatment.

Clomiphene citrate is administered from D2/3 of spontaneous or induced menstrual cycle for a period of 5 days. The starting dose of clomiphene citrate is 50 mg or 100 mg depending on the weight of the women. The clomiphene dose may be increased progressively up to a maximum of 200 mg/day for 5 days. Fewer than 50% of hyporeacting patients will ovulate at that dose. Approximately 50% of normal women ovulate with a dose of 50 mg, and an additional 20% will ovulate with 100 mg/day, the overall ovulation rate ranging from 70–85%. Clomiphene induces an increase in gonadotropins on days 5-9 of the cycle, i.e. when the follicle is selected. Follicular maturation beginning at that time is characterized by the development of a preovulatory follicle, the elevation of circulating estrogens, a preovulatory surge of LH and discharge of LH leading to ovulation with high postovulatory levels of progesterone. Approximately 50% of normal women ovulate with a dose of 50 mg, and an additional 20% will ovulate with 100 mg/day, the overall ovulation rate ranging from 70–85%.[45]

Only 40–50% of ovulatory patients become pregnant. The discrepancy observed between the ovulation index and the fecundity index could be due to many factors. These include the coexistence of a male factor, the existence of other causes of infertility or an antiestrogenic effect of clomiphene on some effectors of the reproductive tract.[46, 47]

This effect is known to arise in cervical mucus and its interaction with spermatozoa, in tubal transport of ova, and in the function and synchronization of the endometrium (Palomino et al., 1998). At times there also could be an abnormal endocrine response in the form of elevated LH levels from D9 resulting in premature luteinization. The efficacy of clomiphene citrate therapy increases with close monitoring by USG, mid-follicular LH levels and PCT.

Treatment is discontinued if 2 consecutive cycles anovulatory or the women fails to conceive despite six ovulatory cycles.

Adverse Effects[107]

Adverse effects include multiple pregnancies in up to 6–8% of cases; most of these are twins, but triplets have been reported in 1%, quadruplets in 0.3% and quintuplets in 0.1% of clomiphene-induced pregnancies.[48]

Furthermore, there is a 23% rate of missed abortions, probably associated with early resumption of oocytic meiosis due to hypersecretion of LH. Ovarian hyperstimulation syndrome is observed in 13% of cases treated with clomiphene but it is usually mild. Other minor effects include visual disorders, flushes, nausea and breast discomfort. Although earlier studies implied that CC was associated with increased ovarian cancer risk after 12 cycles of treatment use, more recent studies have observed no increased ovarian cancer risk related to the use of ovulation-inducing drugs.[49,50]

On the basis of these initial studies (Rossing et al., 1994), the United Kingdom Committee for Medical Safety recommended the use of clomiphene for 6 consecutive cycles only because none of the unexplained infertility trials offers evidence that ovulation stimulation is effective after six cycles.

Letrozole

The new third generation aromatase inhibitors are extremely potent and specific oral inhibitors of estrogen production. Letrozole is an oral, reversible, nonsteroidal aromatase inhibitor.

Mechanism of Action

Inhibition of aromatization will block estrogen production from all sources and release the hypothalamic/pituitary axis from estrogenic negative feedback resulting in increased GnRH and gonadotropin secretion. The resultant increase in gonadotropin secretion will stimulate growth of ovarian follicles. Withdrawal of estrogen centrally also increases activins, which are produced by a wide variety of tissues including the pituitary gland and will stimulate synthesis of FSH by a direct action on the gonadotropes.[51-54]

There is also increased follicular sensitivity to FSH. This could result from temporary accumulation of intraovarian androgens because conversion of androgen substrate to estrogen is blocked by aromatase inhibition.[55] Also, androgen accumulation in the follicle stimulates IGF-I, which may synergize with FSH to promote folliculogenesis.[56-59]

Aromatase inhibition, with suppression of estrogen concentrations in the circulation and peripheral target tissues, results in upregulation of ERs in the endometrium, leading to rapid endometrial growth once estrogen secretion is restored. Estrogen has been shown to decrease the level of its own receptor by stimulating ubiquitination of ERs, resulting in rapid degradation of the receptors. In the absence of estrogen, ubiquitination is decreased allowing upregulation of the ER and increasing sensitivity to subsequent estrogen administration. This could increase endometrial sensitivity to estrogen resulting in more rapid proliferation of endometrial epithelium and stroma and improved blood flow to the uterus and endometrium. As a result, normal endometrial development and thickness should occur by the time of follicular maturation, even in the face of the observed lower-than-normal estradiol concentrations in AI-treated cycles.[60, 61]

The selective nonsteroidal AIs have a relatively short half-life (45 h), compared with CC, and would be ideal for this purpose because they are eliminated from the body rapidly. Because AIs do not deplete ERs, as does CC, normal central feedback mechanisms remain intact. As the dominant follicle grows and estrogen levels rise, normal negative feedback occurs centrally, resulting in suppression of FSH and atresia of the smaller growing follicles. A single dominant follicle, and mono-ovulation, should occur in most cases.[62,63]

Dose

Based on current data, it is likely that the optimal dose of letrozole for a 5-day course of treatment is between 2.5 and 5.0 mg, with higher doses resulting in persistence of aromatase inhibition and estrogen levels too low for normal endometrial development by the time of ovulation.[64] A study using 7.5 mg letrozole from cycle D 3 to 7 showed, for the first time, showed thinning of the endometrium similar to CC.[65] El Helw et al. for the first time compared 20 mg letrozole as a single dose on D3 with 100 mg CC from D3-7. In letrozole group he reported a higher PR (18.2% vs 11.5%).

Side Effects

Aromatase inhibitors are generally well tolerated. It has been seen that there are fewer side effects such as hot flushes and premenstrual syndrome-type symptoms with AIs, compared with CC.

Advantages

The rapid clearance of the aromatase inhibitors (AIs), the reversible nature of enzyme inhibition, and elevated levels of FSH, which induces new expression of aromatase enzyme, are factors that limit accumulation of androgens and likely result in increasing estrogen production that should be relatively normal at the time of ovulation. When used in IVF fertilizable oocytes with normal embryo development were observed.[66-69]

There is improved implantation and pregnancy rate by amelioration of deleterious effects of supraphysiological levels of estrogen during ovarian stimulation. More over a letrozole induced cycle requires minimal monitoring and there is a very low incidence of ovarian hyperstimulation syndrome.

Pregnancy Outcome with AIs

- Ovulation rate: 75%
- PR: 17-20%

Pregnancies conceived after AI treatment was associated with comparable miscarriage and ectopic pregnancy rates, compared with all other groups including the spontaneous conceptions. In addition, letrozole use was associated with a significantly lower rate of multiple gestation, compared with CC (4.3% vs. 22%, respectively), consistent with our hypothesis of an intact negative feedback loop centrally with aromatase inhibition.

AIs plus Gonadotropins

Reducing FSH dose required for optimum controlled ovarian hyperstimulation: Combining an AI with FSH injection reduced the dose of FSH required to achieve optimum controlled ovarian stimulation (COH), without adverse antiestrogenic effects.

There was also a significant reduction in the FSH dose required (from 45% to 55%) with a consequent reduction in the cost of treatment cycle.[70-74]

Gonadotropins

Less extensively studied, but it has been observed that an empiric gonadotropin therapy is an effective therapy for unexplained infertility, especially when combined with IUI.[75] Both cycle fecundity and pregnancy rate per patient were superior when gonadotropin therapy plus IUI was compared with expectant management.[76] Gonadotropins induce multiple follicular development, correct subtle ovulatory defects, improve cervical mucus quality and determine ovulation correctly.

Per cycle pregnancy rate was reported as 7.7% for gonadotropin alone. In a review of 27 studies involving 2,939 cycles, the pregnancy rate per cycle was 8% with gonadotropin treatment alone and 18% when IUI was added to gonadotropin stimulation.[75]

Adverse Effects

Gonadotropin therapy is associated with multiple pregnancy and ovarian hyperstimulation syndrome. In a large multicenter trial in the United States, 33% of live births were multiple pregnancies (3 quadruplet, 4 triplet, and 17 twin pregnancies delivered as 5 triplet births and 19 twin births among the 72 live births).[77] Severe ovarian hyperstimulation occurred in 1.3% (6 of 465 women in the FSH treatment groups required hospitalization).

Artificial Insemination (IUI)

Sperm preparation techniques enhance fertilizing ability of sperm, increases the density of motile sperms and corrects occult seminal defects. It also overcomes subtle unrecognized fertility defects and bypasses the cervical barrier.

When IUI was compared with intercourse, each was performed 40 hours after the detection of a rise in serum LH conceptions occurred in 6 of 145 (4.1%) IUI cycles and 3 of 123 (2.4%) intercourse cycles.[78]

The spontaneous monthly fecundity rate for IUI alone is 3.8%[75] to 7.4%.[79] There is a significant but small effect of IUI therapy.

In the Cochrane review published[80] it was seen that there is no evidence that fallopian tube sperm perfusion (FSP) results in higher pregnancy rates in couples suffering from nontubal subfertility as compared to IUI.

Adverse events after IUI treatment with prepared sperm are reported infrequently.

Controlled Ovarian Hyperstimulation (COH) and Artificial Insemination (IUI)

The IUI is a commonly used treatment strategy for couples with unexplained infertility. Data have indicated a significantly higher live birth rate with IUI plus ovarian stimulation than with IUI alone for unexplained infertility (OR 2.07, 95% CI 1.22–3.50) (Verhulst et al., 2006).[81] IUI brings together multiple oocytes and highly motile sperms in the fallopian tube increasing the likelihood of pregnancy. It is an effective, simple, less invasive, less stressful and cost-effective treatment option for unexplained infertility.

The use of ovarian stimulation in combination with IUI is a controversial and heavily debated topic.[82-84]

Biologically, the use of ovarian stimulation increases the likelihood of a multiple pregnancy because the development of multiple dominant follicles and ovulation of multiple oocytes. A recent systematic literature review of studies of controlled ovarian stimulation and IUI clearly demonstrated that multiple pregnancy rates correlated positively with the number of preovulatory follicles.[85]

Clomiphene Citrate and IUI

In a literature review of eight studies involving 932 cycles, the cycle fecundity rates were 5.6% with CC and 8.3% with CC/IUI.[43]

Although it is logical that two effective treatments would have greater value when combined, the data on CC/IUI are contradictory and the reported effects are compromised by crossover designs and unequal loss to follow-up. The combination of CC with IUI may be useful, but the current evidence indicates only that CC/IUI should be evaluated in a four-arm factorial trial (placebo, CC, IUI, and CC/IUI) with adequate power.

Based on the Deaton et al. trial, the effect of CC/IUI treatment is one additional pregnancy in 16 CC/IUI cycles (95% CI, 9 to 165) compared with untreated control cycles.[86] In 1991, Kirby and colleagues reported a RCT of 73 couples with unexplained infertility who were either randomized to IUI or timed intercourse.[87] Conceptions occurred in 6 of 145 (4.1%) of the IUI cycles and 3 of 123 (2.4%) of the timed intercourse cycles. A large RCT showed that intracervical insemination alone had lower pregnancy rates per couple compared with IUI alone.[88] It has been estimated that 37 cycles of IUI without additional ovarian stimulation would be needed to obtain an additional pregnancy compared with control cycles.[2] A recent Cochrane review on this topic confirmed that IUI with ovulation induction increased the live birth rate compared with IUI alone.[89]

Gonadotropins with IUI

A meta-analysis of 27 studies involving 2939 cycles revealed that the pregnancy rate per cycle was 8% with gonadotropin treatment alone and 18% with gonadotropin treatment combined with IUI.[43] The cumulative pregnancy rate rises with the number of attempted COH/IUI cycles; however, there is some evidence suggesting that the number of COH/IUI cycles prior to treatment with IVF should be limited to 3.[90]

Aboulghar and colleagues performed an observational prospective study on 594 couples with unexplained infertility to determine the optimum number of COH/IUI cycles. They found that 1 to 3 cycles of COH/IUI resulted in 182 pregnancies, with a cycle fecundity of 16.4% and a cumulative pregnancy rate (PR) of 39.2% (total of 1112 cycles with a mean of 1.9 cycles/patient).[90] Up to 3 further trials of COH/IUI in 91 of these women resulted in only 9 more pregnancies, with a cycle fecundity of 5.6%, significantly lower than that in the first 3 attempts (additional 161 cycles with a mean of 1.8 cycles/patient). The cumulative PR rose to 48.5% by cycle 6, a further increase of only 9.3%. A historical comparison group with 131 patients with 3 failed cycles of COH/IUI who underwent 1 cycle of IVF at the same center resulted in 48 pregnancies, with a cycle fecundity of 36.6% per cycle, suggesting that patients should be offered IVF if they fail to conceive after 3 trials of COH and IUI.

In one randomized clinical trial, gonadotropin/IUI was found superior to CC/IUI (cycle fecundity 0.19 vs. 0.04, P = 0.04).[91] The addition of a GnRH agonist to the gonadotropin treatment regimen does not appear to improve fertility.[92]

A systematic review of five randomized controlled trials compared oral (anti-estrogens) and injectable (gonadotropins) drugs for stimulated IUI in couples with unexplained fertility problems and found no significant difference in live birth rates per couple although the pregnancy rate seemed to be higher with gonadotropins.[93] Hence, oral agents may be more suitable for ovarian stimulation, and they are not far from achieving the goals of the procedure.

Single Versus Double IUI

Although some studies suggested marginal benefits of double IUI over single, the most recent randomized trial concluded that among patients undergoing COH/IUI, results of single and double IUI do not statistically differ.[94] Therefore, double IUI is not routinely offered.

Assisted Reproductive Technology

The most expensive but also most successful treatment of unexplained infertility consists of the spectrum of assisted reproductive technology including IVF with or without ICSI. IVF is the treatment of choice for unexplained infertility when the less costly, but also less successful treatment modalities outlined above have failed. ART is advocated by many clinicians based on evidence from retrospective and/or uncontrolled trials. In the Centers for Disease Control and Prevention (CDC), the American Society for Reproductive Medicine (ASRM), and the Society for Assisted Reproductive Technology (SART) report live birth rate among women with unexplained infertility was 30.4%.[95]

In addition to offering the highest success rate, IVF also explains infertility in some of these couples. In some IVF programs ICSI is performed in all couples with unexplained infertility (for an undetected fertilization problem), whereas other programs may perform ICSI in 50% of the retrieved oocytes. There were also publications which showed no advantage to the use of intracytoplasmic sperm injection (ICSI) over conventional fertilization when ART is used for the treatment of unexplained infertility.[96,97]

No differences in live birth rates were demonstrated with IVF or IUI either with (OR 1.15, 95% CI 0.55–2.4) or without (OR 1.96, 95% CI 0.88–4.4) ovarian stimulation in a Cochrane meta-analysis of clinical trials of unexplained infertility.[98]

The ICSI is associated with a significantly lower rate of complete fertilization failure in cases of unexplained infertility than conventional IVF (0.8% versus 19.2%; P, 0.001).[99] However, data from three randomized controlled trials indicate that clinical pregnancy rates are similar following IVF or ICSI: 11% and 28%, respectively, per oocyte retrieval (P ¼ 0.09);[99] 32% and 38% (RR 0.83, 95% CI 0.48–1.45);[100] and 50% for both [not significant (P-value not provided)].[101]

The ICSI would be recommended in patients of unexplained infertility to increase pregnancy rates.

Rationales

1. To increase the number and quality of oocytes available for fertilization.
2. To facilitate the sperm-oocyte interaction and enhance fertilization.
3. To document the occurrence of fertilization, and to evaluate embryo quality.

Cycle Fecundity Rate

- IVF: 25.7% (ESHRE)
- ICSI: 36.2–44.3% (ESHRE)

Moreover, ICSI can also give a clue to the cause of infertility:
- Abnormal eggs
- Abnormal zona pellucida
- Low fertilization rate per egg
- Slow embryo development
- Excessive fragmentation of embryo.

There is no clear evidence that routine administration of peri-implantation glucocorticoids in ART cycles improves the clinical outcome in a non-selected IVF/ ICSI population.[102] This was published by the effectiveness of IVF relative to other treatment options for unexplained infertility remains unproven. Adverse events and the costs associated with the interventions compared have not been adequately assessed. Until more evidence is available IVF may not be the preferred first line of treatment for these couples and it might be appropriate to continue with less invasive options.[103]

Adverse Effects

In vitro firtilization (IVF) is associated with multiple gestation pregnancy, ovarian hyperstimulation and increased pregnancy losses.[104] Multiple pregnancy in the 1996 ASRM/SART report accounted for 38.9% of all IVF/ICSI births, comprising 31.8%, 6.5% and 0.6% twins, triplets and quadruplets, respectively.[105] Ovarian hyperstimulation occurs in approximately 5% of cycles.[106] Preterm delivery rates,[107] ectopic pregnancy rates (5%) and spontaneous abortions (25%) are also higher in part because of multiple pregnancies).[107,108]

Oil Soluble HSG

Tubal flushing with oily media could represent a simple, less invasive and economic alternative to IVF for couples where the woman has normal patent fallopian tubes. It is associated with increased cycle fecundity when compared with water soluble dye.[109]

Comparison of Different Treatments for Unexplained Infertility

A randomized trial comparing each of these treatment alternatives against one another and a nontreated control group has not been performed. The European Society for Human Reproduction and Embryology (ESHRE) Multicenter trial reported in 1991 that pregnancy rates per cycle were 15.2% in gonadotropin-only cycles, 27.4% in gonadotropin and IUI cycles, and 25.7% in IVF cycles.[104] In another trial, live birth rates per cycle initiated in the unexplained subgroup were 6.0% in IUI only cycles, 8.7% in gonadotropin and IUI cycles, and 13.0% in IVF cycles.[79] However, after six cycles, the cumulative success rates associated with IUI, stimulated IUI, and IVF were similar because few couples continued through six cycles of stimulated IUI or IVF treatment, even though the cost of these cycles was not borne by the patients. In a review of unexplained infertility studies, the average cycle fecundity in the untreated control groups was 1.8% in 11 nonrandomized studies and 3.8% in six randomized studies.

The pregnancy rate for IVF cycles has since increased with availability of improved and sequential media, embryo micromanipulation, and extended embryo culture. Depending on the individual couple and their particular clinical situation, COH with IUI may be attempted first, with transition to IVF/ICSI if pregnancy is not achieved in a timely manner.

NICE GUIDELINES : UNEXPLAINED INFERTILITY

The guideline of National Institute for Health and Care Excellence (NICE) on fertility suggests some treatment options regarding unexplained infertility. The age of women and infertility duration are important factors in offering specific therapy to a couple. Expectant management for 2 years is the best choice for good prognosis when the woman's age is less than 30 years. This includes active medical intervention which requires the females to be aware of their ovulation time and the best period for unprotected intercourse. The main advantage of expectant management is avoiding multiple gestations which are accompanied with obstetric and prenatal complications, postnatal disability and the considerable burden on healthcare system can not be neglected in this regard. If the long period of expectant management cannot lead to pregnancy, ovulation induction by clomiphene and letrozole is not effective for these couples. Also insemination cycles without ovarian stimulation (COH) will have little benefit for them. COH/IUI (3-4 cycles) are effective in women under 35, but COH/IUI increase the risk of multiple gestations. However, COH/IUI is ineffective for couples with long duration of infertility.

Couples over 35 years and couples with long duration of infertility are suitable candidates for IVF. In comparison with COH/IUI, IVF shortens time to pregnancy and reduces the risk of multiple pregnancies. Failed fertilization is reported in 8.4–22.7% of IVF cycles for couples with unexplained infertility; therefore, many clinics offer routine ICSI for these couples. It may result in an increase in the costs for each take home baby. However, several studies suggested split IVF/ICSI would be the best option for these couples since its cumulative pregnancy rates are higher than conventional IVF and the costs are less than those in ICSI.

Prognosis of unexplained infertility and its response to above procedures is quite agreeable. However, some problems such as the limited number of these options and high dependence of specialist and couples on ART should not let the physicians offer additional expensive and experimental tests which waste the golden time of couples for pregnancy without any effective results.

SUMMARY AND CONCLUSION

Couples with unexplained infertility suffer from both diminished and delayed fecundity, compared with the normal fertile couples. In the absence of a correctable abnormality, the therapy for unexplained infertility is, by default, empiric. Proposed treatment regimens include intrauterine insemination (IUI), superovulation with oral or injectable medications, combinations of IUI with superovulation and the assisted reproductive technologies (ARTs).

When considering treatment options for couples with unexplained infertility, it is prudent to consider simple treatment before complex treatment and to balance what is known about effectiveness against the cost and adverse effects of different treatments. Diagnosis is made only after the basic infertility evaluation fails to reveal an obvious abnormality.

The basic evaluation should provide evidence of ovulation, adequate sperm production and fallopian tube patency. It remains unclear whether the basic infertility assessment should also test for antisperm antibodies, adequate cervical mucus production, timely development of secretory phase endometrial responses, presence of adhesions and evidence of pelvic endometriosis.

The treatment effects with non-ART treatment for unexplained infertility generally are small. Empiric treatment may do no more than hasten conception in those couples who would conceive eventually without treatment. Level I evidence from randomized clinical trials supports short-term use of IUI, CC, gonadotropins and IUI and ART treatment for unexplained infertility but is insufficient for conclusions regarding CC/IUI treatment. ART therapies are considerably more costly than CC and IUI.

Pregnancy rates are lower with increasing age of the female partner and duration of infertility.

There is a need for appropriately designed controlled trials to evaluate these empiric therapies because conception may occur without therapy.

Pregnancy rates per cycle for comparisons of different treatment modalities should be considered as some interventions, e.g. timed intercourse or natural cycle IUI may be less costly or time-consuming and associated with less patient discomfort and fewer complications.

In summary, evaluation of disease characteristics can help clinicians to select the most appropriate active therapeutic option, thus allowing basic tailoring of treatment modality to the individual.

A better effort should be undertaken to develop reliable tools to diagnose, often undiagnosed conditions like endometriosis, tubal disease, premature ovarian ageing and immunological infertility at the basic evaluation. These may be often misdiagnosed for unexplained infertility if advanced testing is not done. Even the best and most accurate diagnostic approach will leave some patients without a specific diagnosis. Providing information, detailed counseling and education on realistic pregnancy rates are of great value to plan a systemic approach for treatment of this group of patients.

REFERENCES

1. Crosignani PG, Collins J, Cooke ID, et al. The recommendations of the ESHRE workshop on 'Unexplained Infertility'. Human Reproduction. 1993;8(6):977-80.
2. The Practice Committee of the American Society for Reproductive Medicine. Optimal evaluation of the infertile female. Fertil Steril. 2006;86(5 Suppl):S264-67.
3. World Health Organization. WHO laboratory manual for the examination of human semen and sperm-cervical mucus interaction, 2nd edition. New York: Cambridge University Press, 1987.
4. World Health Organization. WHO laboratory manual for the examination of human semen and sperm-cervical mucus interaction, 3rd edition. New York: Cambridge University Press, 1992.

5. Kruger TF, Acosta AA, Simmons KF, et al. Predictive value of abnormal sperm morphology in in vitro fertilization. Fertil Steril. 1988;49:112-7.
6. Exacoustos C, Zupi E, Carusotti C, et al. Hysterosalpingo-contrast sonography compared with hysterosalpingography and laparoscopic dye pertubation to evaluate tubal patency. J Am Assoc Gynecol Laparosc. 2003;10:367-72.
7. Luciano AA, Peluso J, Koch EI, et al. Temporal relationship and reliability of clinical, hormonal, and ultrasonographic indices of ovulation in infertile women. Obstet Gynecol. 1990;75:412-6.
8. Wilcox AJ, Weinberg CR, Baird DD. Timing of sexual intercourse in relation to ovulation. Effects on the probability of conception, survival of the pregnancy, and sex of the baby. N Engl J Med. 1995;333:1517-21.
9. Luciano AA, Peluso J, Koch EI, et al. Temporal relationship and reliability of clinical, hormonal, and ultrasonographic indices of ovulation in infertile women. Obstet Gynecol. 1990;75:412-6.
10. Wathen NC, Perry L, Lilford RJ, et al. Interpretation of single progesterone measurement in diagnosis of anovulation and defective luteal phase: observations on analysis of the normal range. Br Med J. 1984;288:7-9.
11. Jordan J, Craig K, Clifton DK, et al. Luteal phase defect: the sensitivity and specificity of diagnostic methods in common clinical use. Fertil Steril. 1994;62:54-62.
12. Noyes RW, Hertig AW, Rock J. Dating the endometrial biopsy. Fertil Steril. 1950;1:3-9.
13. Shoupe D, Mishell DR Jr, Lacarra M, et al. Correlation of endometrial maturation with four methods of estimating day of ovulation. Obstet Gynecol. 1989;73:88-92.
14. Li T-C, Dockery P, Rogers AW, et al. How precise is histologic dating of endometrium using the standard dating criteria? Fertil Steril. 1989;51:759-63.
15. Batista MC, Cartledge TP, Merino MJ, et al. Midluteal phase endometrial biopsy does not accurately predict luteal function. Fertil Steril. 1993;59:294-300.
16. Coutifaris C, Myers ER, Guzick DS, et al. Histological dating of timed endometrial biopsy tissue is not related to fertility status. Fertil Steril. 2004;82:1264-72.
17. de Crespigny LC, O'Herlihy C, Robinson HP. Ultrasonic observation of the mechanism of human ovulation. Am J Obstet Gynecol. 1981;139:636-9.
18. Roma Dalfó A, Ubeda B, Ubeda A, et al. Diagnostic value of hysterosalpingography in the detection of intrauterine abnormalities: a comparison with hysteroscopy. AJR Am J Roentgenol. 2004;183:1405-09.
19. Wentz AC. Endometrial biopsy in the evaluation of infertility. Fertil Steril. 1980;33:121-4.
20. Hecht BR, Bardawil WA, Khan-Dawood FS, et al. Luteal insufficiency: correlation between endometrial dating and integrated progesterone output in clomiphene citrate-induced cycles. Am J Obstet Gynecol. 1990;163:1986.
21. Davis OK, Berkeley AS, Naus GJ, et al. The incidence of luteal phase defect in normal, fertile women, determined by serial endometrial biopsies. Fertil Steril. 1989;51:582-6.
22. Li T-C, Dockery P, Rogers AW, et al. A quantitative study of endometrial development in the luteal phase: comparison between women with unexplained infertility and normal fertility. Br J Obstet Gynaecol. 1990;97:576-82.
23. Collins JA, So Y, Wilson EH, et al. The postcoital test as a predictor of pregnancy among 355 infertile couples. Fertil Steril. 1984;41:703-8.
24. Glatstein IZ, Best CL, Palumbo A, et al. The reproducibility of the postcoital test: a prospective study. Obstet Gynecol. 1995;85:396-400.
25. Oei SG, Helmerhorst FM, Bloemenkamp KW, et al. Effectiveness of the postcoital test: randomised controlled trial. BMJ. 1998;317:502-5.
26. Glatstein IZ, Harlow BL, Hornstein MD. Practice patterns among reproductive endocrinologists: further aspects of the infertility evaluation. Fertil Steril. 1998;70:263-9.
27. Ayvaliotis B, Bronson R, Rosenfeld D, et al. Conception rates in couples where

autoimmunity to sperm is detected. Fertil Steril. 1985;43:739-42.
28. Fenichel P, Donzeau M, Farahifar D, et al. Dynamics of human sperm acrosome reaction: relation with in vitro fertilization. Fertil Steril. 1991;55:994-9.
29. Liu, DY, Lopata, A , Johnston, WI, et al. Human spermzona pellucida binding, sperm characteristics and in-vitro fertilization. Hum Reprod. 1989;4:696-701.
30. Huszar G, Vigue L, Morshedi M. Sperm creatine phosphokinase Misoform ratios and fertilizing potential of men: a blinded study of 84 couples treated with in vitro fertilization. Fertil Steril. 1992;57:882-8.
31. Kim JG, Parthasarathy S. Oxidation and the spermatozoa. Semin Reprod Endocrinol. 1998;16:235-9.
32. Sartori MT, Danesin C, Saggiorata G, et al. The PAI-1 gene 4G/4G polymorphisms in deep vein thrombosis in patients with inherited thrombophilia. Clin Appl Thromb Hemost. 2003;9:299-307.
33. Coulam CB, Jeyendran RS, Fishel LA, et al. Multiple thrombophilic gene mutations rather than specific gene mutations are risk factors for recurrent miscarriage. Am J Reprod Immunol. 2006;55:360-8.
34. Goodman CS, Coulam CB, Jeyendran RS, et al. Which thrombophilic gene mutations are risk factors for recurrent pregnancy loss? Am J Reprod Immunol. 2006;56:230-6.
35. Coulam CB, Wallis D, Weinstein J, et al. Comparison of thrombophilic gene mutations among patients experiencing recurrent miscarriage and deep vein thrombosis. Am J Reprod Immunol. 2008;60:426-31.
36. Coulam CB, Jeyendran RS, Fishel LA, et al. Multiple thrombophilic gene mutations are risk factors for implantation failure. Reprod Biomed Online. 2006;12:322-7.
37. Rawlins ND, Barrett AJ. Evolutionary families of peptidases. Biochem J. 1993;290:205-18.
38. Botto LD, Yang Q. 5,10-methylenetrtrahydrofolate reductase gene variants and congenital anomalies: a HuGE review. Am J Epidemiol. 2000;151:862-77.
39. Many A, Schrieber L, Rosner S, et al. Pathologic features of the placenta in women with severe pregnancy complications and thrombophilia. Obstet Gynecol. 2001;98:1041-4.
40. Aflalo ED, Sod-Moriah UA, Potashnik G, et al. Differences in the implantation rates of rat embryos developed in vivo and in vitro: possible role for plasminogen activators. Fertil Steril. 2004;81:780-5.
41. Axelrod HR. Altered trophoblast functions in implantation-defective mouse embryos. Dev Biol. 1985;108:185-90.
42. Barbieri RL. The initial fertility consultation: recommendations concerning cigarette smoking, body mass index, and alcohol and caffeine consumption. Am J Obstet Gynecol. 2001;185:1168-73.
43. Guzick DS, Sullivan MW, Adamson GD, et al. Efficacy of treatment for unexplained infertility. Fertil Steril. 1998;70:207-13.
44. Collins JA, Burrows EA, Willan AR. The prognosis for live birth among untreated infertile couples. Fertil Steril. 1995;64:22-28.
45. Imani B, Eijkemans MJC, Te Velde ER, et al. Predictors of patients remaining anovulatory during clomiphene citrate induction in normogonadotropic oligomenorrheic infertility. J Clin End Metab. 1998;83:2361-5.
46. Dickey RP, Olar TT, Taylor SN, et al. Relationship of endometrial thickness and pattern of fecundity in ovulation cycles: effect of clomiphene citrate alone and with human menopausal gonadotropin. Fertil Steril. 1993;59:756-60.
47. Eden JA, Place J, Carter GD, et al. The effect of clomiphene citrate on follicular phase increase in endometrial thickness and uterine volume. Obstet Gynecol. 1989;73:187-90.
48. Tarlatzis B, Grimbizis G. Future use of clomiphene in ovarian stimulation. Will clomiphene persist in the 21st century? Hum Reprod. 1998;13:2356-8.
49. Rossing MA, Tang MT, Flagg EW, et al. A case-control study of ovarian cancer in relation to infertility and the use of ovulation-inducing drugs. Am J Epidemiol. 2004;160:1070-8.
50. Brinton LA, Lamb EJ, Moghissi KS, et al. Ovarian cancer risk after the use of ovulation-stimulating drugs. Obstet Gynecol. 2004;103:1194-203.
51. Kamat A, Hinshelwood MM, Murry BA, et al. Mechanisms in tissue-specific regulation of estrogen biosynthesis in humans. Trends Endocrinol Metab. 2002;133:122-8.

52. Naftolin F, MacLusky NJ. Aromatization hypothesis revisited. In: Serio M (Ed). Differentiation: basic and clinical aspects. New York: Raven Press 1984;79-91.
53. Naftolin F, MacLusky NJ, Leranth CZ, et al. The cellular effects of estrogens on neuroendocrine tissues. J Steroid Biochem. 1988;30:195-7.
54. Naftolin F. Brain aromatization of androgens. J Reprod Med. 1994;39:257-61.
55. Weil SJ, Vendola K, Zhou J, et al. Androgen receptor gene expression in the primate ovary: cellular localization, regulation, and functional correlations. J Clin Endocrinol Metab. 1988;837:2479-85.
56. Vendola K, Zhou J, Wang J, et al. Androgens promote oocyte insulin-like growth factor I expression and initiation of follicle development in the primate ovary. Biol Reprod. 1999;612:353-7.
57. Adashi E. Intraovarian regulation the proposed role of insulin-like growth factors. Ann NY Acad Sci. 1993;687:10-2.
58. Giudice LC. Insulin-like growth factors and ovarian follicular development. Endocr Rev. 1993;13:641-69.
59. Yen SSC, Laughlin GA, Morales AJ. Interface between extra-and intra-ovarian factors in polycystic ovary syndrome PCOS. Ann NY Acad Science. 1993;687:98-111.
60. Nirmala PB, Thampan RV. Ubiquitination of the rat uterine estrogen receptor: dependence on estradiol. Biochem Biophys Res Commun. 1995;213:24-31.
61. Rosenfeld CR, Roy T, Cox BE. Mechanisms modulating estrogen-induced uterine vasodilation. Vascul Pharmacol. 2002;382: 115-25.
62. Sioufi A, Gauducheau N, Pineau V, et al. Absolute bioavailability of letrozole in healthy postmenopausal women. Biopharm Drug Dispos. 1997;18:779-89.
63. Sioufi A, Sandrenan N, Godbillon J, et al. Comparative bioavailability of letrozole under fed and fasting conditions in 12 healthy subjects after a 25 mg single oral administration. Biopharm Drug Dispos. 1997;186:489-97.
64. Al-Omari WR, Sulaiman WR, Al-Hadithi N. Comparison of two AIs in women with clomiphene-resistant polycystic ovary syndrome. Int J Gynaecol Obstet 2004;853:289-91.
65. Al-Fozan H, Al-Khadouri M, Tan SL, et al. A randomized trial of letrozole versus clomiphene citrate in women undergoing superovulation. Fertil Steril. 2004;82:1561-63. [Abstract]
66. Rabinovici J, Blankstein J, Goldman B, et al. In vitro fertilization and primary embryonic cleavage are possible in 17-hydroxylase deficiency despite extremely low intrafollicular 17ß-estradiol. J Clin Endocrinol Metab. 1989;68:693-97. [Abstract].
67. Schoot DC, Coelingh Bennink HJ, Mannaerts BM, et al. Human recombinant FSH induced growth of preovulatory follicles without concomitant increase in androgen and estrogen biosynthesis in a woman with isolated GT deficiency. J Clin Endocrinol Metab. 1992;74:1471-73. [Abstract].
68. Shoham Z, Mannaerts B, Insler V, et al. Induction of follicular growth using recombinant human follicle-stimulating hormone in two volunteer women with hypogonadotropic hypogonadism. Fertil Steril. 1993;59:738-42 [Medline].
69. Mitwally MF, Biljan MM, Casper RF. Pregnancy outcome after the use of an AI for induction of ovulation. Am J Obstet Gynecol. 2005;192:381-6.
70. Mitwally MFM, Casper RF. Aromatase inhibition improves ovarian response to follicle-stimulating hormone in poor responders. Fertil Steril. 2002;774:776-80.
71. Mitwally MF, Casper RF. 2003 Aromatase inhibition reduces gonadotrophin dose required for controlled ovarian stimulation in women with unexplained infertility. Hum Reprod. 2003;188:1588-97.
72. Mitwally MF, Casper RF. Aromatase inhibition reduces the dose of gonadotropin required for controlled ovarian hyperstimulation. J Soc Gynecol Investig. 2004;11:406-15.
73. Biljan MM, Tan SL, Tulandi T. Prospective randomized trial comparing the effects of 2.5 and 5.0 mg of letrozole (LE) on follicular development, endometrial thickness and pregnancy rate in patients undergoing superovulation. Fertil Steril. 2002;78:S55.
74. Healey S, Tan SL, Tulandi T, et al. Effects of letrozole on superovulation with

gonadotropins in women undergoing intrauterine insemination. Fertil Steril. 2003;806:1325-9.
75. Guzick DS, Sullivan MW, Adamson GD, et al. Efficacy of treatment for unexplained infertility. Fertil Steril. 1998;70:207-13.
76. Aboulghar MA, Mansour RT, Serour GI, et al. Ovarian superstimulation and intrauterine insemination for the treatment of unexplained infertility. Fertil Steril. 1993;60:303-6.
77. Guzick DS, Carson SA, Coutifaris C, et al. Efficacy of superovulation and intrauterine insemination in the treatment of infertility. National Cooperative Reproductive Medicine Network. N Engl J Med. 1999;340:177-83.
78. Kirby CA, Flaherty SP, Godfrey BM, et al. A prospective trial of intrauterine insemination of motile spermatozoa versus timed intercourse. Fertil Steril. 1991;56:102-7.
79. Goverde AJ, McDonnell J, Vermeiden JP, et al. Intrauterine insemination or in vitro fertilisation in idiopathic subfertility and male subfertility: a randomised trial and cost-effectiveness analysis. Lancet 2000;355:13-8.
80. Cantineau AEP, Cohlen BJ, Heineman MJ. Intra-uterine insemination versus fallopian tube sperm perfusion for non-tubal infertility. Cochrane Database Syst Rev. 2013;(10).
81. Verhulst SM, Cohlen BJ, Hughes E, et al. Intrauterine insemination for unexplained subfertility. Cochrane Database Syst Rev. 2006;CD001838.
82. Fauser B, Devroey P, Macklon N. Multiple birth resulting from ovarian stimulation for subfertility treatment. The Lancet. 9473(365):1807-16.
83. Goverde AJ, Lambalk CB, McDonnell J, et al. Further considerations on natural or mild hyperstimulation cycles for intrauterine insemination treatment: effects on pregnancy and multiple pregnancy rates. Human Reproduction. 2005;20(11):3141-6.
84. Van Rumste MME, den Hartog JE, Dumoulin JCM, et al. Is controlled ovarian stimulation in intrauterine insemination an acceptable therapy in couples with unexplained non-conception in the perspective of multiple pregnancies? Hum Reprod. 2006;21(11):2941-47.
85. Van Rumste MME, den Hartog JE, Dumoulin JCM, et al. Is controlled ovarian stimulation in intrauterine insemination an acceptable therapy in couples with unexplained non-conception in the perspective of multiple pregnancies? Hum Reprod. Update, 2008;14(6):563-70.
86. Deaton JL, Gibson M, Blackmer KM, et al. A randomized, controlled trial of clomiphene citrate and intrauterine insemination in couples with unexplained infertility or surgically corrected endometriosis. Fertil Steril. 1990;54:1083-8.
87. Kirby CA, Flaherty SP, Godfrey BM, et al. A prospective trial of intrauterine insemination of motile spermatozoa versus timed intercourse. Fertil Steril. 1991;56:102-7.
88. Guzick DS, Carson SA, Coutifaris C, et al. Efficacy of superovulation and intrauterine insemination in the treatment of infertility. National Cooperative Reproductive Medicine Network. N Engl J Med. 1999;340:177-83.
89. Verhulst SM, Cohlen BJ, Hughes E, et al. Intrauterine insemination for unexplained subfertility. Cochrane Database Syst Rev. 2006;CD001838.
90. Aboulghar M, Mansour R, Serour G, et al. Controlled ovarian hyperstimulation and intrauterine insemination for treatment of unexplained infertility should be limited to a maximum of three trials. Fertil Steril. 2001;75:88-91.
91. Karlstrom PO, Bergh T, Lundkvist O. A prospective randomized trial of artificial insemination versus intercourse in cycles stimulated with human menopausal gonadotropin or clomiphene citrate. Fertil Steril. 1993;59:554-9.
92. Sengoku K, Tamate K, Takaoka Y, et al. A randomized prospective study of gonadotrophin with or without gonadotrophin-releasing hormone agonist for treatment of unexplained infertility. Hum Reprod. 1994;9:1043-7.
93. Athaullah N, Proctor M, Johnson NP. Oral versus injectable ovulation induction agents for unexplained subfertility. Cochrane Database Syst Rev. 2002;3:CD003052.
94. Alborzi S, Motazedian S, Parsanezhad ME, et al. Comparison of the effectiveness of single intrauterine insemination (IUI) versus double IUI per cycle in infertile patients. Fertil Steril. 2003;80:595-9.

95. Assisted Reproductive Technology Success rates. National Summary and Fertility Clinic Reports 2003. Accessed June 12, 2006.
96. Bhattacharya S, Hamilton MP, Shaaban M, et al. Conventional in vitro fertilisation versus intracytoplasmic sperm injection for the treatment of non-male-factor infertility: a randomised controlled trial. Lancet. 2001;357:2075-9.
97. Poehl M, Holagschwandtner M, Bichler K, et al. IVF-patients with nonmale factor "to ICSI" or "not to ICSI" that is the question? J Assist Reprod Genet. 2001;18:205-8.
98. Zabeena Pandian, Allan Templeton, Gamal Serour Siladitya Bhattacharya. Number of embryos for transfer after IVF and ICSI: a Cochrane review. Human Reproduction. 2005;20(10):2681-87.
99. Kamal Jaroudi, Saad Al-Hassan, Hamad Al-Sufayan, et al. Intracytoplasmic sperm injection and conventional in vitro fertilization are complementary techniques in management of unexplained infertility. Journal of Assisted Reproduction and Genetics. 2003;20(9):377-81.
100. Bhattacharya S, Hamilton MP, Shaaban M, et al. Conventional in vitro fertilisation versus intracytoplasmic sperm injection for the treatment of non-male-factor infertility: a randomised controlled trial. Lancet. 2001;357:2075-9.
101. Shu C Foong, Judy A Fleetham, Joseph A O'Keane, et al. Greene, A prospective randomized trial of conventional in vitro fertilization versus intracytoplasmic sperm injection in unexplained infertility. J Assist Reprod Genetics. 2006;23(3):137-40.
102. Boomsma CM, Keay SD, Macklon NS. Peri-implantation glucocorticoid administration for assisted reproductive technology cycles in a Cochrane review in 2007.
103. Pandian Z, Bhattacharya S, Vale L, et al. In vitro fertilisation for unexplained subfertility. Cochrane review (Review) 2005.
104. Crosignani PG, Walters DE, Soliani A. The ESHRE multicentre trial on the treatment of unexplained infertility: a preliminary report. European Society of Human Reproduction and Embryology. Hum Reprod. 1991;6:953-8.
105. Society for Assisted Reproductive Technology. The American Society for Reproductive Medicine. Assisted Reproductive Technology in the United States: 1996 results generated from the American Society for Reproductive Medicine/Society for Assisted Reproductive Technology Registry. Fertil Steril. 1999;71:798-807.
106. Navot D, Bergh PA, Laufer N. Ovarian hyperstimulation in novel reproductive technologies: prevention and treatment. Fertil Steril. 1992;58:249-61.
107. Schenker JG, Ezra Y. Complications of assisted reproduction techniques. Fertil Steril. 1994;61:411-22.
108. The American Fertility Society, Society for Assisted Reproductive Technology. Assisted reproductive technology in the United States and Canada: 1992 results generated from The American Fertility Society/Society for Assisted Reproductive Technology Registry. Fertil Steril. 1994;62:1121-8.
109. Johnson N, Vanderkerchove P, Lilford R, et al. Tubal flushing for subfertility. Mol BWJ Cochrane, 2007.

CHAPTER 18

Intrauterine Insemination: At a Glance

Sarat Battina, Madhupriya

Chapter outline

- Pre-intrauterine Insemination Workup
- Various Insemination Techniques
  - Intravaginal Insemination
  - Intracervical Insemination
  - Intrafallopian Insemination
  - Intraperitoneal Insemination
- Intrauterine Insemination Procedure
  - Patient Selection for IUI
  - Center Selection for IUI
  - Steps Involved in Artificial Insemination (AI) Techniques
  - Different Methods for Extraction of Sperm from Seminal Plasma
  - Success Rates of IUI
- Complications of IUI
- RCOG Guidelines on OHSS
- Artificial Insemination of Donor
  - Indications for Use of Donor Semen for IUI
  - Instructions to Prospective Sperm Donor
- Semen Cryopreservation
  - Technique of Cryopreservation of Human Sperm
  - Technique of Human Sperm Thawing
- IUI Procedure Steps at a Glance
- Single versus Dual IUI Treatment Cycles
- IUI–One of the Fertility Options for HIV Patients/HIV Discordant Couple

INTRODUCTION

Intrauterine insemination (IUI) is the least invasive, effective, relatively simple, cheap, first line assisted conception treatment method for infertility couples wherein the washed semen with good sperm quality are inseminated into the uterine cavity of the female partner at the time of ovulation (Fig. 18.1).

Historically, the first successful pregnancy was reported at the end of 18th century when John Hunter advised a man with hypospadias to inject his seminal fluid into his wife's vagina with a syringe that resulted in normal pregnancy.

The first reported case of donor insemination was by Williams Pankhurst in 1884 in Philadelphia, USA.

PRE-INTRAUTERINE INSEMINATION WORKUP

A pre-IUI workup for any couple being considered for IUI should include:
- Thorough clinical history of both partners
- Thorough physical examination of both partners
- Semen sample of male partner for semen analysis,
- Mixed antiglobulin reaction (MAR) test to check for presence or absence of antisperm antibodies

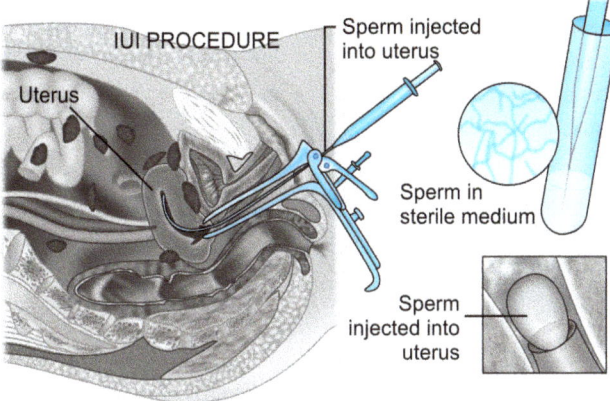

Fig. 18.1: Intrauterine insemination.

- Confirmation of ovulation in female partner by:
  - Follicular Ultrasonography (USG) study
  - Day 21 P2 assay
- Confirmation of tubal patency by:
  - Hysterosalpingogram (HSG)
  - Laparoscopic chromopertubation
  - Hysterosalpingo-contrast-sonography (HyCoSy)
- Ruling out uterine anomalies/cavity abnormalities.

Optional workups

Screen for human immunodeficiency virus (HIV), hepatitis B surface antigen (HBSAG) and heptitis C virus (HCV) in both partners.

Immunity to German measles (Rubella) in both partners.

As careful selection of patients is very important, pre-IUI workup is necessary. Young women with patent fallopian tubes, with no ovulatory disorder, no endometriosis of moderate or severe degree and no severe degree of male factor infertility in their partner are the most benefited.

All couples require indepth advice and counseling about the method and its effectiveness.

VARIOUS INSEMINATION TECHNIQUES

Intravaginal Insemination (IVI)

- Very rarely performed
- Useful in—couples with regularly ovulating female partner
  - Male partner with inability to ejaculate into wife's vagina but can ejaculate by other means (masturbation/penile vibrator) and sperm count or quality are good.

Timing of IVI

- Precise timing is important; to be timed to occur around ovulation
- Is performed about 24 hours after the surge
- Success rates around 5% to 10% per treatment.

Intracervical Insemination (ICI)

- Useful if
  - Female partner does not ovulate regularly and needs to take fertility drugs

- Cycle monitoring by USG/hormones is important to check development of follicles or lining of the endometrium
- Sperm of good count or quality
- No cervical mucus hostility.

Timing of ICI

- When leading follicle measures 18 mm or more, endometrium is well-developed, human chorionic gonadotropin (hCG) injection is given
- Insemination is usually performed about 36 to 44 hours later
- Success rates about 5% to 10% per treatment cycle.

Intrafallopian Insemination (IFI)

- Uncommon
- More invasive
- Steps of treatment are similar to IUI till insemination
- During insemination, for IFI washed sperms is injected into one fallopian tube using a special plastic catheter.

Intraperitoneal Insemination

For intraperitoneal insemination (IPI), washed sperm is injected through top of vagina into peritoneal cavity next to the entrance of fallopian tubes using special needle. Procedure is usually performed under USG guidance. Among the insemination techniques, Cochrane data base systemic review 2008, supports the use of IUI rather than ICI in stimulated cycles.

"Cervical insemination vs intrauterine insemination of donor sperm for subfertility"—A study by Kremer JA, O' Brein, 2000. The study also showed that IUI after 6 cycles significantly improved live birth rates (OR 1.98; 95% CI) and pregnancy rates (OR 3.37; 95% CI) in comparison to cervical insemination.

INTRAUTERINE INSEMINATION PROCEDURE

Patient Selection for IUI

Careful selection of patients for IUI is the cornerstone for achieving good success rates. As inappropriate application of this treatment to the whole of infertile population will obscure its efficacy, patient selection is very important.

IUI with Husband's Semen—Indications

- Ejaculatory failure
- Cervical factor
- Male subfertility
- Immunological
- Idiopathic infertility
- Combined infertility
- Anatomical defects
- Viscous/frozen semen
- Adhesiolysis
- Polycystic Ovary (PCO)
- HIV discordant couple.

Contraindications to IUI

- Bilateral tubal block/tubal infection
- Severe pelvic inflammatory disease
- Severe oligoasthenoteratozoospermia
- Recent pelvic surgery or irradiation
- Failed IUI for more than 6 to 12 times.

Center Selection for IUI

As per the proposed guidelines for assisted reproductive technology (ART) in India, an IUI center has to reach level 2 facility which must have infrastructure for further in depth investigation and advanced treatments of infertility except where oocytes are handled outside the body. The IUI center must have the facilities listed further:

For Investigations

- Immunological tests for infertility
- Sperm function tests
- Assessment of transvaginal sonography (TVS)/follicular growth
- Hysteroscopy/laparoscopy/TV scan.

For Treatment

- Facilities for semen preparation and IUI
- Provision for semen collection on men with a vibrator or electroejaculation
- Conservative surgery either through a hysteroscope, laparoscope or a laparotomy.

Components of an IUI Service in an IUI Center

List of equipments (Fig. 18.2)—Basic:
- Laminar airflow unit
- Sperm counting chambers
- Microscopy
- Incubator
- Centrifuge

Optional:
- Semen analyzer
- Semen freezer
- Semen storage container
- Warmer.

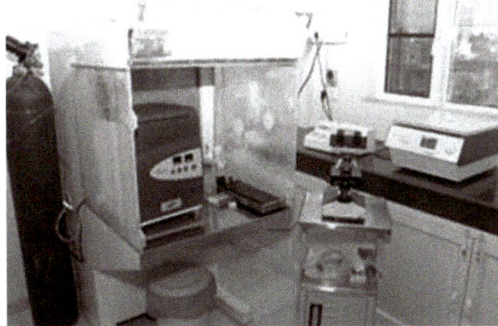

Fig. 18.2: Suggested plan for placing various equipments according to different room dimensions.

Steps Involved in Artificial Insemination (AI) Techniques

1. Proper patient selection
2. Ovarian stimulation
3. Follicular/endometrial thickness (ET) monitoring
4. Timing of insemination
5. Sperm washing and preparation.

Ovarian Stimulation

- AI can be performed either in a unstimulated natural cycle or in a stimulated cycle
- Stimulated cycle involves ovarian stimulation with clomiphene citrate +/- follicle-stimulating hormone (FSH) +/- human menopausal gonodotropin (HMG) (either separately or in combination)
- There is evidence that IUI with ovarian stimulation results in higher success rates than IUI only
- The benefits of increased pregnancy rates and live birth rates achieved with ovarian stimulation must be balanced against the increased cost of fertility drugs, cost of cycle monitoring and potential complications such as multiple pregnancy and ovarian hyperstimulation syndrome.

Follicular/ET Monitoring

- Monitoring of the cycle is essential in stimulated cycles to rule out possibility of ovarian hyperstimulation syndrome (OHSS)/ high order multiple pregnancy
- If more than 4 mature follicles develop, most infertility clinics prefer to either withhold hCG injection or abandon the cycle or abstain from intercourse. Alternatively, the treatment cycle can be converted to in vitro fertilization (IVF) or gamete intrafallopian transfer (GIFT) as appropriate
- Monitoring of follicular development and endometrium is hence done by ultrasound

scans with or without blood hormones tests
- As the dominant follicle reaches >18 mm diameter and endometrium is well-developed, hCG injection is given to time insemination.

Timing of Insemination

- Precise timing of insemination is very important to fetch higher success rates
- IUI is done either when ovulation is imminent or just after
- Methods useful to time insemination in natural cycles are:
  - Ultrasound scans (Most reliable)
  - Detection of luteinizing hormone (LH) surge in urine/blood (Most accurate)
  - Cervical mucus assessment (Not very reliable)
  - Basal body temperature (Least accurate)
- Insemination is usually performed at 24 to 48 hours after urine LH surge
- For stimulated cycles, insemination is usually performed about 40 hours after hCG injection.

Sperm Washing and Preparation

- Male partner produces semen by masturbation or frozen thawed semen is used
- In cases of retrograde ejaculation, sperms are collected from voided urine by centrifugation
- Only washed and prepared sperm are used for IUI because neat semen may cause severe uterine contractions/pains/cramps and even collapse sometimes.
- Aim of washing and preparing sperm
  - Separate sperm from seminal plasma
  - Remove bacteria, other debris and chemicals that may cause infection and irritation
  - To improve sperm capacitation.

Different Methods for Extraction of Sperm from Seminal Plasma

Swim-up Technique (Figs. 18.3A and B)

- Most common
- Convenient method
- Separates good motile sperms by allowing them to swim-up into a large layer of sterile culture medium
- Procedure involves layering sterile culture medium over liquefied semen
- Sperm swim-up into culture medium. Upper part of layered culture medium is removed and centrifuged and pellet is resuspended in a clean sterile medium.

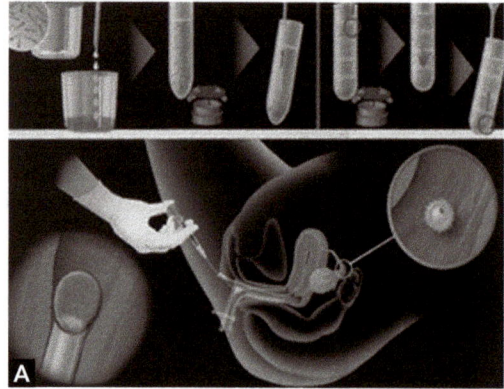

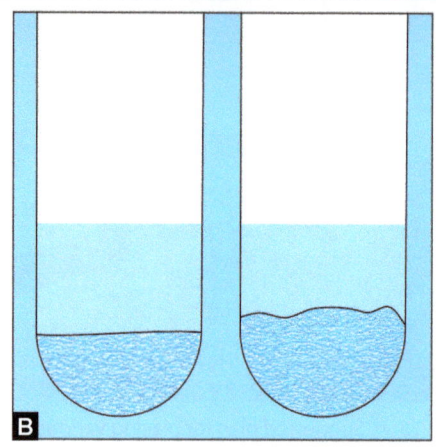

Figs. 18.3A and B: Swim-up technique.

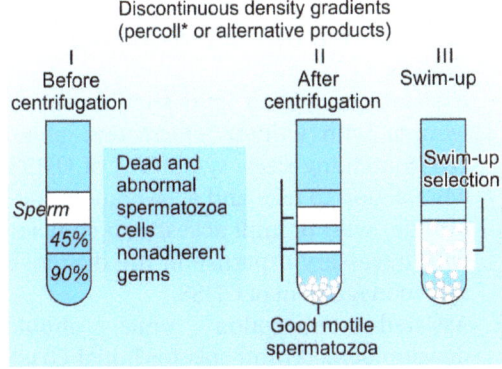

Fig. 18.4: Density gradient technique.
* Percoll is a low viscosity density gradient.

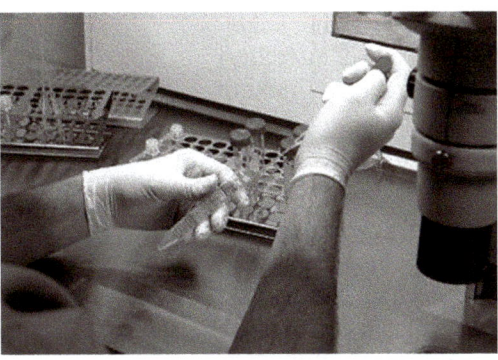

Fig. 18.5: Sperm preparation in progress.

Density Gradient Technique (Fig. 18.4)

- Separates normal live sperm from seminal plasma and other cells and debris
- Procedure involves pipetting semen sample on top of a density gradient column (a layer of fluid containing particles that act as filter) and then centrifuged
- Normal sperm becomes concentrated at the bottom of the layer and can then be removed and washed by centrifugation and resuspension in clean medium.

Wash and Centrifugation

- The procedure involves diluting semen sample with a sterile culture medium (Fig. 18.5) and centrifuge. Following which the pellet is resuspended in culture medium and incubated.
- As per the Cochrane data base, there is no evidence that one technique is superior to other although the trend suggests density gradient is the best.
- Presence of one million motile sperms after preparation seems to provide a realistic cutoff below which pregnancy rates are decreased.
- Morphology of sperm is also important and if the proportion of normal sperm falls below 4%, pregnancy is rarely achieved.
- "Progressive total motile sperm count correlates with pregnancy outcome after IUI" – OWDA, Miller DC, University of Michigan School of Medicine.
- The results of the study have demonstrated that the PTMS count independently predict success with IUI. Alternatives to IUI should be considered for couples when PTMS count is less than 10 million.

Success Rates of IUI

Success rate of insemination varies considerably between infertility clinics and in same clinic between different couples.

Success rate between 5% and 30%, and depend on many factors like:
- Cause of infertility
- *Endometriosis*: Patient with severe endometriosis are not suitable for IUI because of very low success
- *Male factor infertility*: Unstimulated IUI – increases pregnancy rates by 2-fold
- *Stimulated IUI*: increases pregnancy rates by 5-fold
- Unexplained infertility
- Tubal/ovulation factor

- Female partner's age
- Duration of infertility
- Sperm quality/quantity
- Cycle rank.

Complications of IUI

- Failure of treatment
- Possibility of using wrong semen sample
- Infection/bleeding/trauma/pain
- Noninfective salphingitis/allergic reactions
- Antisperm antibodies
- Multiple pregnancy
- Abortion/ectopic pregnancy
- OHSS.

RCOG Guidelines on OHSS

Ovarian hyperstimulation syndrome (OHSS) is a systemic disease resulting from vasoactive products released by hyperstimulated ovaries (Fig. 18.6). The pathophysiology of OHSS is characterized by increased capillary permeability leading to leakage of fluid from vascular compartment with third space fluid accumulation and intravascular dehydration.

- Clinicians need to be aware of the symptoms and signs of OHSS as the diagnosis is based on clinical criteria
- Women with OHSS should have the severity of their condition assessed and documented as an aid to management

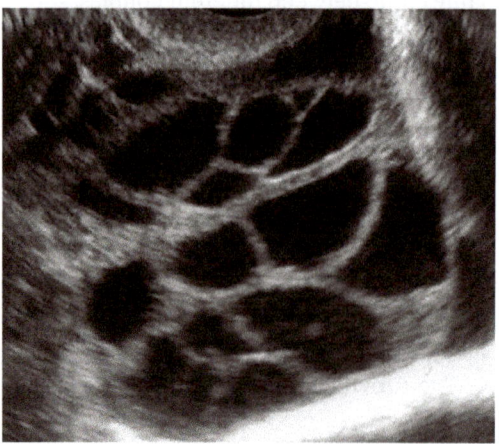

Fig. 18.6: Ovarian hyperstimulation syndrome.

- It should be remembered that the severity could worsen overtime as the condition evolves
- Assisted conception units should provide women with written information about OHSS inclucing risks, symptoms of OHSS, what action to take and a 24-hour contact number with prompt access to a clinician with necessary expertise in the diagnosis and management of OHSS
- Assisted conception units should develop agreed protocols for initial OHSS management and for referral of women with suspected OHSS to hospital care
- Treatment for women with mild OHSS and many with moderate OHSS can be managed on an outpatient basics
- Analgesia using paracetamol or codeine is appropriate. NSAIDS should not be used; antiemetics should be those appropriate for the possibility of early pregnancy
- Women should be encouraged to drink to thirst rather than to excess
- Strenuous excercises and sexual intercourse should be avoided for fear of injury or torsion of hyperstimulated ovaries
- Women should continue progesterone luteal support but hCG luteal support is inappropriate
- Hospital admission should be recommended to women with severe OHSS. Women should be kept under review until resolution of the condition
- Multidisciplinary assistance should be sought for all women with critical or OHSS who have persistent hemoconcentration and dehydration
- Features of critical OHSS should prompt consideration of the need for intensive care
- Pelvic surgery should be restricted to cases with adnexal torsion or coincident problems requiring surgery
- Women should be reassured that pregnancy may continue despite OHSS and there is no increased congenital abnormalities.

ARTIFICIAL INSEMINATION OF DONOR

Indications for Use of Donor Semen for IUI

- Severe oligo-/astheno-/teratozoospermia (in those not willing for IVF/intracytoplasmic sperm injection (ICSI)
- Azoospermia
- Genetic disorders
- These are now relative indications as the newer developments in the field of male infertility such as microsurgical epididymal sperm aspiration (MESA)/testicular sperm aspiration (TESA)/testicular sperm extraction (TESE) male with opportunity for biological parenthood
- Donor screening
- Aims:
  - To prevent disease transmission
  - To increase the chances of pregnancy by selecting appropriate semen parameters
- Hence, complete medical and family history or complete physical examination/appropriate investigations like blood group or typing, urine test, semen analysis (parameters to be judged as per WHO's recent criteria) is important to rule out transmittable diseases, genetically inherited disorders
- In case of attempted sperm banking, the sperm should be checked for good post-thaw recovery and prospective donors should be provided with relevant information and guidelines so that moral/legal implications are understood by them.

Instructions to Prospective Sperm Donor

- Not to supply more than 2 samples per week
- Semen should be collected on site for it to be fresh at laboratory.

SEMEN CRYOPRESERVATION

The only true assessment of the success of the freezing technique is the ability of the thawed sperm to fertilize an oocyte in vitro or the creation of a clinical pregnancy following insemination.

Technique of Cryopreservation of Human Sperm

- Semen sample is allowed to liquefy at room temperature
- Required volume of freezing medium is thawed
- Equal volume of freezing medium is added and mixed slowly dropwise
- Mixture should be placed at 30°C for 10 minutes
- Tube is kept in the refrigerator at 4°C for 90 minutes
- Prepared sample is loaded into the cryovial.

Technique of Human Sperm Thawing (Fig. 18.7)

- The cryovial is identified and removed from the goblet
- Identification details on the removed cryovial is confirmed (Fig. 18.8)
- Vials are put in a waterbath at 37°C
- Vials are swirled gently for 10 minutes
- Complete liquefaction of the sample is confirmed
- Contents are transferred into a round bottomed tube
- A quick count and motility study is performed.

As per the study by the Cleveland clinical center for advanced research in human reproduction, the DI-SQ score (donor insemination semen quality) was an effective predictor of pregnancy and live birth outcomes in IUI patients who underwent AI with anonymous DISQ could also be used by sperm banks to help or select donors.

Insights into Infertility Management

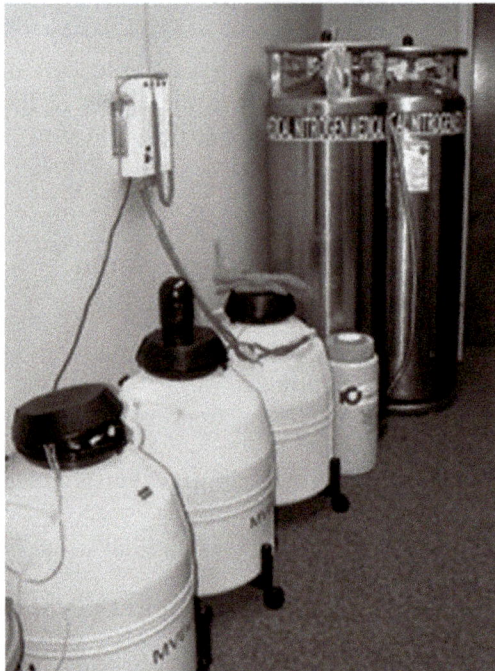

Fig. 18.7: Cryocans for storing semen.

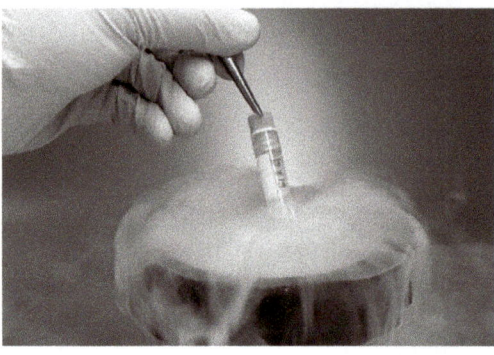

Fig. 18.8: Cryovials being removed from cryocans.

IUI PROCEDURE STEPS AT A GLANCE

- Soon after identification of ovulation by TV can assessment, male partner is instructed to collect semen
- After collection, semen sample is allowed to liquefy
- Rapid semen analysis done to check count and motility
- Sperm wash/preparartion done by appropriate technique
- Patient is given a good preprocedure counseling about the procedure steps
- Patient is asked to void urine
- Placed on an examining table in dorsal or lithotomy position
- It is preferable to elevate the foot end of the table
- Physician should maintain asepsis throughout the procedure
- Vulva and vagina cleaned with warm normal saline
- Cusco's bivalved speculum is inserted into the vagina to expose the cervix
- Vaginal discharge/cervical mucus should be cleaned with cotton swabs
- Prepared and loaded sperm sample is checked for identity
- Sperm loaded tuberculin syringe is attached to insemination cannula after removing air carefully
- Loaded cannula is inserted into uterine cavity
- Sperm gently pushed into uterine cavity
- Pushing air into the uterine cavity should be avoided
- Cannula is removed after keeping it in position for 2 to 3 minutes. In foot end elevated position, patient is advised to rest for 10 to 15 minutes.

SINGLE VERSUS DUAL IUI TREATMENT CYCLES

Two day IUI treatment cycles are more successful than one day IUI cycles when using frozen thawed donor sperm—Matilsky, Geslevich Y, Haernek Medical Centre, Israel.

Such studies support the use of 2 day treatment cycles when using frozen thawed donor sperm while Cochrane database review does not support the difference in pregnancy rates with 1 day vs 2 day IUI treatment cycle especially with fresh semen samples.

IUI–ONE OF THE FERTILITY OPTIONS FOR HIV PATIENTS/HIV DISCORDANT COUPLE

With improved treatment options for HIV patients and the increase in their life expectancy, it is not surprising that many HIV patients desire to have children and discuss the available fertility options. Serodiscordant couples have limited options if they wish to have natural conception as sexual intercourse carries a risk of 1 in 500 times of transmitting virus in semen to the female partner.

The only completely safe option available to HIV discordant couples is adoption or in case of HIV positive males—sperm donation. Nevertheless, many couples desire genetically related offspring.

Intraceterine insemination (IUI) forms one of the treatment options to serodiscordant couples willing for conception without seroconversion of uninfected partners.

In serodiscordant couple, when female partners HIV positive IUI will suffice in order to prevent horizontal infection transmission. However, when male partner is positive, sperm washing technique is used in order to minimize the infection of the healthy partner.

Absence of detectable HIV is verified before insemination using PCR—nucleic acid based sequence amplification assay.

Thus far, worldwide there are more than 3000 such cycles and 497 pregnancies with over 300 deliveries and no infection of female partner or infant.

Pregnancy rate per insemination is 14% based on a European experience of more than 2000 insemination. Though current data from European programs suggest sperm washing to be a safe risk reduction option for heterosexual couples wishing to bear a child, CDC in USA has recommended against insemination of women with semen from men infected from HIV.

"Safety of sperm washing and ART outcome in HIV-1 serodiscordant couples"— Italian study in 2007 concluded sperm washing with a program of reproductive counseling was proved to be safe in a large series of 741 serodiscordant couples. The overall pregnancy rate of about 70.3% independent of the procedure used (IUI or IVF) justifies the effort of medical team in setting up and implementing dedicated centers and individual patient in seeking a safe pregnancy.

Though much more research in the most recent future is compelling, IUI as a reproductive technology provides a logical way to seek baby in many infertility couples desiring pregnancy.

BIBLIOGRAPHY

1. Adams R. In Vitro Fertilization Technique, Monterey, CA 1988.
2. Bagis T, Haydardedeoglu B, Kilicdag EB, et al. Single versus double intrauterine insemination in multi-follicular ovarian hyperstimulation cycles: a randomized trial. Hum Reprod. 2010;25(7):1684-90.
3. Bellver J, Labarta E, Bosch E, et al. GnRH agonist administration at the time of implantation does not improve pregnancy outcome in intrauterine insemination cycles: a randomized controlled trial. Fertil Steril. 2009;94(3):1065-71.
4. Bhattacharya S, Harrild K, Mollison J, et al. Clomifene citrate or unstimulated intrauterine insemination compared with expectant management for unexplained infertility: pragmatic randomised controlled trial. BMJ. 2008;337: a716.
5. Harris I, Missmer S, Hornstein M. Poor success of gonadotropin-induced controlled ovarian hyperstimulation and intrauterine insemination for older women. Fertil and Steril. 2010;94(1):144-8.

6. Hurd WW, Randolph JF, Ansbacher R, et al. Comparison of intracervical, intrauterine, and intratubal techniques for donor insemination. Fertil Steril. 1993;59(2):339-42.
7. Laurie B. Immobilization may improve pregnancy rate after intrauterine insemination. Medscape Medical News. Retrieved October 2009.
8. Leonidas M. Comparison of fallopian tube sperm perfusion and intrauterine tuboperitoneal insemination: a prospective randomized study. Fertil Steril. 2006;85(3):735-40.
9. Marshburn PB, Alanis M, Matthews ML, et al. A short period of ejaculatory abstinence before intrauterine insemination is associated with higher pregnancy rates. Fertil Steril. 2009;93(1):286-8.
10. Merviel P, Heraud MH, Grenier N, et al. Predictive factors for pregnancy after intrauterine insemination (IUI): an analysis of 1038 cycles and a review of the literature. Fertil Steril. 2008;93(1):79-88.

CHAPTER 19

Enhancing IUI Success Rates

Madhuri Patil

Chapter outline

- Progress in IUI
- Literature Search on Use of IUI for Different Etiologies
  - Unexplained Infertility
  - Male Factor Infertility (WHO)
- Success of IUI
  - Success Rates are Contingent Upon Procedure being Performed
  - Factors Affecting Success of IUI
- Trials which Revolutionized IUI

INTRODUCTION

Infertility is a very common condition affecting approximately 13–14% of reproductive-aged couples. Despite a stable prevalence of infertility in this population, the demand for infertility services has increased substantially over the past decade.

Infertility is defined as the inability to conceive after 1 year of properly timed unprotected intercourse. This definition is based on the cumulative probability of pregnancy (Table 19.1).

Assuming a constant monthly probability of conceiving (fecundability) of 20%, the cumulative pregnancy rate after 12 months is 93%. Approximately, 50% of couples should become pregnant after 3 months, but only an additional 25% conceive if attempting pregnancy in additional 2 months. Conventional infertility treatment (excluding *in vitro* fertilization [IVF]) is usually continued until the cumulative pregnancy rate is at least 50%. Because fecundability rates are clearly higher in younger women and lower in older women, counseling a 40-year-old woman to wait 1 year before seeking fertility services is not appropriate. In women older than 35 years, a complete evaluation at 4–6 months is best because their potential response to any therapy may be suboptimal due to diminished ovarian reserve.

The multiple causes of infertility are listed in Table 19.2.

Intrauterine insemination (IUI) is a widely utilized technique for treatment of infertility, indications being extremely varied and has often being used empirically. Though there is serious disagreement about the results of the procedure, it has still become a popular method because of its simplicity, low operational cost and ambulatory character. Although widely used, its effectiveness remains a matter of debate. Although IUI is less invasive and expensive than IVF or gamete intrafallopian transfer (GIFT), it should only be applied if the probability of conception is improved significantly as compared to the natural chance of conceiving. To increase the number of available oocytes

Insights into Infertility Management

Table 19.1: Cumulative probability of pregnancy in couples with normal fertility (All reproductive-aged women).

Month	Monthly probability	Cumulative probability
1	0.2	0.20
2	0.2	0.36
3	0.2	0.49
4	0.2	0.59
5	0.2	0.67
6	0.2	0.74
7	0.2	0.79
8	0.2	0.83
9	0.2	0.86
10	0.2	0.89
11	0.2	0.91
12	0.2	0.93

Table 19.2: Causes of infertility.

Cause	Couples	Women
Male	35%	--
Ovulatory	15%	40%
Tubal	35%	40%
Unexplained	10%	10%
Other	5%	10%

at the site of fertilization, controlled ovarian hyperstimulation (COH) can be applied in conjunction with IUI.

The IUI with partner's sperm can be used as a potentially effective treatment for infertility of all causes in women under 40 years of age except for cases with tubal blockage, severe tubal damage, very poor egg quality, ovarian failure (menopause), and severe male factor infertility.

PROGRESS IN IUI

Progress in IUI is due to advances in IVF and embryo transfer (ET).

- Progress in semen processing and sperm isolation methods
- Improved ovarian stimulation protocols (developed primarily to meet IVF requirements) with less side effects.

If we compare timed intercourse (TI) with IUI the probability of conception is more with IUI. If we compare IUI in an natural cycle and COH cycle it is higher in an stimulated cycle. Table 19.3 clearly explains it.

LITERATURE SEARCH ON USE OF IUI FOR DIFFERENT ETIOLOGIES

Unexplained Infertility

Basic investigations are normal:
1. Ovulation induction and IUI is justified in couples with unexplained infertility (Deaton et al., 1990; Gregoriou et al., 1995).
2. Ovulation induction with IUI is an effective treatment in unexplained infertility, but ovulation induction with TI has negligible impact (Chung et al., 1995).
3. The likelihood of pregnancy is 3 times greater with IUI (22 RCTs, 5214 cycles, Hughes, 1997).

Male Factor Infertility (WHO)

The male factor is classified as shown in Table 19.4.

Mild to Moderate Male Infertility

Intrauterine insemination vs timed intercourse in male infertility (Cochrane library,

Table 19.3: Probability of conception (Cochrane database, 2000).

Ovulation induction (OI)	IUI	Timed intercourse
Clomiphene citrate (CC)	6.3%	2.3%
Gonadotropin therapy (GT)	14.8%	6.7%

Table 19.4: Classification of male factor.

Sub-category	Count million/mL	Motility (%)	Normal morphology (%)
Mild	15–20	40–50	30–40
Moderate	10–15	20–40	10–30
Severe	< 10	< 20	< 10

2000) 17 trials comparing 3775 treatment cycles and they found that:
1. IUI in natural cycles and IUI with COH significantly improved the probability of conception.
2. IUI with COH is superior to TI with COH.
3. IUI overcomes failure to fertilize due to impaired mucus penetration and poor survival in the female reproductive tract (Ford et al., 1997).

Severe Male Factor Infertility

It is not a candidate for IUI but for intracytoplasmic sperm injection (ICSI).

The ICSI is more cost effective than IUI when the mean total motile sperm count is <10 million (Van Voorthis et al., 2001).

Mild Male Infertility or Unexplained Infertility

IUI vs IVF: Goverde et al. (2000): 285 couples
- With at least 1 million progressively motile sperm after sperm preparation.
- The pregnancy rate per started cycle were as follows:
  - 7.4% for IUI
  - 8.7% for IUI with COH
  - 12.2% for IVF
  - No statistically significant difference.

Endometriosis

Minimal endometriosis: Superovulation in combination with IUI is effective in treatment of minimal endometriosis (Iaksson and Tiitinen, 1997).

Minimal and mild endometriosis: Treatment with COH and IUI was associated with superior outcome both by crude live-birth rates and proportional hazard analysis (Tummon et al., 1997).

Cervical Factor Infertility

Postcoital test (PCT) after 8–12 hours.

No sperms with progressive forward motion, IUI in natural cycle is an effective treatment for cervical factor infertility (Check and Spirito, 1995).

Male Immunological Infertility

When mixed antiglobulin reaction to IgG: Positive, IUI is significantly better than timed intercourse with prednisolone.

The IUI is an effective method, results are obtained rapidly and steroid side effects can be avoided (Lahteenmaki et al., 1995).

The IUI significantly improved PR when used as an adjuvant therapy to cyclical dose steroid therapy (Robinson et al., 1995).

Evaluation before initiating therapy is essential.

Three basic tests include:
1. Seminogram
2. Midluteal progesterone
3. Hysterosalpingography (HSG) + laparoscopy

Other tests may be done as indicated and include:
1. Endocrine evaluation on Day 2/3
   - Follicle-stimulation hormone
   - Luteinizing hormone
   - Prolactin
   - Thyroid stimulating hormone
   - Dehydroepiandrosterone
   - Testosterone
   - Androstenedione
   - Alfa hydroxyprogesterone.
2. Baseline USG—TRO ovarian cyst, other potential subfertility factors.
3. Evaluation of utero-tubo-peritoneal factor – HSG, hysterolaparoscopy.
4. Complete workup of infertility.

SUCCESS OF IUI

The review of literature over the past 15 years has shown:
- Wide range of variation
- About 0-26% pregnancy/cycle in different indications.

Take home baby controversial, no evidence-based infertility data.

Success Rates are Contingent Upon Procedure being Performed

- For correct indication.
- Avoiding performance of IUI when CI exist.
- Whether women is ovulating normally on her own.
- The age of women.

Factors Affecting Success of IUI (Table 19.5)

Couple

- Age, duration of infertility, cause of infertility,
- Body mass index.
- Therapies:
  - Semen processing technique

Table 19.5: Pregnancy rate according to female characteristics in IUI treatment.

Age of the patient	
Age in years	% pregnancies
< 30	15
30–35	13.7
36–39	7.8
≥ 40	2.1
$P = 0.007$	
Duration of infertility	
Duration in years	Pregnancies per cycle (%)
≤ 4	14.2
≥ 4	6.1
$P = 0.005$	
(Dunphy et al., Collins et al., Nulsen et al., Tomlinson et al.)	
Pregnancy rate according to etiology	
Infertility etiology	Pregnancies per cycle (%)
UI	63/413 15.3–23
Male factor	27/229 4–13.6
Endometriosis	9/138 5–13
Ovarian dysfunction	3/31 9.7–16
$P = 0.05$	
(Chaffkin et al., Dodson & Haney, Nulsen et al., Collins et al.)	
Pregnancy rates with different OI protocols	
Protocol	PR in %
Natural cycle + IUI	3.3
CC + IUI	9.5
CC + hMG + IUI	13.3
hMG + IUI	19–26

Contd...

Contd...

Number of follicles influencing IUI outcome	
Number of follicles	Pregnancies per cycle (%)
1	5.7
2	13.6
3	16.3
4>	13.9
$P = 0.013$	

Timing of insemination
- Important as viable sperms should be present at the time of ovulation
- Therefore, detection of ovulation is important and can be done by:
  - Serum or urinary LH
  - TVS - leading follicle > 18–20 mm, hCG 10,000 IU given
- Insemination:

TVS after 36 hours of hCG injection:
- 1- Ovulated   IUI once
- 2- Not ovulated   IUI at 36 hr and 48 hr

Semen preparation
- Swim-up semen preparation with test yolk buffer incubation significantly improved the PR in unexplained infertility but not in male factor infertility (Rangi et al.,1998)
- With density gradient one can obtain better quality sperms even in oligospermic patients and those who have a borderline count.

Number of insemination
- Single vs double IUI
  - If correctly timed single insemination is sufficient as sperms remain alive in the female genital tract for 72 hours
  - Cochrane library, 2003 (3 studies, 386 women) published that double IUI showed no significant benefit over single IUI

Inseminated volume
Similar PR for 0.5 mL and 3 mL of inseminated semen, so volume of processed semen does not influence the success rate of IUI
(Do Amaral et al., 2001)

Type of catheter
When comparing the softer Wallace catheter to the less pliable Tomcat catheter during IUI, there was no significant difference in PR when using standard gentle technique that include not touching the top of the catheter
(Smith et al., 2002)

10 minutes bedrest
A 10 minutes bedrest after IUI has a positive effect on PR
(Saleh et al., 2000)

Number of treatment cycles
- Pregnancies resulting from IUI occur during early treatment cycles
  - 71% of IUI pregnancies occurred *in the first-two cycles* (Friedman et al., 1990)
  - 85% of IUI pregnancies occurred during *the first-four cycles* (Isaksson & Titinen, 1997)

Contd...

Contd...

- Continued IUI is not recommended (Kirby et al., 1991)
- The treatment needs careful monitoring in order to prevent the risk of ovarian hyperstimulation and/or multiple pregnancy
- IUI pregnancy outcome is enhanced by shorter intervals from sperm collection to sperm wash, from sperm wash to IUI time and from semen collection to IUI time. Delaying semen processing from 30 minutes to 1 hour and/or delaying IUI from 90 minutes to 2 hours after collection compromises the pregnancy outcome in hMG-IUI cycles (Y Yavas et al.)

- Protocol of COH
- Timing of insemination.

Effect of Maternal Age

As women age, their fertility diminishes. It is a result of the decline in the number and quality of eggs in their ovaries and an increase in the rate of pregnancy loss.

Older women associated with:
- Fewer oocytes per cycle
- Low E2 on day of hCG
- Lower implantation rates
- Increased risk of miscarriage
- Increased chance of chromosomal abnormalities.

TRIALS WHICH REVOLUTIONIZED IUI

In 2010, the "Fast Track and Standard Treatment" Trial (FASTT) (Fertil Steril 2010) studied the best course of treatment in women with unexplained infertility. The study included over 500 women who were between 21 and 39 years old with unexplained infertility. For one arm of the study, patients did "conventional treatment" which involved three cycles of clomiphene citrate (CC) with intrauterine insemination (IUI), followed by three cycles of gonadotropins (GN) with IUI followed by up to six cycles of *in vitro* fertilization (IVF). The "accelerated" arm did three cycles of CC/IUI followed by up to six cycles of IVF—skipping the gonadotropin treatment all together. Pregnancy rates were 8.5% with CC/IUI, 11.4% with GN/IUI, and 38.6% with IVF. However, while we often measure pregnancy rate for success, we also measure "take home baby rates" in discussing live birth rates. Live birth rate (live births plus ongoing pregnancies >20 weeks) during the trial were on average 7.8% in CC/IUI cycles, 9.8% in GN/IUI cycles, and 30.7% in IVF cycles. Overall little loss rate in this under 40 population.

While some patients still may have an indication to pursue gonadotropin therapy, it has become less used mainly because of the extremely high chances of multiples. On average, gonadotropin/IUI treatment results in about 30–35% chance of twins and 3–5% chance of more than twins (multiples). This is unacceptably high for standard treatment.

A follow-up trial, "The Forty and Over Treatment" Trial (FORT-T) (Fertil Steril 2014) was done to answer this question. Approximately 150 women aged 38–42 were randomized to either CC/IUI, GN/IUI, or IVF. If the patients undergoing IUI cycles were not pregnant after two cycles, they would proceed with IVF. Pregnancy rates were 6.9% with CC/IUI, 7.7% with GN/IUI, and 24.7% with IVF. Live birth rates during the trial were 3.4% in CC/IUI cycles, 6.6% in GN/IUI cycles, and 15.3% in IVF cycles. Higher loss rates correlate to the older patient age and expected increase in spontaneous loss and aneuploidy. Time to pregnancy in this study was decreased in the patients who went directly to IVF. It was approximately 12.2 months in the CC and GN arms and decreased to 8.7 in the IVF arm.

CONCLUSION

- IUI is a poor Rx option for women above 40 years
- Cycle fecundity 2 fold higher with GT and 3 fold higher with IUI, thus chance of conception 5 fold higher when both interventions offered
- CC - success rate one half of that achieved with GT
- Almost all pregnancies occurred in first-four treatment cycles of IUI after which PR declined steeply, favoring a maximum of 4 COH + IUI cycles before IVF
- More aggressive stimulation regimens yield higher PR but associated with high rates of multiple pregnancies and OHSS
- Best results with IUI obtained in cases of UI, abnormal ovulation, cervicals mucus hostility unrelated to sperm antibodies, and with DI
- Poorest results with moderate to severe male factor, antisperm antibodies or endometriosis in female reduced treatment effectiveness by half
- An easy and atraumatic transfer is an essence of successful IUI
- Maintenance of equipments and working environment in the lab, good quality consumables and culture media definitely improved pregnancy rate with IUI
- COH + IUI should be considered first approach prior to more expensive and invasive procedure of IVF, with all contraindications ruled out.

CHAPTER 20

IVF and ICSI: Current State of the Art

Christian De Geyter, Alexander Quaas, Maria De Geyter, Katharina Rüther-Wolf

Chapter outline

- Infrastructure and Organization Needed for IVF and ICSI including Quality Assurance
  - Outline of the Diagnostic Workup Prior to ART
  - Controlled Ovarian Hyperstimulation
  - Ovulation Induction
  - Semen Preparation
  - IVF or ICSI?
- Embryo Transfer
- Luteal Phase Support
- The Major Complications of ART
  - Ovarian Hyperstimulation Syndrome
- Monitoring the Outcome of Assisted Reproduction
- Quality Assurance through Data Reporting

INTRODUCTION

Infertility must primarily be seen as a symptom, not as a disease. Therefore, the medical workup of infertility should first include a diagnostic phase, which must essentially include both partners. In most cases, more than one cause of the couple's infertility will be identified and many of the factors involved can be removed with a targeted treatment. Such a cause-related approach should ideally be the first step during the provision of medical assistance to infertile couples. However, many causes of infertility, such as postinflammatory tubal damage or severe male infertility resulting from prenatal testicular dysgenesis or from early childhood testicular maldescent, cannot be overcome by conventional treatment. In those cases, assisted reproductive medical technology (ART), including either *in vitro* fertilization (IVF) or intracytoplasmic sperm injection (ICSI) must be considered. Both methods may assist the couple to achieve successful pregnancy but they do not remove the causal factors of the couple's infertility. In this sense, assisted reproduction must be considered as a symptomatic treatment of the infertility and should therefore be used in second line.

After the first successful deliveries resulting from IVF treatment, starting 1978 with the birth of Louise Brown in the UK, and particularly since the introduction in 1992 of ICSI for the treatment of severe male infertility, ART has rapidly gained ground and is now being offered globally. More than 1 million babies were born worldwide between 2008 and 2010 and the number of treatments being carried out is constantly rising.[1] In some countries in Europe, more than 5% of all newborns arise after IVF or ICSI.[2] In order to cope with the increasing complexity of ART, infertility clinics are now made up of multidisciplinary teams including specialized gynecologists, embryologists, nurses, psychologists and administrators. Those units are supported by a specialized industry, which provides pharmaceuticals, complex culture media, high-quality laboratory infrastructure, special software and sophisticated ultrasound equipment.

INFRASTRUCTURE AND ORGANIZATION NEEDED FOR IVF AND ICSI INCLUDING QUALITY ASSURANCE

Essentially, any ART setting should include at least one surgical room, in which oocyte collections and embryo transfers can be performed, and a laboratory, in which semen is prepared, oocytes are identified and embryo culture is performed. However, in addition to those essential requirements, sufficient working space should be given to all members of the multidisciplinary team. Of course, one should not forget to organize an appropriate, discrete waiting room for the patients, a room for semen collection (with a sufficient amount of discretion as well) and easy access parking facilities in close neighborhood to the treatment unit.

In large institutions, various specialized laboratory techniques are usually carried out in separate rooms, such as semen analysis, semen preparation and cryopreservation, collection of the cumulus-oocyte complexes and oocyte identification, oocyte and embryo freezing and embryo culture. In busy institutions, semen analysis for diagnostic purposes and semen preparation for ART should be separated in order to avoid erroneous mix up of samples. As the culture of embryos tends to be prolonged more often up to the blastocyst stage, the laboratory conditions must fulfil criteria of clean air (Grade A on a background of Grade D)[3] including a constant and controlled ambient temperature. It must be assured that all equipment, particularly in the embryology lab, is adequately connected with electric current and that all systems are secured at least twofold. Particularly when blastocysts are to be cultured, all incubators must be aired with a mixture of three gases, oxygen 5-6%, carbon dioxide 5-6% and nitrogen 88-90%, and the adequate provision of all atmosphere constituents must be secured at all times. The temperature and the gassing of the incubator systems must be checked continuously by dual control systems, one integrated within the incubator and a second independent backup system. All measurements must be recorded continuously allowing for retrospective controls and error detection.

The maintenance and usage of all equipment, not only in the laboratory but also those used for clinical purposes, such as ultrasonography, must be documented together with a written outline of all procedures. This extensive documentation consists of a series of so-called "standard operating procedures" (SOPs) and those should be available to all members of the team at any time. They should be updated regularly (at least once yearly) and repeated controls (so-called audits) should be carried out to check adherence to the rules laid out in the SOPs. Modification of the procedures can only be made through an ongoing validation system and modifications of the SOPs are to be dated and signed by the head of the institution and/or his deputy.

Both the introduction and the organization of such a quality management system (QM system) and their maintenance (Table 20.1) are time consuming and, at least in the beginning, require specific knowledge. During the setup of a QM system, the assistance of qualified and skilled institutions may therefore be helpful. However, the complexity of ART, which includes the close collaboration of many members with sometimes very different training backgrounds, and the constant threat of errors, such as contamination of samples

Table 20.1: In ART a QM-system may be setup based on the guidelines provided by the ISO family of standards (International Organization for Standardization) for either certification or accreditation. QM warrants adherence to formal, established and authorized written protocols. Whereas certification refers to self-imposed standards thereby being more suitable for clinical and nursing programs, accreditation refers to the independent, objective evaluation of both laboratory competence and measuring accuracy of all equipment. For each of both QM-standards a brief overview of the basic requirements is given below.

Certification of infertility counseling in accordance with DIN EN ISO 9001:2000	Accreditation of laboratory activities in ART in accordance with ISO/IEC 17025
Overview of the clinical setting (handbook)	Description of the organization (handbook)
Detailed description of all activities	Detailed description of all laboratory techniques
Description of the organizational network	Description of the validation of all measurements
Description of external interactions	Description of interaction with collaborating units
Training program	Training program
Review program of procedures	Quality assurance in the laboratory
Yearly repeated review-preview	Identification of all documents
Tables with aims set for each year	Staff management
Internal and external auditing system	Internal and external auditing system

from individuals carrying HIV or hepatitis, require the presence of a comprehensive QM system, particularly in the face of rising treatment numbers.

A high throughput ART program together with a sophisticated quality assurance can only be managed with the support of specialized software, which should guarantee to all team members rapid access to all data (Fig. 20.1). Any QM management system should provide the means to identify all incoming and outgoing samples unequivocally with full traceability. Especially busy programs, with many patients being taken care of simultaneously, methods to allow exact identification of the individuals involved in all steps of the process (both the technicians and the patients) should be described in detail in the SOPs and adherence to the SOPs should be followed up at regular intervals. In order to achieve this, devoted quality managers should be appointed, especially in medium-size and large ART institutions.

Outline of the Diagnostic Workup Prior to ART

It is of utmost importance that prior to any treatment with ART, a systematic diagnostic workup is offered to both partners. The details of such workup may vary regionally, but should be based on some basic principles. In the female partner, there are three aims of the diagnostic screening process:

1. To identify the main factors contributing to the couple's infertility
2. To identify any possible risk factors, which may complicate future ART
3. To identify any risk factors which might endanger the subsequent pregnancy.

With respect to the male partner, the diagnostic workup should be based on the following principles:
- Identification of the main factors in the male contributing to the couple's infertility. In the frame of the diagnostic workup, it is sometimes helpful to get

IVF and ICSI: Current State of the Art

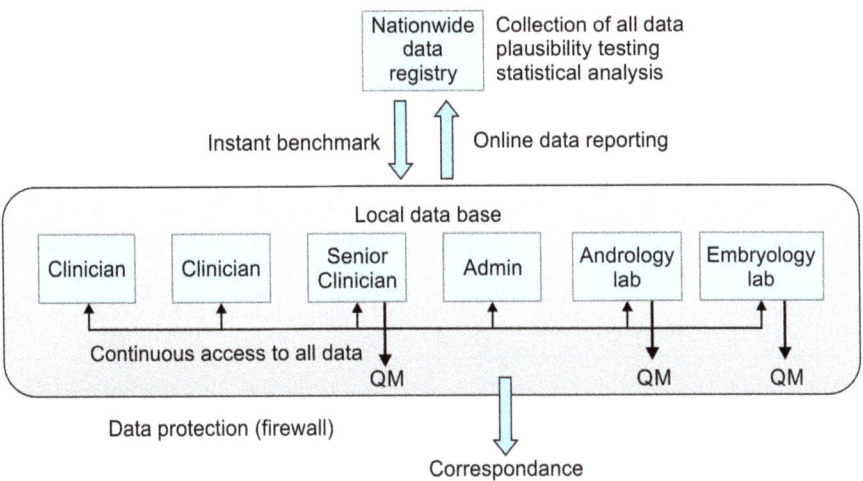

Fig. 20.1: Present-day ART must be considered as a local network of devoted professionals with different educational background working together to assist infertile couples in overcoming/coping with their infertility. This collaboration necessitates close interaction between all members and this is best achieved when all data and results are recorded and validated using a specialized software. A computerized management of all activities not only enables all team members direct access to all data at any time, but also improves the administrative work load and automatizes quality assurance. Online, day-to-day reporting of key data to superstructures, such as nationwide data registries, can be further developed towards instant benchmarking for the purpose of improving and maintaining treatment quality in ART. Of course, confidentiality of the stored data must be secured using all methods of computer protection (firewall, passwords, etc.).

some information about the husband's attitude towards the infertility problem or about his ability to provide the semen sample on demand.
- Male infertility often develops in the context of a major health problem, such as diabetes, hyperprolactinemia or testicular cancer. Such an impairment of the health condition of the male partner should, if present, be diagnosed and cured.
- As severe male infertility may be associated with some specific genetic condition as well, we recommend a targeted genetic screening in cases at risk (Table 20.2).

Current ART still heavily relies on controlled ovarian hyperstimulation. Various studies have demonstrated that the constituents of the most optimal treatment protocol, in particular the daily dose of the gonadotropin preparation to be administered, should be assembled individually:[4-6] despite several attemps, no algorithms presented to date have been demonstrated to be superior to the clinician experience in choosing the starting gonadotropin dose. The following parameters are considered to have the best predictive value: age of the patient, early follicular phase antral follicle count (AFC), anti-muellerian hormone (AMH, in pmol/L), body mass index (BMI, in kg/m^2), and to a lesser extent early menstrual cycle FSH (in the presence of estradiol concentrations below 200 pmol/L) (Figs. 20.2A to D). Due to differences in assay characteristics, the measurement of AMH may be variable among different laboratories, especially at higher concentrations.[7] As ovarian response cannot be predicted reliably there is a need for continued monitoring of follicular development and, whenever needed, the adaptation of the daily dose of gonadotropins.

Table 20.2: Recommended diagnostic tests for the identification of potential genetic causes of severe male infertility.

Genetic test	Complex of symptoms
Chromosomal analysis	Hypergonadotropic azoospermia Severe male infertility with sperm count < 5 million/mL Recurrent miscarriage
Y-chromosome microdeletions	Hypergonadotropic azoospermia Severe male infertility with sperm count < 1 million/mL
CFTR gene mutations	Congenital bilateral absence of the vas deferens (CBAVD) Female partner with known CFTR-mutation

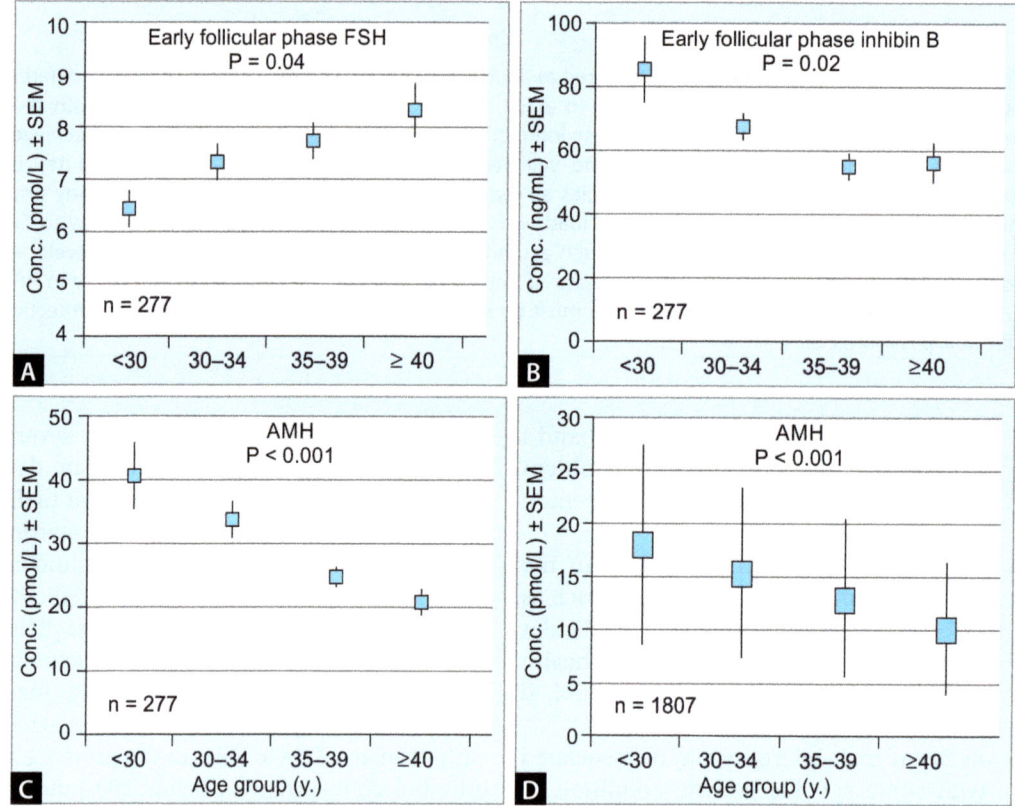

Figs. 20.2A to D: In addition to female age and the number of antral follicles counted in vaginal sonography, various endocrine parameters and the total number of ovarian antral follicles visualized in ultrasound (AFC) correlate with ovarian response to treatment with gonadotropins. The concentration of FSH, as measured between day 3 to 5 of an untreated menstrual cycle (A), rises with age, but this parameter can only be used, when the concentration of estradiol in the same serum sample is lower than 200 pmol/L. The concentration of inhibin B (B), also measured during the early follicular phase, decreases with female age, but this parameter achieves clinical significance only in the presence of very low levels. Finally, the best correlation with ovarian response to treatment with gonadotropins seems to be given both by AMH (C) and by AFC (D).

Controlled Ovarian Hyperstimulation (COH)

In ART, follicular growth is stimulated with exogenous gonadotropins in order to obtain a sufficient number of mature oocytes for fertilization. The optimal number of oocytes needed for high pregnancy rates appears independent of female age[8] and should be a compromise between ensuring a high (cumulative) pregnancy and delivery rate on the one hand and avoidance of complications, such as the ovarian hyperstimulation syndrome (OHSS) and thromboembolic events on the other. The optimal number of oocytes to be collected balancing between treatment efficacy and safety may vary between 11 and 18.[8]

The gonadotropin preparations currently available for ovarian hyperstimulation may be divided into two distinct groups:
1. Those based on gonadotropins extracted from the urine of postmenopausal women (human menopausal gonadotropins, hMG) containing a more acidic type of FSH together with variable amounts of LH and hCG, which is partly endogenous, partly added exogenously to the preparation; 2. Artificially constructed, recombinant gonadotropin preparations produced by genetically modified mammalian cells grown in bioreactors, which usually consist of FSH alone or recombinant FSH mixed with recombinant LH or of recombinant LH alone. The recombinant preparations are produced by immortalized and genetically modified animal or human cells cultured in bioreactors. The pregnancy rates achieved with either type of gonadotropins have not been demonstrated to be significantly different, although this may be due to the design of many of the prospective studies by pharmaceutical companies generally conducting "non-inferiority studies". There may be a slight preponderance in favor of preparations containing both FSH and LH-like activity.[9]

Follicular development during ovarian hyperstimulation entails supraphysiological levels of circulating estrogens, which, if unopposed, triggers the untimely release of endogenous LH in approximately 25% of all cycles, thereby causing premature ovulation and early cancellation of the treatment. Therefore, in addition to the gonadotropins either gonadotropin releasing hormone (GnRH)-agonists or GnRH-antagonists are given to prevent the premature surge of LH. Although in the past, most patients received various combinations of gonadotropins and GnRH-agonists, two major protocols are now used most commonly:
1. Long protocol based on GnRH-agonists
2. GnRH-antagonist protocol.

Due to differences in the pharmacological properties of both GnRH-analogs, the outline of both protocols is completely distinct. After a short-term initial stimulation of the pituitary gland (the so-called "flare up"), continuous administration of a GnRH agonist leads to the downregulation of the GnRH-receptors in the anterior part of the pituitary, thus preventing both synthesis and release of endogenous FSH and LH. The GnRH-agonist is usually given in the luteal phase of the preceding menstrual cycle, but can also be administered very early during menstruation or during intake of a contraceptive pill. The long protocol based on a GnRH-agonist is very reliable, as premature ovulations can be prevented in virtually all cases. Disadvantage is the longer duration of the treatment, the side effects caused by the downregulation (hot flushes, depressive symptoms) and the need for higher doses of gonadotropins.

Instead of GnRH-agonists endogenous preovulatory gonadotropin release may also be prevented by the use of GnRH-antagonists. The GnRH-antagonist competes directly with the physiological GnRH for binding to the pituitary GnRH receptors and provides quicker suppression of gonadotropin release without the initial flare up.

The GnRH-antagonist is administered during follicular growth, usually starting at a follicular diameter of 12 mm.

Compared with the GnRH-agonist long protocol, GnRH-antagonists require a considerably shorter treatment period, less use of exogenous gonadotropins for ovarian hyperstimulation, and are associated with fewer side effects. The prevention of premature ovulation with a GnRH-antagonist may be less reliable than with a long-acting GnRH-agonist. However, the main advantage of GnRH-antagonist based protocols consists of the possibility of avoiding the administration of human chorionic gonadotropins (hCG) for ovulation induction. The flare-up effect of a single administration of a GnRH-agonist causing an upsurge of both LH and FSH may be used to trigger ovulation while avoiding the risk of OHSS (except in few exceptional cases).

Because of the unpredictable interindividual differences in follicular growth and maturation, which often necessitate repeated adaptations of the gonadotropin dosage during the stimulation, the growth process of the ovarian follicles should be monitored. Ovarian follicular development is usually monitored with repeated measurements of the number of growing follicles and their respective diameter. Those measurements are often combined with repeated measurements of the serum concentration of estradiol, which correlates both with the number of growing follicles and their size. Whereas in gonadotropin preparations containing LH-activity, the correlation between the ultrasound findings and the estradiol levels allows good prediction of their developmental status, this is much less so when ovarian hyperstimulation is performed with FSH only. Serial measurements of the progesterone concentration may be helpful as well, particularly when ovarian hyperstimulation is performed with recombinant FSH only. Exaggerate late follicular phase progesterone levels are associated with lower pregnancy rates.[10]

Ovulation Induction

At the end of follicular development, the maturing follicles start to produce higher levels of both estradiol and progesterone.[11] When the follicles reach maturity, (follicular diameter of 17 to 19 mm) ovulation must be induced in order for the oocyte to resume final meiotic maturation.

The appropriate timing of ovulation induction, either with 5000 or 10000 international units of hCG or with a GnRH-agonist (for example 0.2 mg of triptorelin), is crucial for the success of ART. Although the term "ovulation induction" is commonly used, the purpose of this measure is not to induce ovulation, but rather to induce resumption of the meiotic process, which after oogenesis has remained fixed at prophase I of meiosis. Without the upsurge of LH induced by either hCG or by the GnRH-agonist, the retrieved oocytes would not be able to become fertilized. In addition, the LH surge provokes mucification of the cumulus oophorus-oocyte complexes, which is beneficial for their retrieval, which actually takes place few hours before ovulation would occur. Due to its prolonged duration of endocrine action, ovulation induction with hCG has the additional advantage of promoting long-term support of the luteal phase. The disadvantage of the administration of hCG resides in the much higher risk of OHSS, most particularly in those cases in which 15 or more oocytes are recovered. The optimal interval between administration of hCG and oocyte collection is 37 hours.

In GnRH-antagonist cycles (but not in GnRH-agonist cycles), ovulation may be triggered by using the flare up effect of a single dose of a GnRH-agonist. The optimal interval between the administration of the GnRH-agonist and oocyte collection is 36 hours.

The disadvantage of the GnRH-antagonist procol is the occasional occurrence of premature ovulation. In infertile women with irregular menstrual cycles (due to WHO 1 hypogonadotropic anovulation) or in women previously treated with long-acting GnRH-agonists (within three months after the last administration), the LH surge may fail to occur despite the appropriate administration of the GnRH-agonist and oocyte retrieval will fail to be successful. The most important advantage of triggering ovulation with a GnRH-agonist is the near complete avoidance of OHSS.

Semen Preparation

In most cases, semen is collected for ART by masturbation after a recommended period of abstinence of 2 to 7 days. A subsequent washing procedure of the semen is required, because seminal plasma is toxic both for the sperm itself, as well as for the oocytes, even at low concentration. For the washing of semen, various techniques have been described, but the most commonly used are either the swim-up technique or density gradient centrifugation. Whereas the former is more time-consuming, it allows the separation of a highly purified sample of motile spermatozoa. Density gradient centrifugation, however, can be performed faster and has been associated with a lesser risk of damage of the spermatozoa as caused by toxic oxygen radicals through a reduced contact with seminal leukocytes. A recent meta-analysis has not been able to detect differences in the pregnancy rates after intrauterine insemination with respect to both methods of semen preparation.[12]

In men with uncertain ability to produce a semen sample when required, it is wise to cryopreserve one or more semen samples prior to ART. This measure takes away some of the pressure and the men are still free to produce a fresh sample on the day of oocyte collection.

In cases with azoospermia, viable spermatozoa can be retrieved through surgical extraction from the testicular tissue (TESE). For better planning, this procedure may be performed some time before initiation of ART and the tissue can be cryopreserved until thawing. Particulary in cases with hypergonadotropic testicular failure, it is often difficult to identify viable spermatozoa for ICSI. In those cases pentoxiphylline is often used to stimulate mobility of viable spermatozoa.[13,14] In addition, pregnancy rates have been demonstrated to be higher, when the testicular tissue is thawed the day before ICSI and cultured overnight in the presence of recombinant FSH (25 IU/L).[15]

IVF or ICSI?

Whereas the decision to perform ICSI rather than IVF is obvious in cases with severely reduced semen quality, the choice is often difficult in borderline cases. The fertilization rates obtained with IVF have been shown to be similar to those observed after ICSI in couples with normal seminal parameters. However, the frequency of complete failure of fertilization of all oocytes is higher after IVF than after ICSI in some studies,[16] (Figs. 20.3A and B). The dilemma of performing conventional IVF or, alternatively, ICSI, still largely relies on conventional semen analysis, but at present, neither conventional semen analysis nor any other of the available function tests can reliably predict the fertilizing ability of spermatozoa in conventional IVF. For that reason, many institutions tend to perform ICSI indifferently in all cases.[17]

Embryo Transfer (ET)

Although oocytes are now invariably aspirated transvaginally from the mature follicles under ultrasound-guidance, the transfer of embryos into the uterine cavity is still often performed without any visual control.

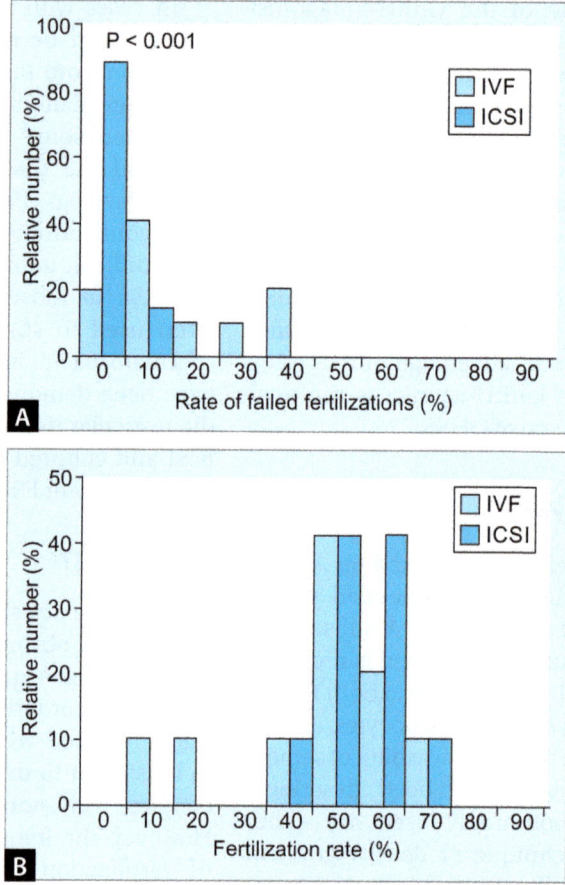

Figs. 20.3A and B: The decision to perform either ICSI or conventional IVF in cases with borderline male infertility or in couples with unexplained infertility is often difficult. A meta-analysis of 10 prospective randomized studies[27] demonstrated that the rate of complete fertilization failures (A) is significantly lower in ICSI as compared to IVF, whereas the number of fertilized oocytes per number of inseminated oocytes (e.g. the fertilization rate) is similar in both treatments (B).

However, compared with clinical touch ultrasound guidance has been demonstrated to significantly improve the chance of live birth/ongoing and clinical pregnancies.[18]

Controversy surrounds both the timing of embryo transfer (with respect to the stage of embryo development) and the number of embryos to be replaced.

Improved and adapted culture media and culture conditions have much improved the culture of human embryos up to the blastocyst stage, which immediately precedes the moment of implantation. Embryo transfer at the blastocyst stage, which is reached on the fifth or the sixth day after oocyte collection, allows the identification of the embryo with the highest developmental capacity. The assessment of embryonic morphology (Figs. 20.4A to C) ideally based on time-lapse technology and possibly also with the help of genetic analysis of the embryos allows for a better discrimination between

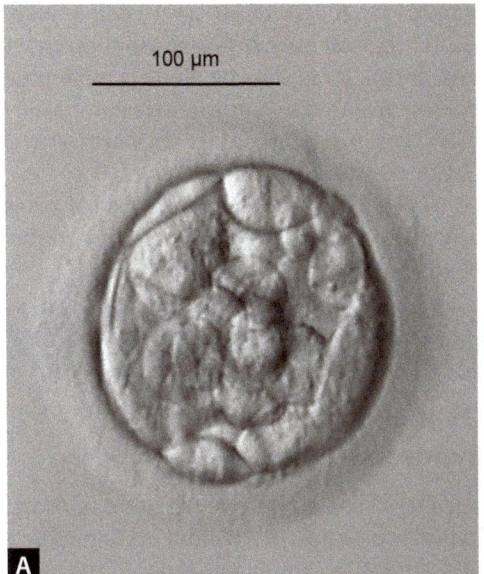
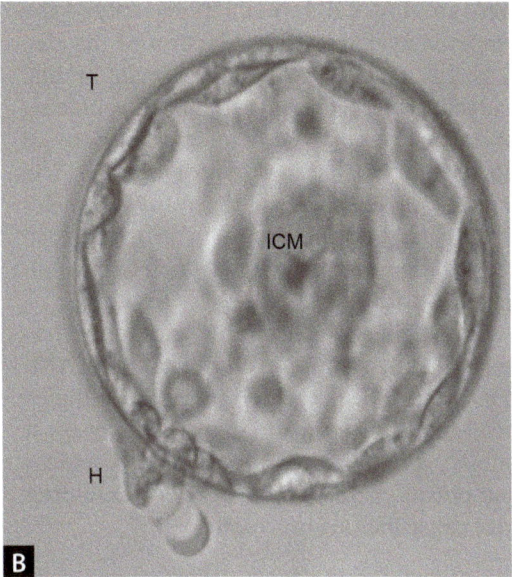
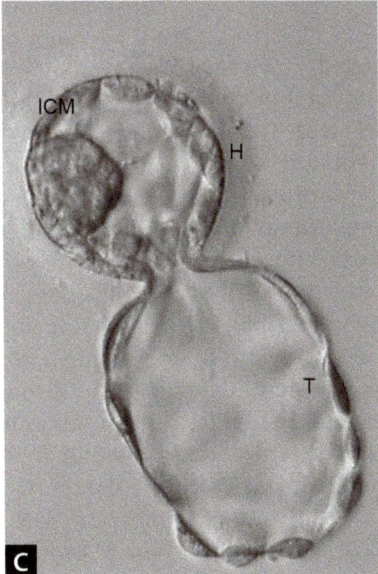

Figs. 20.4A to C: There is an increasing trend to replace embryos to the uterine cavity at the blastocyst stage of development. One of the advantages of such a strategy is that the assessment of the developmental capacity at that particular stage is more reliable. Assessment of blastocyst morphology is based on three characteristics: 1. The size and the compaction of the inner cell mass (ICM).[2] The expansion of the embryo against the zona pellucida resulting in hatching (H).[3] The number and the size of cells in the trophectoderm (T), which should form a closed layer. Whereas the blastocyst in (A) is still undergoing early blastulation, blastocyst in (B) is expanding and blastocyst in (C) is hatching. All blastocysts depicted implanted after transfer and lead to ongoing pregnancies.

high and low developmental capacity of the embryos available. The selection of the one blastocyst with the highest developmental capacity offers the possibility of replacing one single embryo and to cryopreserve all other embryos for later treatment cycles. The strategy of elective single embryo transfer (eSET) has become the main instrument to reduce the number of multiple deliveries on a nation-wide level.[19]

The delivery of multiple gestations has been the most common complication of ART, but can now be prevented by eSET. Multiples may cause obstetric and neonatal risks, most notably prematurity. The risk of neuronal complications in prematurely born children may cause lifelong morbidity.

Luteal Phase Support

All protocols for controlled ovarian hyperstimulation based on a combination of exogenous gonadotropins and GnRH-analogs necessitate medical support of the luteal phase, which can be performed with either hCG or exogenous progesterone. If ovulation is induced with hCG, this hormone will also help to sustain the function of the luteal body due to its prolonged half life. If ovulation is triggered with a GnRH-agonist, even with exogenous progesterone administration, the luteal phase will be deficient and shortened, unless supported by the repeated administration of low dosage hCG (e.g. 1500 IU every third day).[20]

Progesterone for luteal phase support can be administered intramuscularly, subcutaneously or transvaginally. Luteal phase support with progesterone should be initated at the latest within 72 hours after oocyte collection.[21]

Low doses of hCG are required to sustain the luteal phase, but these should be administered with caution. Luteal phase support with hCG lead to a manyfold increase in the risk of the ovarian hyperstimulation syndrome. If ovulation is triggered with a GnRH-agonist only, luteal phase support with exogenous progesterone alone is inadequate. We recommend two or three doses of 1500 IU of hCG at three days intervals, starting on the day of oocyte collection.[20]

The additional administration of exogenous estrogens is without proven beneficial effect.[22]

THE MAJOR COMPLICATIONS OF ART

Ovarian Hyperstimulation Syndrome (OHSS)

The OHSS is a major complication of ovarian hyperstimulation in ART and is characterized by ascites, sometimes accompanied by pleural effusion, hemoconcentration and a massive enlargement of both ovaries. In severe cases, hypovolemia may lead to anuria and renal failure. The hemoconcentration may lead to thromboembolism of deep veins, including the cerebral veins. Although maternal death is a very rare event in ART, OHSS is the major cause of a fatal outcome.

Nowadays, the incidence of OHSS has become less frequent in ART, because the risk factors are now well known and various preventive measures can be taken, most notably through the complete avoidance of the administration of hCG for ovulation induction. In the absence of hCG in the blood circulation, OHSS will not occur (except on very rare cases). The use of GnRH-antagonist-based protocols allows the possibility of triggering ovulation induction with a GnRH-agonist instead of hCG. Instead of cancelling the treatment cycle, oocytes may still be collected, fertilized and cultured up to the embryonic stage. In the presence of high risk of OHSS, embryo transfer may be postponed and all available embryos be cryopreserved. Such a "freeze all strategy" has now become the most effective instrument in preventing OHSS.

In view of "freeze all" the patients at risk should be identified before initiation of the treatment and informed about this option. The risk factors of OHSS include young age of the patient, presence of high numbers of ovarian follicles at the onset of ovarian hyperstimulation, low BMI and high anti-mullerian hormone (AMH) levels.

Particularly in slender women, who are treated with ICSI because of male infertility and in whom intraperitoneal adhesions fail to reduce ovarian mobility, the enlarged ovaries may undergo torsion. Blood circulation from and to the organs may become compromised leading to the organ's infarction. Ovarian torsion occurs in 0.1% to 0.3% of all ART treatments and is observed more often in women carrying multiples.

All women planning ART should be informed about the risk of multiple pregnancies, including the higher incidence of monozygotic multiples, and the risk of both OHSS and ovarian torsion.

MONITORING THE OUTCOME OF ASSISTED REPRODUCTION

A follow-up of the outcome of pregnancies after ART should be part of an overall QM and should reflect concern of the treating crew with their patients beyond the first early positive pregnancy test. It should therefore be mandatory for all institutions offering ART to organize a systematic follow-up of their treatment outcomes. This follow-up should not only include the occurrence or absence of ongoing pregnancies, but also the course of the pregnancies, the deliveries and the health status of the newborns.

Not only is the prevalence of congenital malformations increased in the offspring of previously infertile couples both after natural conception and after infertility treatment, but their pregnancies are also characterized by a higher prevalence of complications both during pregnancy and delivery. Those risks are further enhanced, if the pregnancy was induced with ovarian hyperstimulation followed by ART, as the duration of pregnancy is shortened and neonatal birth weight is reduced.[23] These changes are further aggravated, if a vanishing chorionic sac was observed during early pregnancy,[24] and, even more, in ongoing multiple pregnancies.[25]

QUALITY ASSURANCE THROUGH DATA REPORTING

The continuous follow-up of the various outcome parameters of all treatments is an integral part of all quality assurance. Ideally, the outcome of ART should consist of cumulative live birth data, including the cryopreserved and thawed embryo transfer cycles.[26]

However, those data can only be appreciated if they are compared with those of other data collections. It is best to compare the own results intermittently with the combined results of all other centres in one country or regional area. Such a benchmark may be the starting point for the detection of own weaknesses and to improve treatment quality.

The working conditions in the field of ART may vary much from one country to another, in part due to legislative regulation, but also due to differences in cultural habits, financial reimbursement of treatment costs and the overall population health status. In many countries (such as the United States and Switzerland) and in broader areas (such as the European IVF-Monitoring Group, EIM)[2] large data registries have been organized, which publish their results on a yearly basis.

REFERENCES

1. Dyer S, Chambers GM, de Mouzon J, et al. International Committee for Monitoring Assisted Reproductive Technologies world report: Assisted Reproductive Technology 2008, 2009 and 2010. Hum Reprod. 2016;31: 1588-609.

2. European IVF-Monitoring Consortium (EIM) for the European Society of Human Reproduction and Embryology (ESHRE), Calhaz-Jorge C, de Geyter C, Kupka MS, de Mouzon J, Erb K, Mocanu E, Motrenko T, Scaravelli G, Wyns C, Goossens V. Assisted reproductive technology in Europe, 2012: results generated from European registers by ESHRE. Hum Reprod. 2016; 31:1638-52.
3. ESHRE position paper on the EU tissues and cells directive EC/2004/23 (2007).
4. Popovic-Todorovic B, Loft A, Bredkjaeer HE, et al. A prospective randomized clinical trial comparing an individual dose of recombinant FSH based on predictive factors versus a 'standard' dose of 150 IU/day in 'standard' patients undergoing IVF/ICSI treatment. Hum Reprod. 2003;18:2275-82.
5. Olivennes F, Howles CM, Borini A, et al.; CONSORT study group. Individualizing FSH dose for assisted reproduction using a novel algorithm: the CONSORT study. Reprod Biomed Online. 2009;18:195-204.
6. Nyboe Andersen A, Nelson SM, Fauser BC, et al.; ESTHER-1 study group. Individualized versus conventional ovarian stimulation for in vitro fertilization: a multicenter, randomized, controlled, assessor-blinded, phase 3 noninferiority trial. Fertil Steril. 2017;107:387-96.
7. van Helden J, Weiskirchen R. Performance of the two new fully automated anti-Müllerian hormone immunoassays compared with the clinical standard assay. Hum Reprod. 2015;30:1918-26.
8. De Geyter C, Fehr P, Moffat R, et al. Twenty years' experience with the Swiss data registry for assisted reproductive medicine: outcomes, key trends and recommendations for improved practice. Swiss Med Wkly. 2015;145:w14087.
9. Coomarasamy A, Afnan M, Cheema D, et al. Urinary hMG versus recombinant FSH for controlled ovarian hyperstimulation following an agonist long down-regulation protocol in IVF or ICSI treatment: a systematic review and meta-analysis. Hum Reprod. 2008;23:310-5.
10. Bosch E, Valencia I, Escudero E, et al. Premature luteinization during gonadotropin-releasing hormone antagonist cycles and its relationship with in vitro fertilization outcome. Fertil Steril. 2003;80:1444-9.
11. De Geyter Ch, Steimann S, Huber P, et al. Elaboration of a working model for the involvement of inhibin A as a mediator of the preovulatory rise of progesterone levels. Gynecol Endocrinol. 2007;23:213-21.
12. Boomsma CM, Heineman MJ, Cohlen BJ, Farquhar C. Semen preparation techniques for intrauterine insemination. Cochrane Database Syst Rev. 2007;CD004507.
13. Terriou P, Hans E, Giorgetti C, et al. Pentoxifylline initiates motility in spontaneously immotile epididymal and testicular spermatozoa and allow normal fertilization, pregnancy, and birth after intracytoplasmic sperm injection. J Assist Fert Genet. 2000;17:194-9.
14. Kovačič B, Vlaisavljević V, Reljič M. Clinical use of pentoxifylline for activation of immotile testicular sperm before ICSI in patients with azoospermia. J Androl. 2006;27:45-52.
15. Balaban B, Urman B, Sertac A, et al. In-vitro culture of spermatozoa induces motility and increases implantation and pregnancy rates after testicular sperm extraction and intracytoplasmic sperm injection. Hum Reprod. 1999;14:2808-11.
16. Jain T, Gupta RS. Trends in the use of intracytoplasmic sperm injection in the United States. N Engl J Med. 2007;357:251-7.
17. De Geyter Ch, De Geyter M, Behre HM. Assisted reproduction. In: Nieschlag E, Behre HM, Nieschlag S (Eds). Andrology, 3nd edition Berlin, Heidelberg, New York: Springer; 2009. pp. 469-504.
18. Brown J, Buckingham K, Buckett W, et al. Ultrasound versus 'clinical touch' for catheter guidance during embryo transfer in women. Cochrane Database Syst Rev. 2016;3:CD006107.
19. Karlström PO, Bergh C. Reducing the number of embryos transferred in Sweden – impact on delivery and multiple birth rates. Hum Reprod. 2007;22:2202-7.
20. Humaidan P, Polyzos NP, Alsbjerg B, et al. GnRHa trigger and individualized luteal phase hCG support according to ovarian

response to stimulation: two prospective randomized controlled multi-centre studies in IVF patients. Hum Reprod. 2013;28:2511-21.
21. Connell MT, Szatkowski JM, Terry N, et al. Timing luteal support in assisted reproductive technology: a systematic review. Fertil Steril. 2015;103: 939-46.
22. Van der Linden M, Buckingham K, Farquhar C, et al. Luteal phase support for assisted reproduction cycles. Cochrane Database Syst Rev. 2015;7:CD009154.
23. De Geyter Ch, De Geyter M, Steimann S, et al. Comparative birth weights of singletons born after assisted reproduction and natural conception in previously infertile women. Hum Reprod. 2006;21:705-12.
24. Pinborg A, Lidegaard O, Freiesleben NC, Andersen AN. Vanishing twins: a predictor of small-for-gestational age in IVF singletons. Hum Reprod. 2007;22:2707-14.
25. Bergh T, Ericson A, Hillensjö T, et al. Deliveries and children born after in-vitro fertilisation in Sweden 1982-95: a retrospective cohort study. Lancet. 1999;354:1579-85.
26. De Geyter Ch, Wyns C, Mocanu E, et al. Data collection systems in ART must follow the pace of change in clinical practice. Hum Reprod. 2016;31:2160-3.
27. De Geyter Ch, De Geyter M, Behre HM. Assisted fertilization. In: Nieschlag E, Behre HM (Eds). Andrology, 3rd edition. Springer-Verlag; Berlin, Heidelberg, New York: 2009.

CHAPTER 21

Embryo Culture Systems

Judith Menezes

Chapter outline

- Physiology and Metabolism of the Preimplantation Embryo
- pH Control
- Temperature and Osmolarity
- Oxygen Concentration
- Oil
- Culture Media

INTRODUCTION

It is the aim of every *in vitro* fertilization (IVF) clinic to set-up a successful IVF program. How can this be achieved? Does success merely depends on owning sophisticated equipment such as incubators, microscopes, etc., buying a particular brand of culture media and using certain types of consumables? How does one ensure top quality embryos that have a high chance of implanting? How can one minimize or eliminate the complications associated with multiple pregnancy as a result of transferring more than one embryo?

Embryo culture system is the answer. They are in fact a crucial step influencing the potential for success in IVF programs and comprise of a whole gamble of things (Fig. 21.1). Central to this system are the two main players—the embryologist who is the immediate service provider and of course the customer who is the most important and must come first—the embryo! Depending on the duration of culture practiced by a particular clinic, the corresponding embryos must fulfill established milestones (Fig. 21.2). It is evident that an embryologist cannot make a good embryo from a bad egg. However, one can certainly make a good embryo bad by stressing it. Stress to the precompaction embryo causes alterations in metabolism, homeostasis and epigenetic control. This leads to perturbed development, reduced placental function, impaired fetal development and increased susceptibility to adult onset disease (Khosla et al., 2001; Watkins et al., 2007, Dumoulin et al., 2010). Suboptimal conditions also cause altered gene expression via altered methylation

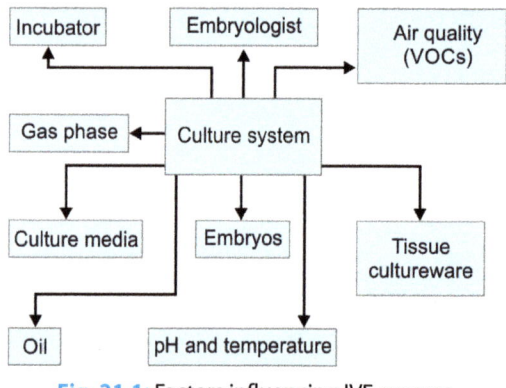

Fig. 21.1: Factors influencing IVF success.

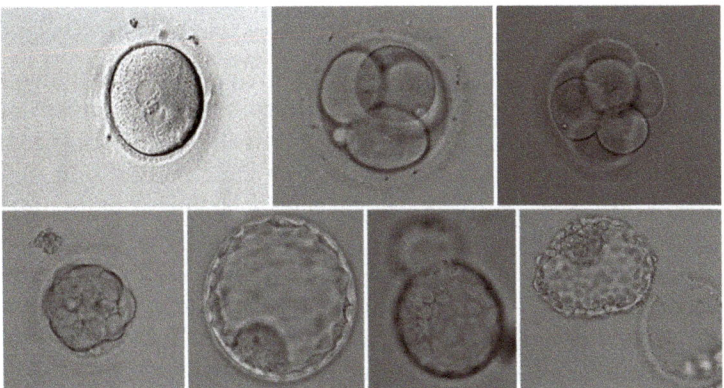
Fig. 21.2: Embryo development from Day 1 to 5.

patterns; assisted reproductive technology (ART) is associated with an increased incidence of gene imprinting disorders such as Beckwith-Wiedmann syndrome and Angelman's syndrome (Huntriss and Picton, 2008). The goal of embryo culture systems therefore, is to maintain embryo cellular physiology, normal developmental regulation, gene expression and minimize stress.

PHYSIOLOGY AND METABOLISM OF THE PREIMPLANTATION EMBRYO

In order to establish good embryo culture systems, it is essential to understand the differences in physiology of the embryo from the zygote to the blastocyst stage. The precompaction embryo (prior to the eight-cell stage) is characterized by low oxygen consumption and biosynthetic activity. Metabolism is pyruvate based, there is a low requirement for glucose and energy is produced via oxidative phosphorylation. The maternal genome is operative at this stage. Since the ability for cellular homeostasis is low, the embryo is very suspectible to trauma. The switchover to the embryonic genome occurs during the postcompaction stage, which is characterized by high oxygen consumption and biosynthetic activity. Nutrient preference shifts to glucose; metabolism is via oxidative phosphorylation and aerobic glycolysis. Differentiation into inner cell mass and trophectoderm also occur postcompaction. The ICM cells are dependent on glycolysis whereas the trophectoderm cells are dependent on oxidative phosphorylation (Lane and Gardner, 2007).

If precompaction embryos *in vitro* are exposed to high concentrations of glucose, oxidative phosphorylation is depressed due to stimulation of glycolysis (Crabtree effect). On the other hand, total absence of glucose leads to decreased glycosylation and cell survival and altered levels of key transcription factors. A low but finite concentration of glucose is required which is metabolized via the pentose phosphate pathway for the production of reduced glutathione (a potent antioxidant), biosynthesis of nucleic acids and lipids and O-linked glycosylation. Glucose acts as a signal to activate gene expression, differentiation and development, via this pathway (Pantaleon et al., 2008).

The importance of the malate-aspartate shuttle (MAS) in embryos also needs to be emphasized. The MAS transfers NADH from the cytoplasm to the mitochondria. This is essential for cells to metabolize glucose and lactate. Disruption of the MAS does not inhibit blastocyst formation. However, it reduces the number of inner cell mass (ICM) and trophectoderm cells, causes reduced implantation and fetal growth via altered placental development (Mitchell et al., 2009).

Currently, there is a global effort to find effective means of selecting a single viable embryo for transfer, from a cohort. Elective transfer of a single embryo eliminates all the complications involved with multiple embryo transfer (Adashi et al., 2003). The most common grading of embryo quality is based on development stage and morphology (Sjoblom et al., 2006) but cellular disturbances that occur as a result of embryo exposure to suboptimal environments cannot be determined using morphology. In such cases, morphologically normal blastocysts can develop but they are severely compromised at the cellular level (Khosla et al., 2001; Watkins et al., 2007). Therefore, other biomarkers of embryo viability are urgently required. Leese et al., 2008 have proposed that embryos with a quieter metabolism are more viable. In response to environmental stress such as elevated ammonium or high oxygen concentrations, there may be upregulation of metabolism. ICM cells of the blastocyst are known to be metabolically quieter than those of the trophectoderm (Houghton, 2006). Research is also underway to address the question as to whether quieter ICM cells are more likely to give rise to stem cells. Culture of embryos in low oxygen, which promotes a low level of energy metabolism, also helps in maintaining the pluripotent state of human ES cell lines (Ezashi et al., 2005). Noninvasive methods for determining viable embryos include measurement of respiration or metabolic profiling such as amino acid turnover. In keeping with the quiet embryo hypothesis, Sturmey et al. (2009) have shown that viable human embryos with the lowest DNA damage had the lowest amino acid turnover. What is striking is the fact that there is extremely poor correlation between embryo morphology grade and DNA damage.

pH CONTROL

Maintenance of intracellular pH (pHi) of early embryos is of fundamental importance. Let us begin with somatic cells to understand how this system functions. In the latter, pH in the acid range is regulated by the Na^+/H^+ antiporter with Na^+ moving into the cell and H^+ moving out. In the alkaline range, it is the HCO_3^-/Cl^- exchanger which moves an HCO_3^- out in exchange for a Cl^-. Oocytes and early zygotes however have no transport systems for pHi regulation. These are activated only around the time of fertilization (pronuclei formation). The Na^+/H^+ antiporter activity is variable and not robust for removing acid loads, while the HCO_3^-/Cl^- system becomes active in later stage embryos. There is an increased ability to regulate pH after compaction has occurred due to the formation of a transporting epithelium. The pHi is reportedly in the range of 7.2 (Gardner, 2008). Hence, most commercially available media have a pH of 7.27 ± 0.5. Earlier culture media had pH values between 7.3 and 7.4, as it was believed that the embryo was meant to work against this gradient. It is now known that such high pH levels stress the oocyte and embryo. While handling oocytes and embryos one must be careful to avoid fluctuations in pH and 'out of range' pH as they not only disrupt protein and enzyme function, but mitochondria and microfilament organization as well (Van Blerkom et al., 2000).

In vitro, embryos are dependent on HCO_3^-/CO_2 for pHi regulation. This is provided by the bicarbonate present in the medium and the appropriate concentration of carbon dioxide, CO_2 in the incubator, to maintain pH in the range 7.2-7.3. Accurate monitoring of pH or CO_2 levels within incubators is needed continually in order to obtain consistent outcomes. Exposure outside the incubator should be minimal as pH increases beyond 7.4 within two minutes of atmospheric exposure. Many of the commercially available media do not contain the pH indicator, phenol red. Hence, one can remain blissfully ignorant of the rapid pH changes occurring as the media remain colorless.

When exposed to the atmosphere for longer periods such as oocyte pickup and intracytoplasmic sperm (ICSI), buffers such as HEPES or MOPS should be included to maintain physiological pH. The use of the latter is also recommended for denudation both prior to ICSI and prior to fertilization check for IVF. A recent study by Swain and Pool, 2009, has reported the utilization of multibuffered media containing a mixture of HEPES, MOPS and DIPSO to have better pH buffering capacity while handling gametes and embryos outside the incubator. Most of these buffers require just warming to 37°C before use without pre-equilibration in carbon dioxide atmosphere. One must therefore carefully read the specifications and instructions provided by the manufacturer. Accidental equilibration of these buffers in carbon dioxide will cause a drop in pH to the neutral or acidic range, thereby stressing the embryo.

TEMPERATURE AND OSMOLARITY

Besides pH, temperature regulation is another crucial factor. Exposure of oocytes and embryos to room temperature for a few minutes irreversibly disrupts microtubules in oocytes and embryos, thus risking aneuploidy in the resulting embryos (Almeida and Bolton, 1995). Exposure to high temperatures (39°C) is also detrimental to microtubule organization. Temperature shifts can affect transmembrane transport and metabolism. Exposure to suboptimal temperatures is believed to slow down development and decrease embryo viability. It is important to see that the oocytes and embryos are maintained at a stable 37°C both within and outside the incubator. This demands proper quality assurance procedures in the laboratory. Oocytes and embryos must be examined on warmed stages. Care must be taken to see that the oocytes right from the time of collection to the moment of transfer are constantly exposed to physiological temperature. Temperatures of all warming stages and tube warmers must be frequently checked with certified calibrated thermometers. It is important to note that the temperature of the medium within the dish or tube should be measured and not the surface temperature of the warming device. If one resorts to the latter, then one does not take into account the thermal conductivity of the tissue culture dish or tube as well as the air gap between the dish and the warming device, which results in an insulation effect. While working on warmed stages, one must be cautious with open dishes containing oocytes and embryos, as the osmolarity of the medium will increase rapidly, due to evaporation in a nonhumidified environment.

The culture of gametes and embryos at 37°C (body temperature) has recently been debated. Temperature within mammalian ovarian follicles is reported to be about 2°C lower than body temperature. Besides, temperature gradients exist in the fallopian tube. The reduced temperature in the isthmus may be responsible for sperm being maintained in a quiescent state prior to hyperactivation at fertilization in the ampulla. The question has therefore been raised as to whether IVF should be done at 35.5–36°C instead of 37°C, since the metabolism of embryos will be around 15% lower in this temperature range, thus making the embryos more quiet in terms of metabolism and hence more viable. However, before reducing the incubation temperature for human IVF, it is necessary to study the effects of temperature reduction on animal embryos (Leese et al., 2008).

It is therefore imperative to have stringent control over both temperature and pH. The incubators chosen for embryo culture should be able to precisely provide these requirements. In addition, there should be minimal door openings in order to prevent fluctuation of both parameters, which would

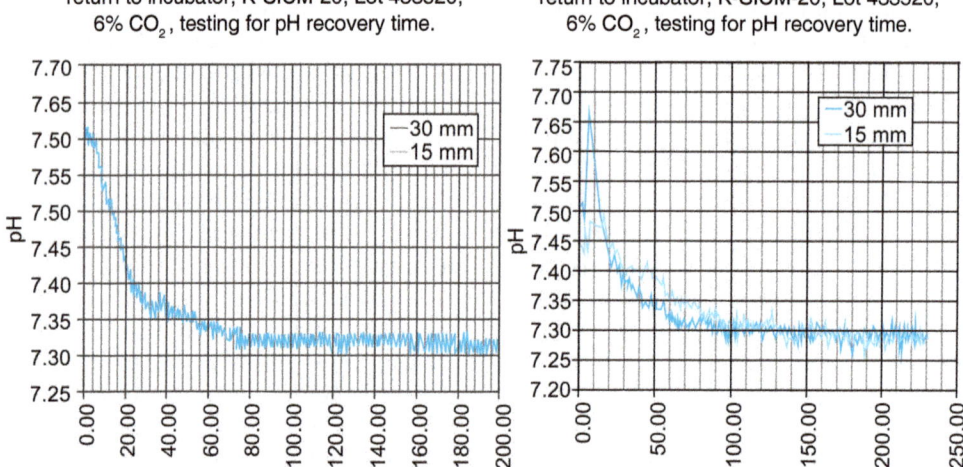

Fig. 21.3A: Slow pH recovery time in a large volume incubator (left) compared to a mini-incubator (Wiemerm, 2006).
(Courtesy: Cook Medical)

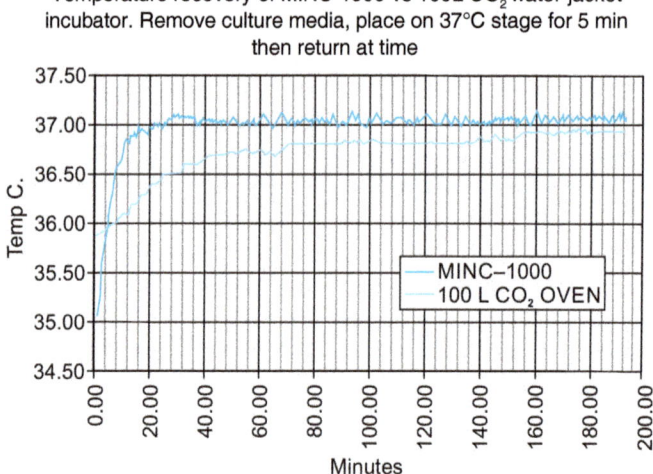

Fig. 21.3B: Slow temperature recovery in a large incubator (blue) compared to a mini-incubator (red) (Wiemerm, 2006).
(Courtesy: Cook Medical)

negatively influence embryo quality and subsequent results. Since an IVF laboratory caters to several patients, each laboratory needs to ensure that it has sufficient incubators to meet the workload. Small volume gas incubators or mini incubators are preferable to the large volume ones as both temperature and pH recovery are more rapid (Figs. 21.3A and B). Mini-incubators have a distinct advantage in this regard as they provide rapid heat transfer (as there is no gap between the bottom of the dishes and incubation surface) and the gas purge function operates immediately after door opening which makes pH recovery rapid (Fujiwara et al., 2007). The ideal way to maintain physiological conditions would be to use complete gas, temperature and humidity controlled environments such as the 'EMcell' and 'Active IVF'.

OXYGEN CONCENTRATION

While 5-6% CO_2 is universally used for embryo culture with a view to providing physiological pH, oxygen, O_2, concentration used by the majority of the laboratories worldwide is 20%. The oviductal oxygen tension in several mammalian species studied to date varies between 1% and 9% (Fisher and Bavister, 1993), so the question arises whether the use of atmospheric O_2 (20%) is physiological. There is ample evidence to prove the detrimental effects of high O_2. I will cite a few of the most important. Pabon et al., 1989 were the first to show that exposure of mouse embryos to 20% O_2 for just one hour did not affect development till the four-cell stage, but subsequent development to blastocysts and their ICM number were significantly decreased in comparison with controls cultured throughout in low (5%) O_2. This has implications for IVF performing transfers on Day 2 when embryos are at the four-cell stage. Many of these embryos would be nonviable if they have been cultured under high oxygen. Gardner et al., 1996, too reported similar results when embryos were transferred to dishes prequilibrated in high oxygen and then cultured in low oxygen. Mosaicism in human embryos has been reported to be lower in laboratories culturing embryos in low oxygen (Munne et al., 1997). A study on sibling oocyte development in human IVF revealed a significantly higher pregnancy and implantation rate with 5% O_2 compared to 20% O_2 (Kovacic et al., 2008). In a recent RCT comparing culture in high and low O_2, both clinical pregnancy and live birth rate were significantly higher in the low O_2 group, irrespective of the day of transfer (Meintjes et al., 2009). The global pattern of gene expression of mouse embryos cultured in low O_2 resembles more closely that of *in vivo* control embryos, compared to embryos cultured in 20% (Rinaudo et al., 2006). With the available evidence to date, the inconvenient truth is that there is no justification to continue culturing embryos in high oxygen.

Why is atmospheric oxygen considered a villain for embryo culture? The answer lies in the overproduction of reactive oxygen species (ROS). ROS which are highly reactive are generated as a byproduct of respiration in the mitochondria. Overproduction leads to loss of calcium homeostasis within the cells and oxidation of proteins (enzymes) in the inner mitochondrial membrane. This causes collapse of mitochondrial membrane potential and hence ATP synthesis, which ultimately leads to necrosis, apoptosis and fragmentation. ROS levels seem to be a good marker for early embryonic growth as they are inversely correlated with fertilization, blastocyst development and pregnancy (Bedaiwy et al., 2004).

With the evidence available regarding the benefits of a low oxygen environment for culture, multigas incubators should be used. These can be constant flow incubators where premixed gas (6% CO_2, 5% O_2, 89% N_2) is used or those with infrared carbon dioxide sensors to minimize fluctuations in gas concentrations as well as to ensure rapid recovery after door opening.

OIL

In vitro embryo culture is usually performed in two ways, either open culture in a large volume of medium (0.5-1 mL) or in microdroplets overlaid with oil. The latter is believed to have many advantages, namely prevention of water from the medium which would affect osmolarity, reduction of gas (and hence pH) and temperature fluctuations in the medium, protection from microbial contamination, ease of embryo examination and neutralization of toxins. Oil overlay has also been reported to significantly influence development to blastocysts with subsequent improvement in freezability (Van Soom et al., 2001). Mineral oil has been extensively used for embryo culture in IVF. Most commercial suppliers usually test oil for microbial contamination, endotoxin and also perform a mouse embryo test. However, the fact that mineral oil is less stable due to the presence of increased unsaturated bonds and hence prone to attack by free oxygen radicals and photo-oxidation, is ignored. There is now evidence gathering that peroxidation of mineral oil used in droplet culture is detrimental to fertilization and embryo development. It is recommended that mineral oils with a peroxide value (POV) of more than 0.02 mEq/kg should not be used for embryo culture. It is likely that the free radicals produced by peroxidation of the oil attach to albumin which is an essential ingredient of culture medium and are transported across the zona pellucida, thus causing embryo damage (Otzuki et al., 2009). Paraffin oil on the other hand has been shown to yield better embryo development since it has more saturated bonds than mineral oil (Tae et al., 2006). However, one must be cautious even with the latter and make sure that the oil has been maintained at low temperature (4°C) during transport by the supplier and subsequent storage by the user. It should become mandatory for suppliers to provide the POV values of every batch of oil supplied as well as the POV profiles of the oil with time.

CULTURE MEDIA

Culture media used for IVF have evolved from primitive media, which ranged from simple balanced salt solutions such as Earles, T6 and HTF containing glucose, pyruvate, lactate, supplemented with patient's own serum to complex media such as Ham's F10, MEM, TC199 meant for tissue culture and cell lines. The modern sequential media were developed to support the changing metabolic needs of the embryo as well as to support homeostasis and minimize intracellular stress. In the ampulla, pyruvate and lactate concentrations are the highest and decrease down the tract, reaching the lowest concentrations in the uterus. Glucose concentration however is low in the ampulla and high in the uterus. The composition of sequential media have therefore been formulated to reflect these physiological conditions within the female reproductive tract.

Important ingredients in currently used media are buffers of intracellular pH, osmolytes, biosynthetic precursors, energy sources, regulators of energy metabolism, antioxidants, chelators, etc. Fertilization medium is characterized by the presence of high glucose, which is required as an energy source for cumulus cells. Glucose in fertilization medium is taken up by cumulus cells and converted via glycolysis to pyruvate in order to generate ATP. The latter is generated by oxidative phosphorylation in the mitochondria. Cleavage medium, which contains low glucose must be introduced following removal of cumulus cells after ICSI or at fertilization check in standard IVF. This medium is used till the compaction (8-cell stage). Following this, blastocyst medium which is high in glucose and is the most complex of the three media in the sequential medium series is used.

Ethylene-diamine-tetra-acetic-acid (EDTA) is an essential ingredient of cleavage (pre-compaction) media, as it inhibits glycolysis in the cleavage stage embryo, thus enhancing development. EDTA acts by chelating magnesium, thus reducing the availability of this cofactor to the glycolytic kinases (Lane and Gardner, 2007). Since the ICM exclusively uses glycolysis, EDTA is excluded from postcompaction media, as its inclusion could adversely affect fetal development. Other components include hyaluronan, which is the major glycosaminoglycan present in the reproductive tract and appears to help in sperm selection, embryonic cell proliferation and implantation. Hyaluronan has also been reported to significantly improve embryo cryosurvivability (Balaban and Urman, 2005). Pantothenate, which is a component of coenzyme A, is included in some formulations of cleavage media as it helps the crucial third cell cycle (cleavage from 4 to 8 cells when the activation of the embryonic genome takes place).

Antioxidants in the media are necessary for counteracting excessive ROS production from gametes and embryos during culture. Lipoate, which is the most potent known antioxidant, is an ingredient in certain commercially available media. It is synthesized in the mitochondria and is soluble in both aqueous and lipid phases, which is unique. Lipoate is also capable of regenerating other antioxidants including glutathione (Bilska and Wlodek, 2005). Simply using antioxidants in culture media to counteract the damaging effects of free oxygen radicals on embryos, seems to be a cheap and easy strategy, instead of using expensive incubators that provide low oxygen for culture. However, it is only the combination of such antioxidant containing media and culture in low oxygen that results in a significant increase in livebirth rate (Meintjes et al., 2009, Waldenström et al., 2009). The carry home message is to prevent the formation of damaging agents in the vicinity of developing embryos instead of attempting to neutralize these agents after they have been formed. Hence, the recommendation and enforcement of incubation environments containing low oxygen is fully justified.

Use of patient's serum in the medium has been discontinued due to reports of its adverse effects such as fetal overgrowth in bovine species as well as epigenetic alterations in imprinted genes (Huntriss and Picton, 2008). Human serum albumin (HSA) or recombinant albumin is used instead of serum. HSA prevents gametes and embryos from becoming sticky, facilitates manipulation by altering surface tension, negates the effects of toxins and contributes to colloidal osmotic pressure.

All culture media contain albumin as well as amino acids. The reproductive tract fluids contain significant amounts of amino acids while oocytes and embryos have specific transport systems for amino acids as well as an endogenous pool of amino acids. Nonessential amino acids and glutamine stimulate cleavage rates, blastocyst formation and hatching. Following compaction, essential amino acids stimulate cleavage and development of the ICM in the blastocyst. The beneficial effects of amino acids are their use as energy substrates but more importantly their role as intracellular osmolytes and regulators of internal pH. Other attributed roles of amino acids during early embryo development are biosynthetic precursors, regulators of metabolism, antioxidants, chelators, signaling and regulation of differentiation. The presence or absence of nonessential amino acids and glutamine in the oocyte collection medium at follicle aspiration, has a significant effect on subsequent embryo development. When zygotes were exposed to media, which lacked amino acids for less than 5 minutes, there was a sudden efflux of the endogenous pool of amino acids. This caused stress to the zygotes and even if they were replaced in medium containing amino acids, development to the blastocyst stage was impaired (Gardner and Lane, 1996). In view of these findings, oocytes are now collected in media containing nonessential amino acids. In an attempt to cut costs, phosphate buffered saline, phosphate buffered saline (PBS) should not be used for oocyte collection.

As a result of amino acid metabolism as well as breakdown at 37°C, ammonium ions are released into the surrounding culture medium, the majority of it being derived from glutamine. Increasing ammonium production leads to reduction of intracellular pH. The adverse effects of this are retarded ICM and fetal development, alteration of gene expression and imprinting status of H19. Neural tube defects, which is the worse case scenario has been reported only in the mouse (Gardner and Lane, 1993). Ammonium has therefore been termed the silent demon. Its adverse effects have been alleviated to a large extent by replacing the most labile amino acid, glutamine, with dipeptide forms such as alanylglutamine or glycylglutamine which are more stable. Besides albumin concentration in the newer versions of media has been reduced in order to limit breakdown into ammonium. It is also mandatory to change the culture medium every 48 hours to prevent ammonium buildup.

Recently, global medium has been launched into the IVF market. It is claimed to fully support human embryo development from Day 1 to 6, without intermittent media changes. This medium, which is based on KSOM (potassium supplemented simplex Optimization medium), is albumin free and contains glucose, lactate, pyruvate, EDTA and amino acids. The medium must be supplemented with human serum albumin or synthetic serum substitute prior to use. The developers of this medium claim that it reduces stresses on the embryo caused by intermittent media changes. The proportions of blastocysts and ongoing pregnancies have been reported to be significantly higher than that obtained with sequential medium (Angus et al., 2006). The rationale behind use of this medium is completely in conflict with the earlier doctrine of the changing needs of the embryo. Besides no prospective randomized trials comparing this medium with sequential media have been reported to date.

Since culture medium is labile, one must be sure that the cold chain has been maintained right from dispatch till arrival. The user must also ensure that the culture media are refrigerated and that there is minimal exposure out of the refrigerator during preparation of dishes, tubes, etc. for the following day. Temperatures within the refrigerators should be strictly monitored. Media containers once opened should be used within a week or two, as bioburden is likely to increase with time. The volume of individual media containers used should depend on the workload of the particular clinic. It may also be appropriate to aliquot media after opening but the containers used for this purpose must be sterile and embryo tested. Use of 'home made' media is highly discouraged unless one has the resources to use ingredients of the highest quality and conduct extensive and appropriate quality control tests to confirm its eligibility for use.

Several aspects must be taken into account in order to ensure an efficient culture system. Everything that comes in contact with the gametes and embryos should be considered. This begins with the tissue cultureware (dishes, tubes, pipettes, etc.) which must be of tissue culture grade, pyrogen tested and mouse embryo assay tested. Quality control documentation supplied by the manufacturer should be preserved for an appropriate period of time and batch numbers must be recorded to provide for traceability. This is very useful in case of any suboptimal outcomes when it becomes necessary to do a root cause analysis. Use of suboptimal tissue cultureware can and will lead to impaired embryo development.

Air quality is another essential component of embryo culture systems. Poor air quality, high in volatile organic carbons (VOCs) and other environmental pollutants can affect any stage of embryo development from fertilization to viability of embryos, which may or may not be evident from their morphology (Cohen et al., 1997). Air within the embryo laboratory must undergo filtration via HEPA and carbon filters. The quality of the air should be checked at routine intervals to make sure that the required standards are being maintained. Hygiene control is also important. Work benches and other areas in the laboratory and operating areas must also be routinely checked for bioburden. The source and quality of the gases used in the incubators is of prime importance. Only medicinal grade gases should be used and gas lines should contain carbon filters where appropriate to adsorb the volatile agents. Access to the laboratory should be restricted and special clothing and footwear is mandatory.

In spite of the advancements in embryo culture techniques, the third dimension is not available for surface chemistry. *In vivo* in the oviduct and uterus, the embryo is surrounded by oriented glycoproteins as they are moved by ciliated epithelia, thus creating a constricted moist environment. The female tract constantly modifies the environment providing gradients of nutrients required by the embryo and removing toxins. *In vitro* however, the embryo is in a 'static' environment, placed on inert synthetic polymers in the petri dish and bathed in a relative large ocean of media. To overcome these drawbacks, microfluidics seems to be underway to usher in a new era in embryo culture, where conditions are more physiologic and there is minimal handling and hence stress to both gametes and embryos (Smith and Takayama, 2007). In the future, the lab on a chip technology could provide for automation of embryo culture, inclusive of noninvasive diagnostic assays of embryo quality.

In all this, the pivotal role of the immediate service provider—the embryologist should not be underestimated. The embryologist holds the greatest responsibility in helping to provide the most physiological possible milieu for the embryo. He or she must have a thorough knowledge of basic physiology and chemistry in order to understand the basic needs of the embryo and monitor the adequacy and reliability of the culture system. Practical training, experience and constant upgrading of knowledge and skills are equally important. The European Society of Human Reproduction (ESHRE) has implemented a program for Certification of Clinical Embryologists with the aim of defining the concept of qualified embryologists and contributing to the assurance of good laboratory practice (Magli et al., 2008).

Postgraduate degree courses in Clinical Embryology are now available in some countries. These however, of high standard, are extremely expensive for young aspirants coming from a middleclass background. Recently a Masters course has been initiated at one of the universities in India and such courses should be encouraged and supported by well-established Indian embryologists. There is also an urgent need for strictly implementing directives in addition to guidelines, for the practice of ART in India.

In conclusion, one can achieve an efficient culture system only through continuous analysis and improvement. This can be achieved through a good quality management system, which covers both quality control and quality assurance, as well as continual monitoring of outcomes such as fertilization rates, cleavage rates, percentage of good quality embryos, blastocyst development, etc. (Mortimer and Mortimer, 2005). This demands setting up of benchmarks for the various parameters as well as very thorough and methodical documentation. The simplest way to document would be to use an Excel sheet. However, with the expertise in information technology that India boasts of, there should be no problem in setting up user friendly programs to record and analyze data.

The ultimate goal of the IVF clinic is healthy babies, hence the most essential component of the culture system is to ensure the quality and consistency of the environment that the gametes and embryos are exposed to. With the static nature of the current practice of embryo culture being questioned, microfluidics is likely to drastically alter embryo culture systems in a far more physiological direction. Finally, successful embryo culture systems cannot be established without good embryologists.

BIBLIOGRAPHY

1. Adashi EY, Barri PN, Berkowitz R. Infertility therapy-associated multiple pregnancies (births): an ongoing epidemic. Reprod Biomed Online. 2003;7:515-42.
2. Almeida P, Bolton V. The effect of temperature fluctuations on the cytoskeletal organisation and chromosomal constitution of the human oocyte. Zygote. 1995;3:357-65.
3. Angus S, Grunert GM, Dunn RC, et al. No advantage of using the sequential GIII media versus the single media Global. Fertil Steril. 2006;86 Suppl 2: S22 (Abstr P-254).
4. Balaban B, Urman B. Comparison of two sequential media for culturing cleavage stage embryos and blastocysts: embryo characteristics and clinical outcome. RBM Online. 2005;10(4):485-91.
5. Bedaiwy MA, Falcone T, Mohamed MS, et al. Differential growth of human embryos *in vitro*: role of reactive oxygen species. Fertil Steril. 2004;82(3):593-600.
6. Bilska A, Wlodek L. Lipoic acid – the drug of the future? Pharmacol Rep. 2005;57(5):570-7.
7. Cohen J, Gilligan A, Esposito W, et al. Ambient air and its potential effects on conception *in vitro*. Hum Reprod. 1997; 2:1742-9.
8. Dumoulin JC, Land JA, Van Montfoort AP, et al. Effect of *in vitro* culture of human embryos on birthweight of newborns. Hum Reprod. 2010;25: 605-12.
9. Ezashi T, Das P, Roberts RM. Low O_2 tensions and the prevention of differentiation of hES cells. Proc Natl Acad Sci USA. 2005;102:4783-8.
10. Fisher B, Bavister BD. Oxygen tension in the oviduct and uterus of rhesus monkeys, hamsters and rabbits. J Reprod Fertil. 1993;99:673-9.
11. Fujiwara M, Takahasi K, Izuno M, et al. Effect of microenvironment maintenance on embryo culture after *in vitro* fertilisation: comparison of top-load mini incubator and conventional front-load incubator. J Assist Reprod Genet. 2007;24:5-9.
12. Gardner DK. Dissection of culture media for embryos: the most important and less important components and characteristics. Reprod Fertil Dev. 2008;20:9-18.
13. Gardner DK, Lane M. Alleviation of the 2 cell block and development to the blastocyst of CF1 mouse embryos: role of amino acids, EDTA and physical parameters. Hum. Reprod. 1996;11(12):2703-12.
14. Gardner DK, Lane M. Amino acids and ammonium regulate mouse embryo development in culture. Biol Reprod. 1993;48:377-85.
15. Houghton FD. Energy metabolism of the inner cell mass and trophectoderm of the mouse blastocyst. Differentiation. 2006;74:11-8.
16. Huntriss J, Picton HM. Epigenetic consequences of assisted reproduction and infertility on the human preimplantation embryo. Human Fertility. 2008;11(2)85-94.
17. Khosla S, Dean W, Reik W, Feil R. Culture of preimplantation embryos and its long term effects on gene expression and phenotype. Hum Reprod Update. 2001;7:419-27.
18. Kovacic B, Vlaisavljevic V. Influence of atmospheric versus reduced oxygen concentration on development of human blastocysts *in vitro*: a prospective study on sibling oocytes. Reprod Biomedicine Online. 2008;17(2):229-36.
19. Lane M, Gardner DK. Embryo culture medium: which is the best? Best Practice and Research Clinical Obstetrics and Gynaecology. 2007;1: 83-100.
20. Leese HJ, Baumann CG, Brison DR, et al. Metabolism of the viable mammalian embryo: quietness revisited. Mol Hum Reprod. 2008;14(12)667-72.
21. Magli MC, Van den Abbeel E, Lundin K, et al. Revised guidelines for good practice in IVF laboratories. Hum Reprod. 2008;23(6):1253-62.
22. Meintjes M, Chantilis SJ, Douglas JD, et al. A controlled randomized trial evaluating the effect of lowered incubator oxygen tension on live births in a predominantly

blastocyst transfer program. Hum Reprod. 2009;24(2):300-7.
23. Mitchell M, Cashman KS, Gardner DK, et al. Disruption of mitochondrial malate-aspartate shuttle activity in mouse blastocysts impairs viability and fetal growth. Biol Reprod. 2009;80:295-301.
24. Mortimer DM, Mortimer S. Quality and Risk Management in the IVF Laboratory. Cambridge: Cambridge University Press; 2005.
25. Munne S, Magli C, Adler A, et al. Treatment related chromosome abnormalities in human embryos. Hum Reprod. 1997;12(4): 780-4.
26. Otzuki J, Nagai Y, Chiba K. Damage of embryo development caused by peroxidized mineral oil and its association with albumin in culture. Fertil Steril. 2009;91(5):1745- 9.
27. Pabon JE, Findley WE, Gibbons WE. The toxic effect of short exposures to the atmospheric oxygen concentration on early mouse embryonic development. Fertil Steril. 1989; 51:896-900.
28. Pantaleon M, Kaye PL. Nutrient sensing by the early mouse embryo: hexosamine biosynthesis and glucose signalling during preimplantation development. Reprod Fertil Dev. 2008; 78(4):595-600.
29. Rinaudo PF, Giritharan G, Talbi S, et al. Effects of oxygen tension on gene expression in preimplantation mouse embryos. Fertil Steril. 2006;86(4 Suppl):1252-65.
30. Sjoblom P, Menezes J, Cummins L, et al. Prediction of embryo developmental potential and pregnancy based on early stage morphological characteristics. Fertil Steril. 2006;86(4):848-61.
31. Smith GD, Takayama S. Gamete and embryo isolation and culture with microfluidics. Theriogenology. 2007; 68 Suppl 1:190-5.
32. Sturmey RG, Hawkhead JA, Barker A, Leese HJ. DNA damage and metabolic activity in the preimplantion embryo. Hum Reprod. 2009;24(1):81-91.
33. Swain JE, Pool TB. New pH-buffering system for media utilized during gamete and embryo manipulations for assisted reproduction. Reprod Biomed Online. 2009;18(6):799-810.
34. Tae JC, Kim EY, Lee WD, et al. Sterile filtered paraffin oil supports in vitro developmental competence in bovine embryos comparable to coculture. J Assist Reprod Genet. 2006; 23(3):121-7.
35. Van Blerkom J, Davis P, Alexander S. Differential mitochondrial distribution in human pronuclear embryos leads to disproportionate inheritance between blastomeres: relationship to mitotubular organisation, ATP content and competence. Hum Reprod. 2000;15:2621-33.
36. Van Soom A, Mahmoudzadeb A, Christophe A, et al. Silicone oil used in microdrop culture can affect bovine embryonic development and freezability. Reprod Domest Anim. 2001;36:169-76.
37. Waldenström U, Engstrom A, Hellberg D, Nilsson S. Low oxygen compared with high oxygen atmosphere in blastocyst culture, a prospective randomised study. Fertil Steril. 2009; 91(6): 2461-5.
38. Watkins AJ, Platt D, Papenbrock T, et al. Mouse embryo culture induce changes in postnatal phenotype including raised systolic blood pressure. Proc Natl Acad Sci USA. 2007;104:5449-54.

CHAPTER 22

Laboratory Set-up for IVF-ICSI

Vijay Mangoli, Ranjana Mangoli,

Chapter outline

- Location of the Laboratory
- Structural Requirements
- Layout
  - Reception Area
  - Nurse's Work Area
  - Changing Room
  - Semen Collection Room
  - General Laboratory
  - Sterilization Area
  - Scrubbing Area
  - Operation Theater
  - Culture Room
  - Administration Office
- Embryologist and Staff Rest Room and Discussion Room
- Storage Space
- Gas Cylinders and Liquid Nitrogen Tanks
- Electricity Control Room
- Instruments
  - Instruments for Operation Theater
  - Instruments and Materials for Laboratory
  - Instruments and Materials for Culture Room
  - Laboratory Personnel
- Record Keeping
- Quality Control

INTRODUCTION

In 1978, Dr Robert Edwards—an embryologist and Dr Patrick Steptoe- a gynecologist from UK made history by creating implantable human embryo in a test tube.[1] The procedure known as '*in vitro* fertilization' (IVF) was basically aimed for the indication of tubal factor where both the fallopian tubes were damaged beyond repair thus making natural conception impossible. IVF was the first treatment modality where basic science was equally involved along with clinical science in getting a successful outcome while treating infertility. Over a period of time, many more indications apart from tubal factor like endometriosis, male factor, repeated failed intra uterine insemination, and unexplained infertility were found to be benefitted through IVF. Though it appears as a simple method of dispersing motile sperms around the oocyte and transferring resulted embryo into the uterine cavity, it require lots of scientific efforts to achieve the goal.

As a matter of fact, there can be vast differences between IVF laboratories from infrastructure, material, and methodology point of view; still all of them can result in acceptable pregnancy rates. IVF laboratory is a place where male and female gametes are manipulated to achieve successful fertilization and to get viable embryos. Other supportive techniques like micromanipulation, cryopreservation including sperm, oocyte and embryo freezing, pre-implantation genetic diagnosis, and research activities are also carried out in the laboratory. IVF laboratory has to be looked upon with a great sense of responsibility as it is a place where pre-implanting human embryos are created. Setting up an IVF laboratory involves— planning defined areas for specific purposes, maintaining clean and sterile environment, setting up high quality instruments, getting proper disposables, maintaining quality control, appointing qualified personnel, and making provisions for proper record keeping.

LOCATION OF THE LABORATORY

Though ideally, a quiet, isolated place is more suitable, nowadays IVF centers are located in city centers keeping patient's convenience in mind. This may impose additional precautionary measures in terms of maintaining 'dust and particulate free' sterile areas. Locations like one near petrol pump, chemical godown, factories emitting fine particles or with heavy traffic are always at risk of becoming unsuitable for cell tissue culture.[2]

STRUCTURAL REQUIREMENTS

Some buildings like stone walled with vary rough outer and inner surfaces may be intrinsically harmful for IVF laboratory from infrastructure point of view. The inner wall surface of the laboratory and culture room should be of hard material with non-porous texture like granite or specially treated marble. Such surfaces are easy to clean, to keep free from contaminations and also longer lasting with minimum maintenance. Hard POP walls painted with minimum emitting odors are another alternative but needs frequent maintenance. Paints should be water based with acrylic latex polymers rather than epoxy. Epoxy paints emit amine catalysts over a long period of time. Therefore, if such paints are applied, the walls must be 'cured' for about 3 months.[3]

From disturbance point of view, it is advantageous to have IVF laboratory on upper floor. Attention also should be given to water seepage and accumulation of rain water near the outer surfaces that may damage walls and cause fungal contamination. A survey of any new constructions nearby or demolition of existing structures helps as, such civil works has negative effect on IVF outcome.[4] Basic environmental evaluation like particulates, volatile organic compounds, organics and aldehydes should be done to decide preventive measures like air changes per hour under positive pressure. However, we should remember that due to anesthetic and cleaning activities, sometimes outer air may be more 'pure' than laboratory.[5] There should be minimum penetrations with all electrical, gas and air conditioning fittings concealed but with provisions for easy maintenance. Window air conditioners should be avoided. Gases required in operation theater (OT) and culture room if brought in from centralized location, the quality of tubing used plays an important role. Oxidation of copper tubing may become toxic over a period of time. Either a high grade stainless steel (SS) or Teflon coated tubing is preferred particularly for CO_2 used in the incubators. Even those tubing should be cleaned using inert gases frequently once in 6 months. In many places, IVF centers are located in residential premises. Extra care has to be taken for water storage tanks. Separate stainless steel tanks should be installed for laboratory and water should not be used from building's common storage tanks, which are regularly disinfected using strong chemicals like chlorine. As a general rule, minimum wood material should be used in laboratory. If unavoidable, longer lasting, high density, termite proof, treated marine plywood should be used. It is better to coat it with SS. For flooring, vinyl and rubber are discouraged due to their off gassing effect.[6] Large vitrified tiles or treated marble is preferred. After completion of the culture room, OT and laboratory, to make it practically usable, fumigation and UV sterilization is done. All the surfaces and walls are thoroughly cleaned with 70% ethyl alcohol and then with sterile water. The traces of VOCs and other gases are blown out using hot air blowers raising room air temperature by about 20°C.

LAYOUT

It is very important to plan layout of the Assisted reproductive technology (ART) laboratory carefully after consulting an experienced architect and engineer. Space allocation depends upon volume of patients, staff and activities of the center. Always there should be provision for future expansions as ART is changing with a lightning pace demanding more working place. IVF laboratory carries activities like semen analysis, hormonal evaluations (can be outsourced), *in vitro* fertilization, intracytoplasmic sperm injection (ICSI), cryopreservation, and may be pre-implantation genetic diagnosis. It is advisable to have culture room adjacent to the operation theater, where ovum pickup and embryo transfer takes place. This is to minimize exposure of the gametes and embryos to outer environment and also to save time of handling.[7] An ideal IVF laboratory should have following sections (Fig. 22.1).

Reception Area

Patients and their accompanying persons should have a comfortable sitting arrangement with basic facilities. Because depending upon number of patients and type of treatments, it may take hours before procedure starts (Fig. 22.2).

Nurse's Work Area

An important place where patient interacts with nurse for taking preliminary instructions, filling up the necessary consent forms, changing outdoor clothes to OT gowns.

Changing Room

Changing room should have attached toilets and lockers for the clinic staff and the visitors.

Semen Collection Room

Often a neglected area but needs detail planning. It should be isolated from main reception area, should have enough privacy, space for a small bed, a chair, a clean platform to keep collection jars, a wash basin, a urinal, provisions like vibrator, magazines and videos that help patient getting psychologically prepared to give sample.

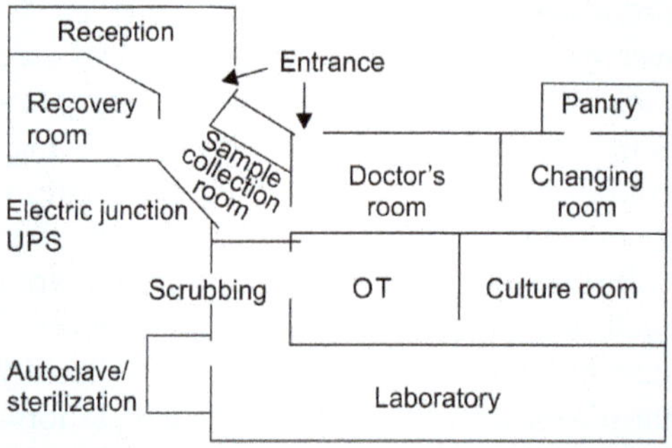

Fig. 22.1: *In vitro* fertilization laboratory layout.

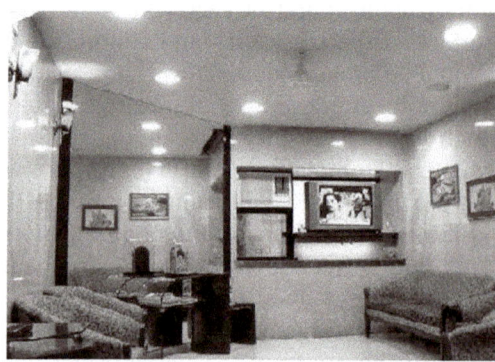

Fig. 22.2: Reception area.

General Laboratory

Used for in house media preparation, intrauterine insemination (IUI) semen preparations. Storing part of disposables and media, and cryopreservation. This part comes under sterile area.

Sterilization Area

Used for autoclave, boilers and hot air ovens for dry sterilization.

Scrubbing Area

Located opposite to OT. Used for hand scrubbing. It should be a general practice to wash hands and forearms with antiseptic, odorless soap and then rinsing thoroughly with sterile soft water before entering culture room.

Operation Theater

Should be well equipped to handle emergencies and routine instruments for anesthesia, Ovum pick up, embryo transfer and surgical retrieval of sperms (Fig. 22.3).

Culture Room

It is the heart of an IVF laboratory. It should be adjacent to OT and its entrance should be through OT. It should be under positive pressure so that air will flow unidirectional from culture room to OT and then outwards. The positions of incubators and other instruments like laminar airflow hood, centrifuge, stereomicroscope, and inverted microscope should be planned carefully to avoid collision during movements. Culture room should not be uncomfortably compact, but at the same time, it should not be too large or elongated. Area wise, it should be square, semi-circular or rectangle so that embryologist does not have to move more than three meters to complete any single procedure. An automatic system of turning on UV light late in the night and switching it off four to five hours before procedure helps in keeping culture room sterile. However, the intensity of UV light should be determined by an expert to avoid excessive ionization of air borne particles, which can be toxic to the medium and embryos kept in the incubator[8] (Fig. 22.4).

Administration Office

Again a very important aspect of an IVF laboratory. Administration includes patient's contact and payment details, consent formalities, and record keeping. All the laboratory details of the patients, the stock books, the AMC records for all the instruments, pest control and air conditioners should be maintained in the files. Patient's records

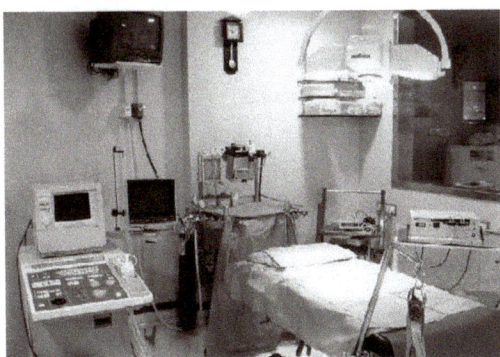

Fig. 22.3: Operation theater/Ovum pickup-embryo transfer room.

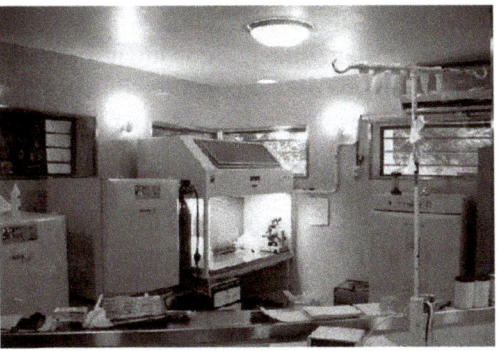

Fig. 22.4: Culture room.

should be entered in the computer and a backup should be taken on a safe media.

Embryologist and Staff Rest Room and Discussion Room

A separate area is to be allocated for laboratory staff to relax, to discuss cases and to interact with clinicians. Same room can be used to talk to patients giving them general information on embryology using animated or recorded clippings, in case they have any difficulties like semen collection problem, failed fertilization, queries related to embryo freezing, etc.

Storage Space

Separate storage place for quarterly stock of consumables is a must as one should not keep all these materials in the general laboratory. This place should be kept clean, dry, disinfected and should be easily accessible. Poorly maintained storage area can become a major source of contamination, as many times, the disposables are directly brought into the culture room.

Gas Cylinders and Liquid Nitrogen Tanks

Depending upon volume of patients, categories of surgical procedures and number of incubators, CO_2 and other gases can be piped from the central source to the work station or alternately individual cylinders can be placed near incubators. Either inline or external charcoal filters for CO_2 helps in absorbing volatile gases and filter particulate matter.

Electricity Control Room

From the safety point, one should be able to monitor electric switches, particularly those of heavy duty appliances like air conditioners, refrigerators, autoclave and sterilizers from a control room. All other instruments that must run continuously should be connected to a suitable uninterrupted power supply (UPS) system. The batteries for such systems should be kept away from culture room, in a well ventilated and easily accessible area.

INSTRUMENTS

In IVF, instruments play pivotal role in achieving pregnancies. It is always better to have backup of all instruments ready. This becomes more obvious in non-metros, where it is difficult to get service or spares in emergencies for imported instruments. Each instrument should be covered under annual maintenance contract (AMC) for its smooth working. One cannot give an excuse of non-working instrument for an incomplete or abandoned treatment.

Instruments for Operation Theater

1. Sonography machine with vaginal and abdominal probe for scanning follicles during daily monitoring and during the ovum pick-up procedure (Fig. 22.5).
2. Aspiration pump with adjustable foot pressure control for oocyte aspiration (Fig. 22.6).
3. Boyle's machine for general anesthesia, oxygen and nitrogen cylinders.

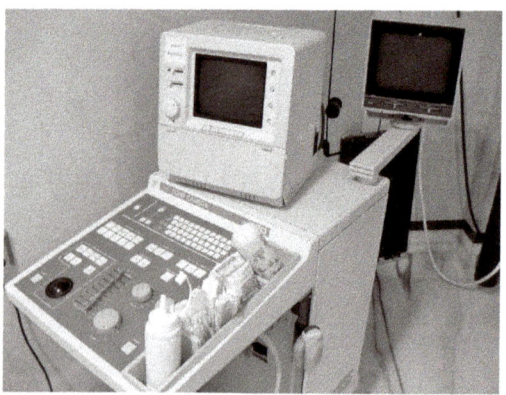

Fig. 22.5: Ultrasound machine.

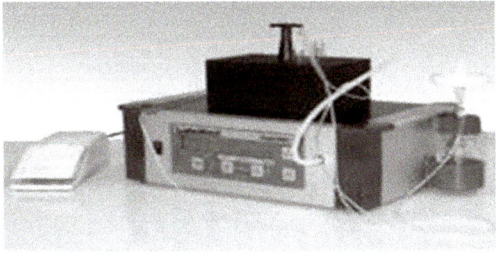

Fig. 22.6: Follicle aspiration pump.

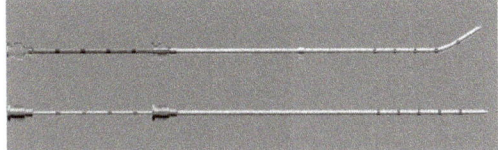

Fig. 22.7: Embryo transfer catheters.

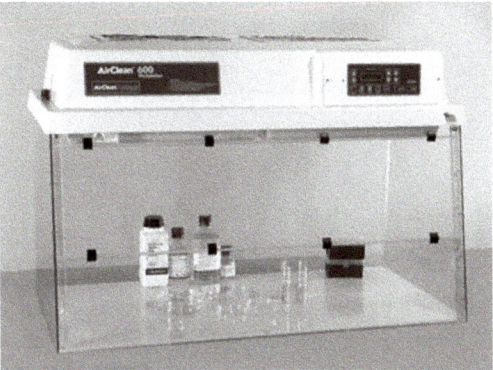

Fig. 22.8: Laminar airflow hood.

4. Pulse-oximeter.
5. Operation table with proper OT light.
6. Suction machine.
7. Oocyte aspiration set.
8. ET catheters (Fig. 22.7).
9. Drums with sterile instruments.
10. Heating blocks to keep test tubes at 37°C.
11. Dustbins with properly labeled degradable plastic bags separate for sharp objects and other materials.

Instruments and Materials for Laboratory

A general laboratory in the vicinity of culture room can be used for Andrology and cryopreservation. It should have:

1. Laminar airflow (Fig. 22.8).
2. CO_2 incubator for keeping sperm preparation media and processed sperm samples.
3. Compound microscope for semen analysis (Fig. 22.9).
4. Centrifuge machine displaying speed and time with suitable rotor head to accumulate different tubes for semen preparation (Fig. 22.10).

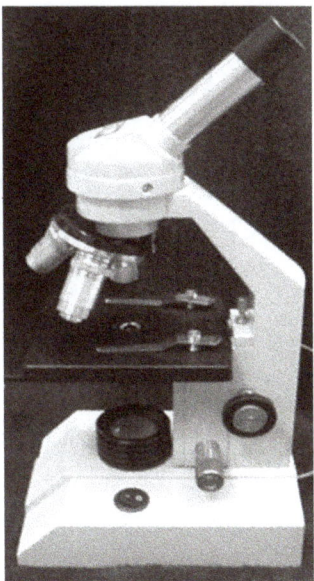

Fig. 22.9: Compound microscope.

5. A suitable device like Makler's chamber or hemocytometer to assess sperm count and motility (Fig. 22.11).
6. Refrigerator for media storage.
7. Programmable freezing machine for cryopreservation of sperm, oocyte and embryos is an essential part of an IVF laboratory. Other materials for cryopreservation include liquid nitrogen storage Dewars with canisters, cryocans, cryovials and straws (Fig. 22.12).

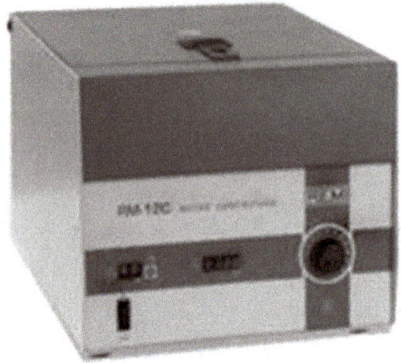

Fig. 22.10: Centrifuge.

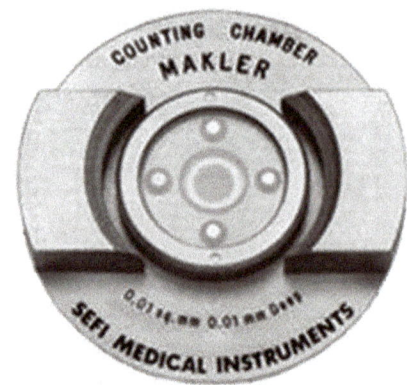

Fig. 22.11: Makler chamber.

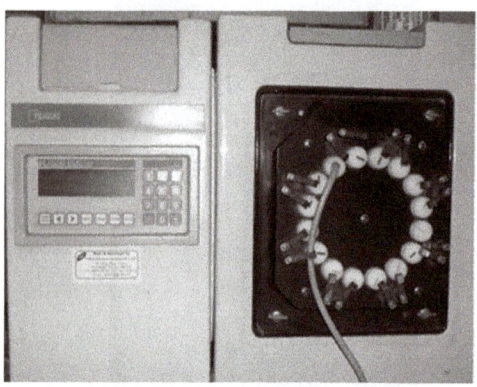
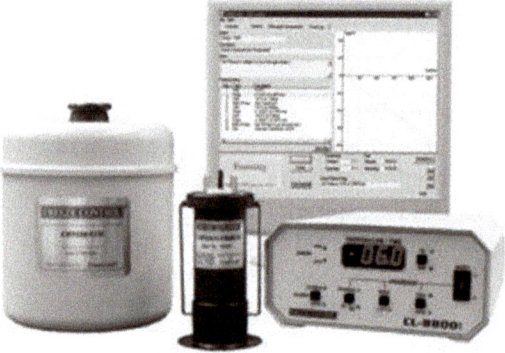

Fig. 22.12: Programmable freezing machines.

8. Tissue culture grade tubes and pipettes for handling semen samples, glass beakers, test-tube stands, rubber bulbs, permanent markers.

Instruments and Materials for Culture Room

1. *Laminar airflow hood:* A vertical laminar flow is preferred over horizontal one from efficiency point of view. UV lamp may be fitted inside the hood for sterilization.
2. *Air purifier system:* Generally, incubators maintaining 5-6% CO_2 is used for culturing gametes and embryos. These incubators are supplied 100% CO_2 gas, which is reduced to desired concentration using, built in sensors. As rest of the air is taken into the incubators from the surrounding area of the culture room, it becomes necessary to maintain clean, sterile and embryo-friendly air quality around the incubators. There are many procedures and materials that may contribute to air pollution. Those include anesthetic gases; ethylene oxide sterilized disposables that emit toxicity through 'off-gassing' effect, paints, alcohol, etc. There has to be an effective system to absorb all these toxic components. The filtration system should consist of HEPA filter which removes 99.97%

of contaminants including volatile organic compounds (VOCs) and chemical air contaminants (CACs). It should have activated carbon together with alumina impregnated with potassium permanganate for optimum absorption and oxidation of a wide variety of gases and particulate contaminants[9] (Fig. 22.13).

3. Carbon dioxide incubators with accurate CO_2 and temperature control. Number of incubators should be directly proportional to number of procedures. To maintain minimum fluctuations, one incubator is suitable for handling maximum three OPU procedures. A Separate incubator is desirable for equilibrating culture media. The quality of the gas is the key factor in getting good outcome. Therefore, medical grade gases should be obtained with proper certification of purity (Fig. 22.14).

4. To check the efficacy of incubators, the displayed values on the panel should be daily counterchecked using calibrated digital instruments like pH meter, thermometer, and CO_2 analyzer (Fig. 22.15).

5. *IVF chamber:* It is a workstation either on the laminar airflow hood or as separate isolate with fitted stereozoom microscope and warm working platform at 37°C for handling oocytes and embryos. A provision of triple gas mixture in the enclosed chamber is highly effective in minimizing temperature, pH, and humidity fluctuations[10] (Fig. 22.16).

6. Stereozoom microscope for scanning of the aspirated follicular fluid for

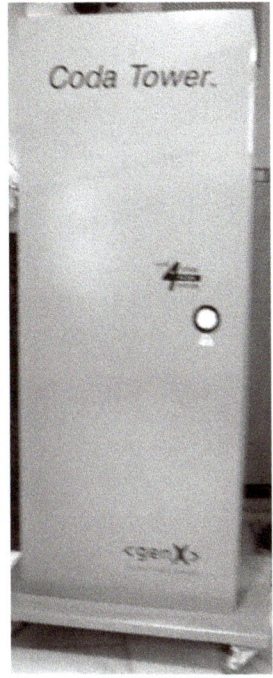

Fig. 22.13: Air purification system.

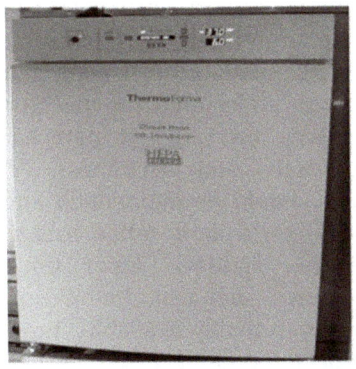 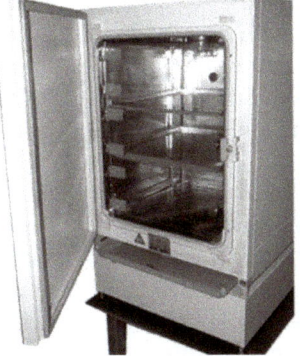 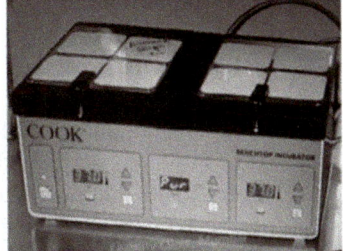

Fig. 22.14: Carbon dioxide incubators.

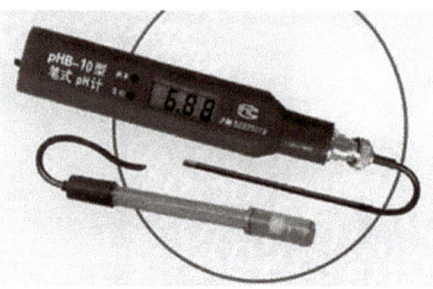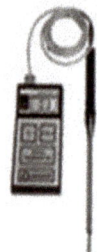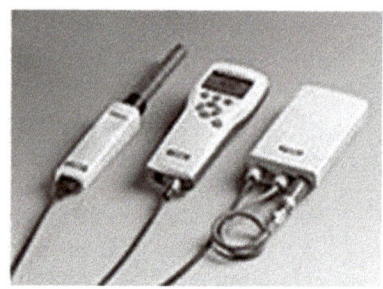

Fig. 22.15: pH meter, digital thermometer, and digital CO_2 analyzer.

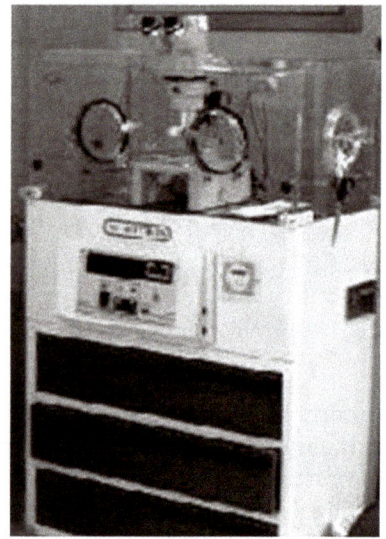

Fig. 22.16: *In vitro* fertilization chamber.

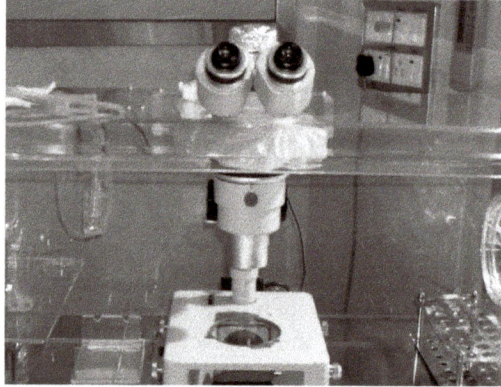

Fig. 22.17: Stereozoom microscope.

the presence of the oocytes and for quick evaluations of fertilization and embryonic growth (Fig. 22.17).

7. Inverted microscope with good optics like Hoffmann's modulation or Nomarski's is required to study the oocyte and embryo in detail and help in grading them.
8. Micromanipulator has become an indispensible part of an IVF laboratory. Not only it is useful in treating sever male factors like obstructive, nonobstructive azoospermia, and asthenoteratozoospermia, many times even good motile sperms fail to fertilize mature oocytes due to immunological factors or without any obvious reason. In such cases, intracytoplasmic sperm injection (ICSI) is the only technique available today to achieve fertilization. ICSI workstation is a part of IVF culture room. It should be placed in a corner with minimum disturbance on a vibration free platform. It is extremely important to understand the machine because even the smallest part has its significance and usefulness. All the spares should be maintained and kept ready, particularly teflon tubing, silicon seals, syringes, inner rings, power source, halogen bulbs, etc. which are not readily available. These may appear minor accessories but they are responsible for controlling

the movement of sperm and oocyte. Micromanipulator is also used for preimplantation genetic diagnosis (PGD), somatic cell nuclear transfer (SCNT), and stem cell research. A micromanipulator is extremely delicate assembly and should be handled with great care. A single handed instrument lasts much longer than if used by many users. The choice depends upon embryologist's training, availability, service, spares and budget (Fig. 22.18).
9. Microscope stage warmer for maintaining the temperature of the culture plates throughout the procedures, e.g. oocyte screening, oocyte denudation, insemination, assessing fertilization, cleavage and during embryo transfer.
10. It is recommended to have microscope fitted with still camera, video camera and a monitor for recording details of oocytes, embryos and training new embryologist.
11. Laser for assisted hatching and pre-implantation genetic diagnosis (PGD) (Fig. 22.19).

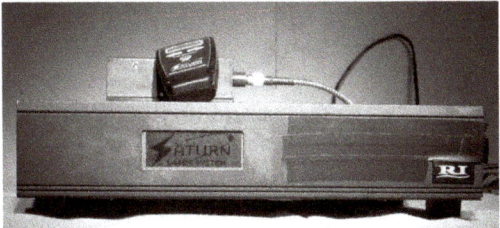

Fig. 22.19 : Laser machine.

Laboratory Personnel

Though money can set-up best IVF center with latest equipments and instruments, the success in terms of consistent pregnancy outcome depends upon people of all categories working in the IVF center. As far as laboratory part is concerned, an efficient, experienced, knowledgeable and skilled laboratory director can change the scenario. At the same time, junior embryologists and nurses are key factors because IVF is a team effort. In many parts of the world, there is no certified training course as "embryologist". The experience is passed on to colleagues. As science progresses continuously in the field of ART, the laboratory director should keep pace with the latest update and try to implement changes. It may happen that the new findings and discoveries may be completely contradictory to current practice of many years. But they should be implemented with open mind without any bias or prejudice. According to Indian Council of Medical Research (ICMR) guidelines, laboratory director should be a senior person who has had considerable experience in all aspects of ART. He/she should be a postgraduate - preferably PhD—in an appropriate medical or biological science. He/she should be able to coordinate the activities of the rest of the team and take care of staff administrative matters, stock keeping, finance, maintenance of patient records, statutory requirements and public relations.

Junior embryologists can be science graduate or postgraduate with adequate knowledge about laboratory procedures, sterility and quality control measures. They should have keen interest in the field, ability to learn new techniques, and sense of responsibility of working with human life.

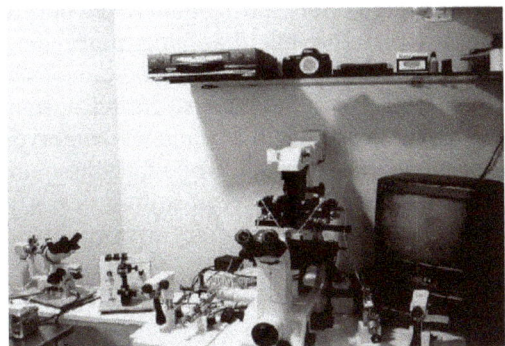

Fig. 22.18: Intracytoplasmic sperm injection workstation.

Nurses are very important personnel of an IVF center. Though they are not directly involved in laboratory procedures, they can always help in maintaining coordination between patient and laboratory.

Counselor should be a qualified and professional person can talk to patient at length giving details about the center, staff, treatment, success rate, expenses and how to deal in case of failure.

RECORD KEEPING

In IVF, we deal with genetic material of the couples. It is entirely their property and they have all the rights to know about each and every oocyte, embryo and sperm handled by the laboratory staff. Therefore, keeping proper records of gametes and embryos is as important as the actual treatment. In cases like oocyte, sperm recipient and surrogacy, issue may become further complicated ethically and legally. Proper records, and duly signed consent forms can help both the couple and the clinicians. Records of disposable, materials, and AMCs are important from the laboratory point for a smooth day-to-day working. In many countries, including India, now all records will be collected online for a central registry that will make treatment transparent and data retrieval and compiling easy from all centers for a centralized registry. Of course, care should be taken to avoid exposure of patient's identity.

QUALITY CONTROL

In ART, it is easier to start an IVF center, but equally tough to maintain consistent acceptable pregnancy rate. There are many variables that can account for either unexpectedly higher pregnancy rate or disappointingly lower outcomes. It is maintaining a strict quality control program that gives steady pregnancy rates per embryo transfer. Quality control in IVF is a continuous process that monitors all aspects of ART laboratory to function within acceptable limits. To discuss details about quality control measures is beyond the scope of this article. Briefly, quality control in IVF laboratory involves:

- Upgrading skills and knowledge of laboratory personnel
- Maintaining environment, equipments and instruments to optimum working condition
- Steps to eliminate infections and contaminations[11]
- Record keeping
- Preparing and updating written protocols
- Daily monitoring temperature, CO_2, humidity, pH and sterility of incubators
- Checking the staff following standardized procedures.

These are some precautionary measures to improve pregnancy rates. However, most important point we have to remember that in IVF, there is no scope for correction of certain mistakes. It is not like general pathology laboratory, where, if an error is observed one can repeat the test. In IVF, once the pregnancy is established, the issue becomes much complicated—socially, emotionally, ethically and legally. So, the other aspect of quality control is to avoid mixing of genetic materials from different couples. There should be always at least two persons involved during following stages to countercheck possible errors like wrong naming on semen sample containers and pipettes, on oocyte storing plates, while handling more than four to five ovum pick-ups simultaneously, while preparing ICSI plates, during normal insemination, loading patient's embryos during embryo transfer, while freezing more than one patient's embryos, storing straws in correct canisters with proper entry in registers and computers, etc.[12]

In assisted reproductive technology, IVF laboratory plays crucial role in achieving final goal of the treatment—clinical pregnancy. To achieve and maintain acceptable pregnancy rate, the laboratory should be scientifically set and the methodologies be followed as per world standards. The layout and materials may vary but the quality control measures should be strictly observed. A good laboratory, a good team work and an able guidance can certainly achieve excellent pregnancy rates.

REFERENCES

1. Steptoe PC, Edwards RG. Birth after reimplantation of a human embryo. Lancet. 1978;2(8085):366.
2. von Wyl S, Bersinger NA. Air quality in the IVF laboratory: results and survey. J Assist Reprod Genet. 2004;(10):347-8.
3. Hall J, Gilligan A, Schimmel T, et al. The origin, effects and control of air pollution in laboratories used for human embryo culture. Hum Reprod. 1998;13 (Suppl 4):146-55.
4. Compendium of methods for determination of toxic organic compounds in ambient air, US EPA 600/4-84-041, April 1984/1988.
5. Cohen J, Gilligan A, Esposito W, et al. Ambient air and its potential effects on conception *in vitro*. Hum Reprod. 1997;12:1742-9.
6. Achour-Frydman N. Improvements of results and optimization of quality control. J Gynecol Obstet Biol Reprod (Paris). 2008;37 Suppl 1:S1-3.
7. Zhang JQ, Li XL, Peng Y, et al. Reduction in exposure of human embryos outside the incubator enhances embryo quality and blastulation rate. Reprod Biomed Online. 2010;20:510-4.
8. Magli MC, Van den Abbeel E, Lundin K, Royere D, Van der Elst J, Gianaroli L; Committee of the Special Interest Group on Embryology. Revised guidelines for good practice in IVF laboratories. Hum Reprod. 2008;23(6):1253-62.
9. Lane M, Mitchell M, Cashman KS, et al. To QC or not to QC: the key to a consistent laboratory? Reprod Fertil Dev. 2008;20(1):23-32.
10. Gardner DK, Reed L, Linck D, et al. Quality control in human *in vitro* fertilization. Semin Reprod Med. 2005;23(4):319-24. Review.
11. Coccia ME, Cammilli F, Ginocchioni L, et al. Role of infection in *in vitro* fertilization treatment. Ann N Y Acad Sci. 2004;1034:219-35.
12. Cutting R, Pritchard J, Clarke H, et al. Establishing quality control in the new IVF laboratory. Hum Fertil (Camb). 2004;7(2):119-25.

CHAPTER 23

Noninvasive Strategies for Selection of Human Oocytes and Embryos

Simone Palini, Silvia de Stefani, Raffaella Depalo

Chapter outline

- Noninvasive Strategies for Selection of Human Oocytes and Embryos
- Oocytes
- Oocyte Investigation: New Approaches
- Embryos
- Embryos Investigation: New Approaches

INTRODUCTION

Despite numerous progresses in the practice of assisted reproductive technology (ART) in the past three decades, implantation rates following the transfer of *in vitro* produced embryos have remained <30%. Implantation failure is believed to be due to a range of factors, including oocyte competence and embryo health. In this perspective, the trouble-shooting in *in vitro* fertilization (IVF) laboratory is related:

- To design a noninvasive viability assay to assist in the selection of oocytes for insemination and of embryos for transfer.
- To optimize the oocytes cryopreservation method.
- To improve the *in vitro* maturation (IVM) of immature oocytes.

NONINVASIVE STRATEGIES FOR SELECTION OF HUMAN OOCYTES AND EMBRYOS

Gametes are the key to any ART treatment success, and it is well accepted that the developmental fate of the embryo is largely dictated by the "quality" of the oocyte. Oocyte quality is reflected in an oocyte's intrinsic developmental potential that refers to the biochemical and molecular state allowing a mature oocyte to be fertilized and to develop to an embryo.[1]

Quality or developmental competence is acquired during folliculogenesis as the oocyte grows and is deeply affected by multiple endocrine, paracrine and autocrine factors during oogenesis and follicular development.[2]

Locally produced growth factors as IGF 9, KL and BMP15 work in concert with gonadotropins and other extraovarian factors contributing to coordinate oocyte maturation through ovulation. Contact between oocyte and granulosa cells make possible that hormones as insulin, glucacon, leptin, growth hormone (GH), thyroid hormones, and hepatic insulin-like growth factor (IGF) and their binding proteins as well as metabolic fuels, such as glucose, fatty acids, and low- and high-density lipoprotein are involved in mediating these nutritionally induced changes in follicle dynamics and oocyte quality.[2-3] There is a growing awareness in the field of reproductive medicine that oocyte quality is a key limiting factor in female fertility and that oocyte quality impacts early embryonic survival, thus, alterations to the oocyte contribute significantly to the reduced conception and pregnancy rates. Hence, utilization of the most competent oocytes during IVF is crucial to ensure the derivation of high-quality embryos and successful pregnancy.[4]

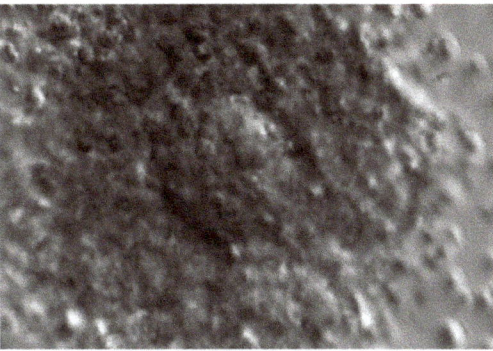

Fig. 23.1: Apparently mature oocyte surrounded by a radiant corona which consisting of many layers.

OOCYTES

In standard IVF cycles, the quality and maturity of oocyte are usually evaluated according to the expansion and radiance of cumulus-corona complex. Oocytes are scored as "mature" when they possess an expanded cumulus matrix and a radiant corona, and a transparent and homogeneous cytoplasm (Fig. 23.1); a less expanded corona complex and a dark, slightly granular cytoplasm denotes an intermediate stage maturity; the absence of an expanded cumulus and an oocyte with dark granular cytoplasm were generally associated with immaturity.[5]

In intracytoplasmic sperm injection (ICSI) cycles, after that oocytes are denudated, the evaluation is based on the characteristic structure of oocyte cytoplasm, polar body, perivitelline space, zona pellucida (ZP) and meiotic spindle. Classically, a human oocyte is considered "normal" when under light microscopy it shows a round clear ZP, a small perivitelline space containing a single unfragmented first polar body (1st PB) and a pale moderating granular cytoplasm that does not contain inclusions (Fig. 23.2).

A great variety of oocyte dysmorphism can be observed in *in vitro* culture. The oocyte's morphological characteristics were classified as extracytoplasmic abnormalities, including fragmented first polar body (1st PB), large and/or degenerated 1st PB, thick

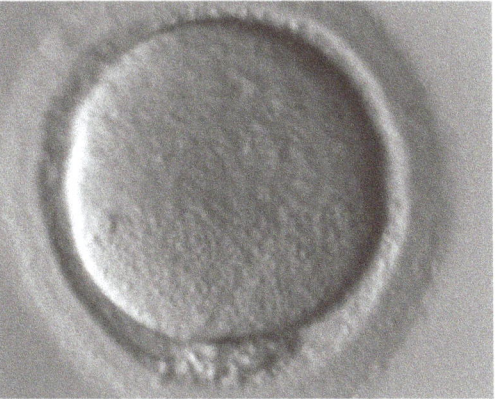

Fig. 23.2: Fully mature oocyte at metaphase II of meiosis, with granular cytoplasm without inclusion and first polar body.

and/or dark zona pellucida (ZP), large perivitelline space and abnormal shape and cytoplasmic abnormalities as granular cytoplasm (Fig. 23.3), centrally located granular area, vacuoles (Fig. 23.4), refractile bodies and smooth endoplasmic reticulum cluster (SER).[6]

Several studies have correlated oocyte features and developmental potential of embryo. Visualizing the presence of the 1st PB in the perivitelline space is a sign of nuclear maturity. Some morphological criteria of the 1st PB, such as the shape (round or ovoid), size (large or small), surface (smoth or rough) and

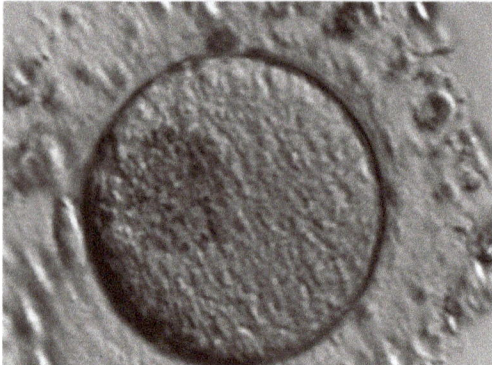

Fig. 23.3: Oocyte with cytoplasmic granularity.

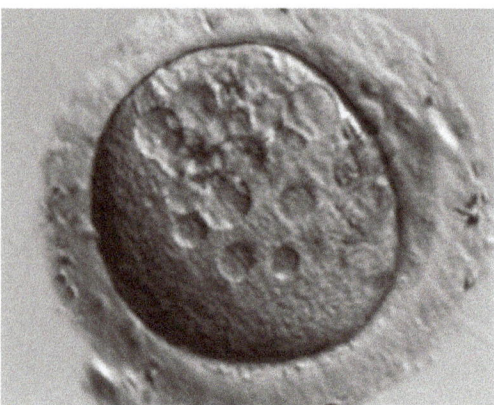

Fig. 23.4: Oocyte with vacuoles.

integrity of cytoplasm (intact or fragmented) can be used to predict the oocyte quality. Ebner et al. (2000), reported that normal morphology of the 1st polar body results in a higher fertilization rate and better quality embryos with an increased implantation and ongoing pregnancy rates.[7] Ciotti et al. (2004), observed that since polar body has a short half-time, morphological degeneration of the first polar body indicates the postovulatory age of the human oocyte, however embryo quality, pregnancy rate and implantation rate are not related to the 1st PB fragmentation.[8] Furthermore, PB morphology does not show a correlation with the genotype analyzed for aneuploidy in patients who underwent preimplanation genetic diagnosis.[9] Also the perivitelline space of human oocytes may vary in size (enlarged or not) and content (presence or absence of the grain). It was estimated that oocytes with a large perivitelline space or containing large grains in the perivitelline space, negatively correlate with fertilization rate and embryo quality.[10] Appearance of zona pellucida is another sign of oocyte quality. The tickness of the zona pellucida, varies from 10 to 31 µm and it is not related to the cytoplasm diameter. Its thickness influences sperm penetration. The oocytes are best fertilized in vitro when the thickness of the zona pellucida is less than 18.6 µm.[11] The recovery of sporadic giant oocytes (mean diameter 200 µm, versus 155 µm) appears to be possible after hormonal stimulation. The occurrence of giant in human is 0.3% of oocytes retrieved during IVF. These giant cells are believed to be produced by a lack of cytokinesis during meiotic divisions of oogonia or by cell fusion of two adjacent oogonia or oocytes. Giant fertilized oocytes, obtained after standard in vitro insemination and showing normal or atypical polyploid number of pronuclei, may be a possible source of human digynic triploidy.[12] To conclude, two anomalies remain that should be handled with caution: (i) 'giant' oocytes because of their likely abnormal genetic constitution and (ii) smooth endoplasmic reticulum (SER) clusters because of their potentially lethal outcomes.

Oocytes Investigations: New Approaches

Meiotic Spindle

Morphology is today the only parameter useful to identify the best oocytes. Other approaches are under study. In recent years, it has been possible support to the morphological study an additional parameter, the meiotic spindle. The meiotic spindle can be viewed using techniques such as immunohistochemistry or electron microscopy, but in these ways, samples must undergo a process of fixing, making the results useful for research but not for clinical practice, then serving noninvasive methods that allow this study. Inouè[13] was the first to use a polarized light microscope to observe the meiotic spindle in cells using birefringence of microtubules. Conventional polarized light microscopes have a limited sensitivity caused mainly by using a system orientament-dependent. A new and particularly microscope, Polscope (Cambridge Research and Instrumentation, Inc. [CRI], USA), overcomes these limitations because it allows the display of macromolecular structures ordered in a orientament-indipendent way. We must remember also that this system is not invasive and has no toxic effects on the cell, this was demonstrated by previous studies carried out on mice.[14-15] Several studies show that there is a correlation between the presence of meiotic spindle in metaphase II oocytes and a good percentage of fertilization. A normal spindle is crucial to allow a correct alignment of chromosomes and a correct separation. The destruction of this structure can lead to loss of chromosomes and can contribute to numerical chromosomal aberrations as the aneuploidie.[16-17] One study[18] has verified that on a total of 533 oocytes analyzed through Polscope, 39% did not have a meiotic spindle visible. Of these, only 44% showed a normal fertilization compared to 62% of oocytes that possessed a spindle visible. A work by the same author[19] shows that the presence of a birefringent spindle in human egg can not only increase the fertilization but also increased the probability of a good embryonic development. These results are confirmed by further study[20]: the percentage of high-quality embryos that developed from oocytes with visible spindle is significantly greater than percentage of high-quality embryos that developed from oocytes without visible spindle (64.2% versus 35.9%). Similar data were obtained from Rienzi et al.,[21] 9% of oocytes analyzed has not a visible spindle; these oocytes showed a lower fertilization rate of 33.3%.

Cumulus Cells

Cumulus cells that surround oocytes are investigated to identify noninvasive markers of oocyte chromosome status and competence.[22] Fragouli et al. used microarray comparative genomic hybridization to assess oocyte ploidy.[22] In this study, *SPSB2* gene involved in intracellular signaling and *TP53I3* gene involved in carbohydrate metabolism and apoptosis, exhibited highly significant differences in their expression between cumulus cells of normal and chromosomally abnormal oocytes. These genes might have the potential to serve as indirect markers of oocyte aneuploidy. The use of new instrument as Next Generation Sequencing to study the transcriptomic analysis of granulosa cells is likely to be of clinical value as noninvasive methods to detect the best competent oocyte. Unfortunately, this technology is not so frequently used due to its high cost and complex bioinformatic analysis.

Follicular Fluid

Another approch in oocyte investigation involved follicular fluid (FF) that provides a very important microenvironment for the development of oocytes. FF is a product of both the transfer of blood plasma constituents that cross the blood follicular barrier and of the secretory activity of granulosa and thecal cells. It is reasonable to think that some biochemical characteristics of the FF surrounding the oocyte may play a critical role in determining oocyte quality and the subsequent potential to achieve fertilization and embryo development. In a recent article, the authors demonstrate the influence of

FF antioxidant system on pregnancy after stimulation.[23] The FF chemical constituents that influenced oocyte and embryo quality can be grouped in the following categories: (a) hormones; (b) growth factors of the transforming growth factor-beta (TGF-beta) superfamily; (c) other growth factors and interleukins; (d) reactive oxygen species (ROS); (e) antiapoptotic factors; (f) proteins, peptides and amino acids; (g) sugars; (h) prostanoids.[24] Among these components, steroid hormones have emerged as important elements in reproductive outcomes. A follicular environment rich in estradiol, progesterone, and testosterone is key to good oocyte development. Among the oocytes immersed in a follicular environment rich in progesterone and testosterone, those with higher levels of estradiol obtained higher pregnancy rates. In the future, analysis of follicular hormone composition could be considered as an additional tool in oocyte selection.[25]

All the studies aiming to find a good molecular predictor of oocyte quality in FF are not performed on large scale, and correlate few molecules with oocyte quality. Other multivariate and multicenter studies are necessary to find the right FF mixture that positive influenced an IVF cycle.

EMBRYOS

Morphological criteria are routinely used to select the "best" embryos for transfer including pronuclear morphology, scoring system for days 2 to 3 embryos, and grading system for blastocyst.

As the spermatozoon enters, the oocyte is released from the meiotic block, the second polar body is extruded in a highly asynchronous division to limit the amount of cytoplasm lost, the female pronucleus begins to form, and the sperm head decondenses, forming the male pronucleus. At 16 to 18 hours after insemination (about 50–60 hours after hCG) the oocyte should have two centrally located pronuclei of approximately the same size (Fig. 23.5). Oocytes presenting with pronuclei that are not centrally located may have disruptions in the cytoskeleton and those with very disparate size pronuclei are predominant aneuploid. Nucleoli are present in all mitotically active cells and in number between two and seven in human cell nuclei. Nucleoli develop on DNA site known as the Nucleolar Organizing Regions (NOR) and are located at the points where the ribosomal genes are. The nucleoli are the sites of protein synthesis and also of certain mitogenic and growth regulatory proteins, which are involved in cell-cycle control.[1]

Scott L et al. (2000)[26] identified five pronuclear categories based on both the number and the distribution of nucleoli and pronuclei (Fig. 23.6). Zygote grade 1 had equal numbers of nucleoli (between three and seven) aligned at the pronuclear junction. Zygote grade 2 had equal numbers/sizes of nucleoli, but one nucleus having alignment at the pronuclear junction and the other with scattered nucleoli. Grade 3 zygotes had equal numbers and sizes of nucleoli, which were equally scattered in two nucleoli. Grade 4 zygote had unequal numbers and/or sizes of nucleoli. Grade 5 zygotes had pronuclei not aligned, with grossly different sizes or

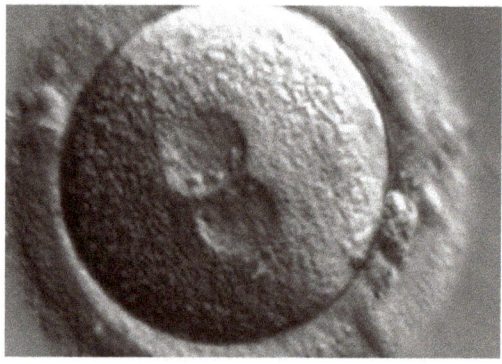

Fig. 23.5: Fertilized oocyte with two pronuclei, nucleoli aligned at adjacent poles, and two polar bodies.

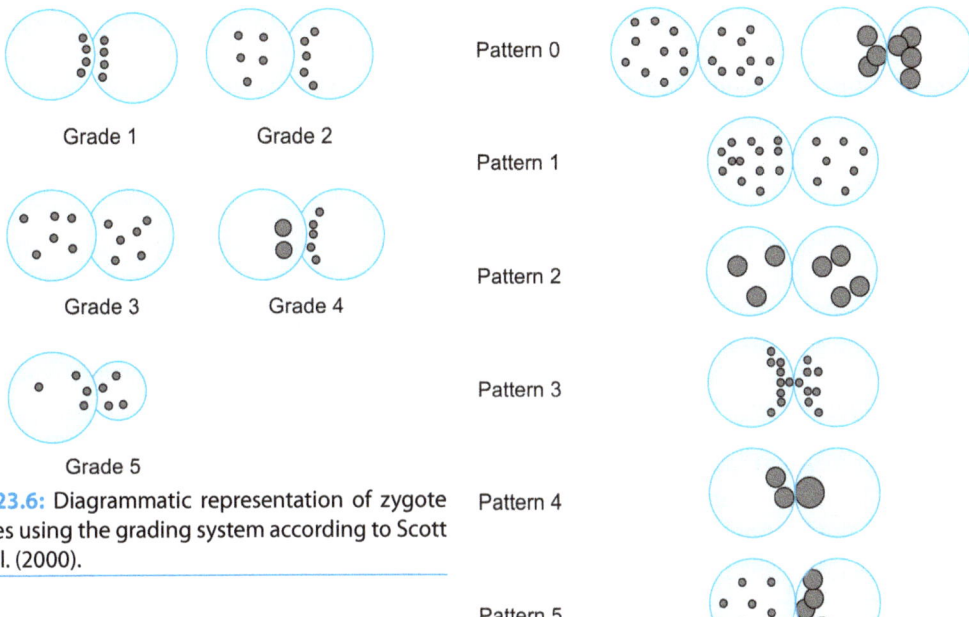

Fig. 23.6: Diagrammatic representation of zygote grades using the grading system according to Scott L et al. (2000).

Fig. 23.7: Schematic representation of pronuclear morphology, according to Tesarik and Greco (1999).

not located in the central part of the zygote.[26] The zygote scoring system was further revised after a review of the results from the first series, taking into account the zygote grade, day 3 morphology and ability to growth to the blastocyst stage.

Tesarik and Greco (1999) reported a modified grading system in which the nucleoli size, number and distribution were utilized in a single-observation scoring (Fig. 23.7).[27] In a retrospective analysis of their data, they found a strong association between implantation rates and the equality of nucleoli within each nucleus of the pronuclear embryos.

The advantages of the Tesarik zygote-grading system over the Scott system are the single observation and fewer parameters to take into account. A further indicator of normal development at the pronuclear oocyte stage is the appearance of a clearing or "halo" on the periphery of the oocyte. The clearing has been associated with the redistribution of mitochondria during meiosis and mitosis, and it is an indication that the cell/oocyte is functioning normally. The lack of halo has been associated with slowed development and low blastocyst formation.[1,28]

Alpha Scientists in Reproductive Medicine and ESHRE Special Interest Group of Embryology in 2011 published a paper that reports the proceedings of an international consensus meeting on oocyte and embryo morphology assessment. The consensus on pronuclear scoring was that there should be three categories: symmetrical; non-symmetrical; and abnormal. The abnormal category includes pronuclei with no NPBs (so-called 'ghost pronuclei'), and those with a single nucleolar precursor body ('bulls-eye pronuclei"), which have been associated with abnormal outcomes in animal models. Furthermore at present, there is insufficient evidence to support a prognostic value for the observation of a peripheral cytoplasmic translucency in the fertilized oocyte (a 'halo').[29]

Morphological criteria for embryo selection are assessed on the day of transfer including: number of blastomeres, degree of fragmentation, variation in blastomeres size, symmetry of the cleavage. The degree of fragmentation was scored as 0 (no fragments), 1 (<10% fragmentation), 2 (>10 to <25%), 3 (>25 to >50%) and 4 (>50% fragmentation). Fragmentation in some instances may be due to a poor culture conditions, which induces multinucleation and cell death or apoptosis.[30]

At 60 to 64 hours post hCG (40–42 hours post-insemination), the embryo should be at the 2- to 4-cell stage. Each cell should only have a single nucleus; multinucleation results from nuclei fragmentation with a total disintegration of the mitotic spindle (Fig. 23.8). It could also be the result of an abnormal mitotic event involving the spindle such as duplication of the microtubule organizing center. Multinucleation has been correlated with decreased in vitro development, decreased or not implantation and increased rate of aneuploidy.[13]

At the 8- to16-cell stage, the embryo will begin to compact itself and to form tight junctions; differentiation begins with the formation of two cell lines, the inside and outside. A good grade blastocyst needs to have: (i) from 16 cell to compacted morula on day 4; (ii) on day 5 the presence of a blastocoel, defined trophectoderm with enough cells to form a continuous layer and a well-defined and organized inner cell mass (>60).[31]

The ALPHA and ESHRE consensus opinion was that an optimal day-2 embryo (44 + 1 h post-insemination) would have 4 equally sized mononucleated blastomeres in a three-dimensional tetrahedral arrangement, with, 10% fragmentation, and an optimal day-3 embryo (68 + 1 h post-insemination) would have 8 equally sized mononucleated blastomeres, with, 10% fragmentation. The scoring system for day 2 and day 3 embryos for ALPHA and ESHRE consensus were: cell number, and grade as in Table 23.1.

It was the consensus that an optimal embryo at this developmental stage (116 + 2 h) will be a fully expanded through to hatched blastocyst with an ICM that is prominent, easily discernible and consisting of many cells, with the cells compacted and tightly adhered together, and with a TE that comprises many cells forming a cohesive epithelium. It was agreed that while the ICM has a high prognostic value for implantation and fetal development, a functional TE is also essential.

Scoring system for blastocyst checked blastocoel expansion (1–4), ICM grade (1–3) and TE grade (1–3) (Table 23.2). The consensus agreed that the ICM and TE should be graded relative to the Gardner A–C scale, but that a grade of 1–3 (rather than A–C)

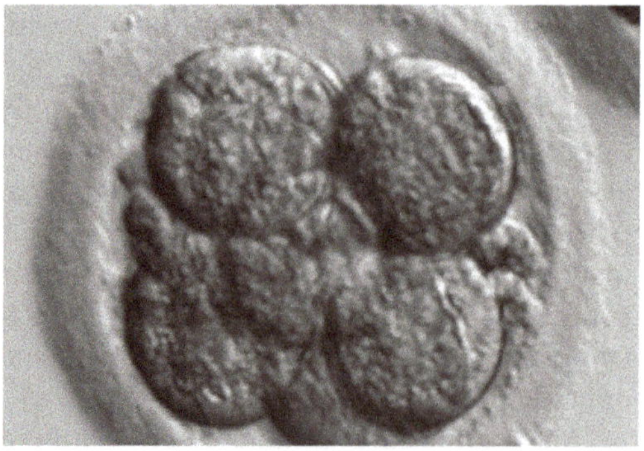

Fig. 23.8: Eight-cell embryo with equal size blastomeres.

Table 23.1: Scoring system for cleavage embryos.[30]

Grade	Rating	Description
1	Good	<10% Fragmentation Stage-specific cell size No multinucleation
2	Fair	10–25% Fragmentation Stage-specific cell size for majority of cells No evidene of multinucleation
3	Poor	Severe fragmentation (>25%) Cell-size not stage-specific Evidence of multinucleation

Table 23.2: Scoring system for blastocyst.[30]

	Grade	Rating	Description
Stage of development	1		Early
	2		Blastocyst
	3		Expanded
	4		Hatched/hatching
ICM	1	Good	Prominent, easily discernible, with many cells that are compacted and tightly adhered together
	2	Fair	Easily discernible, with many cells that are loosely grouped together
	3	Poor	Difficult to discern, with few cells
TE	1	Good	Many cells forming a cohesive epithelium
	2	Fair	Few cells forming a loose epithellum
	3	Poor	Very few cells

The scoring system for blastocysts is a combination of the stage of development, and of the grade of the ICM and of the TE (e.g. an expanded blastocyst with a good ICM and fair TE would be scored as 312). It is a numerical interpretation of the Gardner scale (Gardner and Schoolcraft, 1999a.b).

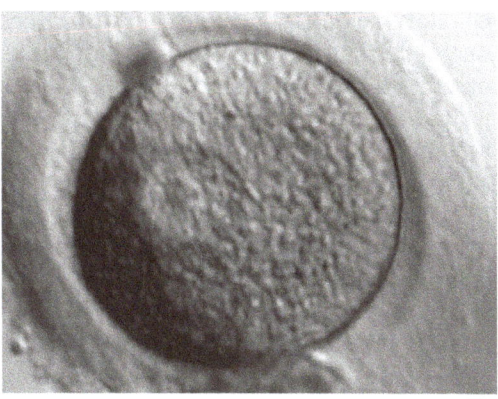

Fig. 23.9: Blastocyst score system example: 3.1.1.

should be given—with Grade 1 equivalent to Gardner A (Fig. 23.9). The rationale for this change is to support the entry of scores into numeric databases and facilitate statistical analysis.[29]

Embryos Investigations: New Approaches

Time Lapse Technologies

Usually the embryologists remove embryos from the incubator to assess morphology, but this type of monitoring only gives them a snapshot of a dynamic process and also the embryos do not tolerate removal from optimal culturing conditions. Time lapse technology can give an optimal solution to avoid these problems because give to embryologist the possibility to monitor embryo development inside the incubator ambient and in a continuated way. This type of monitoring allows for the collection of much more information on the timing of the cleavages and the dynamics of the morphologic changes.[32]

There is also a long way to go before the method's routine application for embryo selection can be recommended.

Certain parameters have already been identified that are associated with blastocyst formation and implantation potential. Campbell and colleagues published two papers[33-34] about their findings regarding embryo morphokinetic parameters and genetic health. The observations made by Campbell and colleagues were criticized by

Ottolini et al.[35] in their commentary in which they note that the conclusions were drawn based on small number of cases without taking age as a confounding factor into account. All these studies are retrospective and used different markers, then the predictive ability of the same markers has to be tested prospectively and using the same clinically endpoints.

In summary, time-lapse technology provides to embryologist an option to observe embryos in a undisturbed and continuous way, however, the clinical benefit of the technology remains to be determined.

Culture Media and Blastocoel Fluid Study

Recent technologic advances in translational research have now enabled the proteomic and metabolic status of embryos to be noninvasively determined in the embryo secretome, reflecting its biochemical status. Several biomarkers include: hCG, apolipoprotein-A1, human leukocyte antigen G, granulocyte-macrophage colony-stimulating factor (GM-CSF), pregnancy-specific β1-glycoprotein, interferon (IFN) α2, and platelet-activating factor.

Using mass spectrometry (MS) Cortezzi et al. (2011) identified 25 proteins in the secretome, of which 15 predicted positive pregnancy outcome and 10 were associated with negative pregnancy outcome.[36]

A third category of molecules detected in culture media were microRNA (miRNA), small (18–22 nucleotides), non-coding RNA molecules that are mostly considered to be negative regulators of gene expression as they can destabilize or repress translation of messenger RNA (mRNA).[37]

One type of miRNA can potentially regulate more than a hundred different target genes. Extracellular miRNA is very stable and resistant to degradation, this might be due to its encapsulation in small membrane-derived vesicles called exosomes, which can be delivered to other cells and thereby impact the gene expression in those cells.[38]

Rosenbluth et al. studied 754 human miRNA and found that three (miR-372, miR-191 and miR-645) were differentially expressed on day 5 between the spent culture medium of embryos that had successful pregnancy outcomes and spent culture medium from embryos that did not lead to pregnancy.[39]

The search for miRNA in culture media is an interesting tool in noninvasive embryo analysis, but further studies on a larger number of samples, on different culture media and on the same miRNA panel, are needed. The aim is to get a fast, inexpensive and standardized technique useful in clinical routine.

Another important source useful in embryo investigation is blastocoel fluid. Recent developments in mass spectrometry techniques allow the identification and characterization of thousands of metabolites and proteins from low nanoliters of samples. Approaches relying on both optical and nonoptical spectroscopy have been proposed to noninvasively monitor fluctuations of metabolic intermediates in culture media of developing blastocysts.[40] In this article, metabolites included were: (i) ATP; (ii) glucose-6-phosphate; (iii) lactate; (iv) NAD+; (v) NADH; (vi) NADPH; (vii) 6-phosphogluconic acid; (viii) glutamic acid and (ix) α-ketoglutarate.

Jensen PL et al. using highly sensitive nano-high-pressure liquid chromatography-tandem mass spectrometry, have identified 286 proteins in the blastocoel fluid and 1,307 proteins in the corresponding cells of the blastocyst. Furthermore, several heat shock proteins (Hsp27, Hsp60, Hsc70, and Hsp90) were identified in blastocoel fluid together with zona pellucida proteins (ZP2-4), vitamin D-binding protein, and retinol-binding protein 4. Proteins that regulate ciliary assembly and function were also identified.[41]

Blastocoel fluid is the colture media of ICM cells that are exposed to via this liquid to several proteins and metabolites.

Another important biomarker present in blastocoel fluid and in culture media is genomic DNA.[42-43] These studies showed using real-time PCR that genomic DNA was present in about 90% of blastocoel fluid samples harvested during the vitrification procedure. Moreover, the potential for determining embryo sex directly from blastocoele fluid is demonstrated by amplifying the multicopy genes *TSPY1* (on the Y chromosome) and *TBC1D3* (on chromosome 17). This opens up the possibility of screening embryos from couples carrying an X-linked disorder to identify male embryos at high risk of disease.

The same authors in a second paper evaluated the possibility to genotype the *MTHFR* polymorphism *C677T* from media at day 5/6 and blastocoele fluids by direct sequencing. The *C677T* polymorphism detection rate was 62.5% and 44.4% in medium and fluid, respectively.

These studies demonstrated that a noninvasive approach for embryo genotyping (Preimplantation Genetic Diagnosis) and for the detection of healthy status of the embryos was possible but other studies are needed to confirm its usefulness in the clinic.

CONCLUSION

To date, there are many methods that are developing in the research of noninvasive parameters to match with morphology study of embryos.

Probably there is not a single parameters but a panel of biomarkers useful in the identification of the best embryo, because we can image embryo as a dinamic structure and not in a snapshot.

In addition, it is vital to ensure that the necessary research and development is conducted before bringing new techniques into clinical practice.

ACKNOWLEDGMENT

Authors would like to thank to Margherita Vacca, BSc for providing the pictures used in this review.

REFERENCES

1. Scott L. The biological basis of non-invasive strategies for selection of human oocytes and embryos. Hum Reprod Update. 2003;9(3):237-49.
2. Sanfins A, Plancha CE, Overstrom EW, et al. Meiotic spindle morphogenesis in in vivo and in vitro matured mouse oocytes: insights into the relationship between nuclear and cytoplasmic quality. Hum Reprod. 2004;19(12):2889-99.
3. Gilchrist RB, Ritter LJ, Armstrong DT. Oocyte-somatic cell interactions during follicle development in mammals. Anim Reprod Sci. 2004;82-83:431-46.
4. Li Q, McKenzie LJ, Mathzuk MM. Revisiting oocyte-somatic cell interactions: in serch of novel intrafollicular predictors and regulators of oocyte developmental competence. Mol Hum Reprod. 2008;14(12):673-8.
5. Lasiene K, Vitkus A, Valaneiute A, et al. Morphological criteria of oocyte quality. Medicina (Kaunas). 2000;45(7):509-15.
6. Ubaldi F, Rienzi L. Morphological selection of gametes. Placenta. 2008;29 Suppl B:115-20.
7. Ebner T, Yaman C, Moser M, et al. Prognostic value of first polar body morphology on fertilization rate and embryo quality in intracytoplasmic sperm injection. Hum Reprod. 2000;15(2):427-30.
8. Ciotti PM, Notarangelo L, Morselli-Labate AM, et al. First polar body morphology before ICSI is not related to embryo quality or pregnancy rate. Hum Reprod. 2004;19(10):2334-9.
9. Verlinsky Y, Lerner S, Illkevitch N, et al. Is there any predictive value of first polar body morphology for embryo genotype or developmental potential? Reprod Biomed Online. 2003;7(3):336-41.
10. Xia P. Intracytoplasmic sperm injection: correlation of oocyte grade based on polar body, perivitelline space and cytoplasmic

inclusions with fertilization rate and embryo quality. Hum Reprod. 1997;12(8):1750-5.
11. Montag M, Schimming T, Köster M, et al. Oocyte zona birefringence intensity is associated with embryonic implantation potential in ICSI cycles. Reprod Biomed Online. 2008;16(2):239-44.
12. Balakier H, Bouman D, Sojecki A, et al. Morphological and cytogenetic analysis of human giant oocytes and giant embryos. Hum Reprod. 2002;17(9):2394-01.
13. Inouè S. Polarization optical studies of the mitotic spindle. The demonstration of spindle fibers in living cells. Chromosoma. 1953;5:487-500.
14. Liu L, Oldenbourg R, Trimarchi JR. A reliable, non-invasive technique for spindle imaging and enucleation of mammalian oocytes. Nat Biotechnol. 2000a;18:223-5.
15. Keefe D, Tran P, Pellegrini C. Polarized light microscopy and digital image processing identify a multilaminar structure of the hamster zona pellucida. Hum Reprod. 1997;12:1250-2.
16. Wang W, Keefe DL. Prediction of chromosome misalignment among in vitro matured human oocytes by spindle imaging with the polscope. Fertil Steril. 2002;78:1077-81.
17. Korkmaz C, Cinar O, Akyol M. The relationship between meiotic spindle imaging and outcome of intracytoplasmic sperm injection: a retrospective study. Gynecol Endocrinol. 2011;27(10):737-41.
18. Wang W, Meng L, Hackett RJ. The spindle observation and its relationship with fertilization after intracytoplasmic sperm injection in living human oocytes. Fertil Steril. 2001c;75:348-53.
19. Wang WH, Meng L, Hackett RJ. Developmental ability of human oocytes with or without birefringent spindles imaged by Polscope before insemination Hum Reprod. 2001a;16(7):1464-8.
20. Moon JH, Hyun CS, Lee SW. Visualization of the metaphase II meiotic spindle in living human oocytes using the PolScope enables the prediction of embryonic developmental competence after ICSI. Hum Reprod. 2003;18:187-20.
21. Rienzi L, Ubaldi F, Martinez F. Relationship between meiotic spindle location with regard to the polar body position and oocyte developmental potential after ICSI. Hum Reprod. 2003;18:1289-93.
22. Fragouli E, Wells D, Iager AE, et al. Alteration of gene expression in human cumulus cells as a potential indicator of oocyte aneuploidy. Hum Reprod. 2012;27(8):2559-68.
23. Palini S, Benedetti S, Tagliamonte MC, et al. Influence of ovarian stimulation for IVF/ICSI on the antioxidant defence system and relationship to outcome. Reprod Biomed Online. 2014;29(1):65-71.
24. Revelli A, Delle Piane L, Casano S, et al. Follicular fluid content and oocyte quality: from single biochemical markers to metabolomics Reprod Biol Endocrinol. 2009;4;7:40.
25. Carpintero NL, Suárez OA, Mangas CC, Follicular steroid hormones as markers of oocyte quality and oocyte development potential. J Hum Reprod Sci. 2014;7(3):187-93.
26. Scott L, Alvero R, Leondires M, Miller B. The morphology of human pronuclear embryos is positively related to blastocyst development and implantation. Hum Reprod. 2000;15(11):2394-03.
27. Tesarik J, Greco E. The probability of abnormal preimplantation development can be predicted by a single static observation on pronuclear stage morphology. Hum Reprod. 1999;14(5):1318-23.
28. Ebner T, Moser M, Sommergruber M, et al. Presence, but not type or degree of extension, of a cytoplasmic halo has a significant influence on preimplantation development and implantation behaviour. Hum Reprod. 2003;18(11):2406-12.
29. Alpha Scientists in Reproductive Medicine and ESHRE Special Interest Group of Embryology. The Istanbul consensus workshop on embryo assessment: proceedings of an expert meeting. Hum Reprod. 2011;26(6):1270-83.
30. Holte J, Berglund L, Milton K, et al. Construction of an evidence-based integrated morphology cleavage embryo score for implantation potential of embryos

scored and transferred on day 2 after oocyte retrieval. Hum Reprod. 2007;22(2):548-57.
31. Scott L, Finn A, O'Leary T, et al. Morphologic parameters of early cleavage-stage embryos that correlate with fetal developmental and delivery: prospective and applied data for increased pregnancy rates. Hum Reprod. 2007;22(1):230-40.
32. Meseguer M, Herrero J, Tejera A, et al. The use of morphokinetics as a predictor of embryo implantation. Hum Reprod. 2011;26:2658-71.
33. Campbell A, Fishel S, Bowman N, et al. Modelling a risk classification of aneuploidy in human embryos using non-invasive morphokinetics. Reprod Biomed Online. 2013;26:477-85.
34. Campbell A, Fishel S, Bowman N, et al. Retrospective analysis of outcomes after IVF using an aneuploidy risk model derived from time-lapse imaging without PGS. Reprod Biomed Online. 2013;27:140-6.
35. Ottolini C, Rienzi L, Capalbo A. A cautionary note against embryo aneuploidy risk assessment using time-lapse imaging. Reprod Biomed Online. 2014;28:273-5.
36. Cortezzi SS, Garcia JS, Ferreira CR, et al. Secretome of the preimplantation human embryo by bottom-up label-free proteomics. Anal Bioanal Chem. 2011;401:1331-9.
37. Bagga S, Bracht J, Hunter S, et al. Regulation by let-7 and lin-4 miRNAs results in target mRNA degradation. Cell. 2005;122:553-63.
38. Valadi H, Ekström K, Bossios A, et al. Exosome-mediated transfer of mRNAs and microRNAs is a novel mechanism of genetic exchange between cells. Nat Cell Biol. 2007;9:654-9.
39. Rosenbluth EM, Shelton DN, Wells LM, et al. Human embryos secrete microRNAs into culture media-a potential biomarker for implantation. Fertil Steril. 2014;101:1493-500.
40. D'Alessandro A, Federica G, Palini S, et al. A mass spectrometry-based targeted metabolomics strategy of human blastocoele fluid: a promising tool in fertility research. Mol Biosyst. 2012;8(4):953-8.
41. Jensen PL, Beck HC, Petersen J, et al. Proteomic analysis of human blastocoel fluid and blastocyst cells. Stem Cells Dev. 2013;1;22(7):1126-35.
42. Palini S, Galluzzi L, De Stefani S, et al. Genomic DNA in human blastocoel fluid. Reprod Biomed Online. 2013;26(6):603-10.
43. Galluzzi L, Palini S, Stefani S, et al. Extracellular embryo genomic DNA and its potential for genotyping applications. Future Sci OA. 2015;1(4):FSO62.

CHAPTER 24

Fertility Preservation in Women with Gynecologic Cancer

Ava Desai

Chapter outline

- Fertility and Ovarian Cancer
  - Fertility Preservation in Invasive Epithelial Ovarian Cancer
  - Fertility Preservation in Borderline Epithelial Ovarian Cancer
  - Pregnancy and Epithelial Ovarian Cancer
  - Fertility Preservation in Germ Cell Ovarian Tumors
  - Pregnancy and Germ Cell Tumors
  - Fertility Preservation in Granulosa Cell Tumors
- Fertility and Cervical Cancer
  - Cone Biopsy in Stage IA1 Microinvasive Disease
  - Stage IA2 Microinvasive Disease
  - Ovarian Transposition
  - Pregnancy and Cervical Cancer
- Fertility and Endometrial Cancer
  - Ovarian Preservation in Endometrial Cancer
- Fertility and Gestational Trophoblastic Disease
- Preservation of Ovarian Function in Cancer Patients
  - Cryopreservation of Embryos/Oocytes or Ovarian Tissue

INTRODUCTION

Once a gynecological cancer occurs, the patient is often rendered infertile: either due to the lesion itself or due to extirpative surgery, radiation or chemotherapy. In the past, cancer was always treated with the most radical therapy. Conservative treatment was not considered to be curative in any situation. Nowadays, with a better understanding of tumor biology, identification of prognostic factors and availability of effective therapy, fertility can be preserved in certain selected cases. However, the caveat must always be: *fertility preservation can only be considered if there is no compromise to cure.*

FERTILITY AND OVARIAN CANCER

Fertility Preservation in Invasive Epithelial Ovarian Cancer

The majority of cases of epithelial ovarian cancer are seen in the perimenopausal and postmenopausal age. Many occur bilaterally. Most are diagnosed in advanced stages where radical surgery is essential for cure. Hence, fertility preservation is usually not possible in epithelial ovarian cancer. However, in a few younger patients with early stage invasive disease, and many cases of borderline cancer, fertility can be preserved.

Standard surgical management for invasive epithelial ovarian cancer includes hysterectomy and removal of the opposite ovary, even if normal; along with all staging or cytoreductive procedures, including omentectomy, peritoneal biopsies, pelvic and para-aortic lymphadenectomy. The rationale for removal of the apparently normal contralateral ovary is (a) the possibility of occult, microscopic disease and (b) risk of recurrence in the contralateral ovary later on. Bilaterality is seen in 30% of serous, 15% of endometrioid and 5–10% of mucinous tumors in Stage I. The incidence of microscopic metastases in a normal looking opposite ovary has been variously reported as between 6–43% in different stages. Munnel[1] described a 12% incidence of microscopic metastases in the contralateral ovary, with serous lesions being seven times more often bilateral than mucinous ones. The uterus is usually removed because the uterine serosa and endometrium may have occult metastases, or an endometrial malignancy may co-exist or develop later on.

Some cases of epithelial ovarian cancer are seen in the reproductive age group. Often these cases are diagnosed during a workup for infertility. Even if the patient is young and desires children, fertility preservation can only be considered in Stage I, preferably Stage IA. Stage is the single most important prognostic factor. Grade and histological type of tumor are also important. Fertility preservation is best considered in low grade serous, mucinous or endometrioid tumors. It was formerly not recommended in IC, grade 3 and those with clear cell/undifferentiated histology. However, recent evidence shows non-impaired survival rates with fertility preserving surgery followed by chemotherapy in higher-risk early stage ovarian cancer (1AG3 or higher).[2] The evidence on fertility sparing in high-risk cases is still, however, sparse, with data from small series only.

Counseling and informed consent of patient and her family is essential when fertility preserving surgery is being considered. All the potential risks must be explained and only then should decisions be taken. The patient must be explained that a grossly normal opposite ovary may be harboring a microscopic lesion, which will be missed with conservative surgery. Also, she may be harboring a synchronous endometrial malignancy. This is especially important with endometrioid ovarian cancer. Kottmeir et al.[3] found endometrial endometrioid cancers to co-exist with endometrioid ovarian cancers in 14% of cases. Hence, if conservative surgery is being considered, a preoperative endometrial biopsy is essential. If the tumor ruptures, or if there is ascites, the chance of peritoneal spread is increased. (In such cases complete surgery is preferable.) The patient must also be counseled that after staging laparotomy, all further decisions depend on the final histopathological reports. If any of the staging biopsies reveal extra-ovarian microscopic tumor, then fertility preservation is not to be considered. A second surgery for completion is indicated. The need for close and regular follow-up to detect recurrence must also be explained to the patient.

Often these tumors are diagnosed in young women during inadvertent laparoscopy/laparotomy for infertility or for suspected "adnexal mass" or "endometriosis". Frozen section can be very helpful in the management of an indeterminate adnexal mass, especially when fertility preservation is an issue. If frozen section reveals a malignant epithelial tumor, and if surgical expertise is available, then the unilateral adnexectomy should be accompanied by full staging procedures. If no oncology specialist is available, then the tumor should be removed without rupture, and peritoneal washings should be obtained. As soon as the final histopathology report confirms malignancy, she must be appropriately referred for thorough staging laparotomy, preferably within two to three weeks of the first surgery. Staging to rule out extra-ovarian disease becomes even more important with conservative surgery. Again, the patient must be counseled that if extra-ovarian disease is discovered, then fertility sparing is no longer an option.

Fertility preserving surgery must include full staging procedures as recommended by International Federation at Gynecology and Obstetrics (FIGO), including:
- Four quadrant peritoneal washings for cytology
- Meticulous inspection and palpation of abdominal cavity and retroperitoneum
- Close inspection of uterus and opposite ovary
- Removal of ovarian tumor without rupture
- Infracolic omentectomy
- Target peritoneal biopsies/biopsy of suspicious areas
- Pelvic and para-aortic lymphadenectomy.

Wedge biopsy of the contralateral normal appearing ovary is currently not recommended, as it may produce hemorrhage/mechanical infertility. A biopsy should be performed only for a suspicious area. In this case, the biopsied ovary should be protected from adhesions, e.g. by wrapping with interceed.

There is enough evidence in the literature to support fertility preservation if recommendations are followed. Munnel[1] demonstrated the same (75%) 5 years survival in both conservative and radically treated groups. Brown et al.[4] performed conservative surgery in 16 of 127 Stage I patients. 37% required platinum based chemotherapy. After a median follow-up of 66 months, 88% were alive without disease. However, 2 patients (13%) recurred in the preserved ovary and both of them died of disease.

In some series, the indications for fertility sparing have been extended to include unfavorable factors such as stage IC and grade 3. Schilder et al.[5] reported on 52 patients if IA/IC, grades 1 to 3, who were conservatively managed. Fruscio et al.[6] showed that the outcome of G3 tumors was not worsened with conservative surgery. In such cases, chemotherapy is a necessary adjunct to fertility sparing surgery. Patients of Stage IC, higher grade, or those with dense adhesions, rupture or ascites, i.e. "high-risk early stage" should be given chemotherapy even if fertility preserving surgery has been performed. The risk of gonadal damage is probably not high. Brown[4] reported 8 pregnancies among 16 women, 2 after chemotherapy.

However, ovarian cancer is an aggressive disease, and fertility sparing must always be approached with caution and complete understanding of the inherent risks. Morice et al.[7] demonstrated recurrence in 7 of 25 conservatively treated patients. Five of these seven recurred in the contralateral ovary. Three of 19 Stage IA and all with Stage IC recurred. Only three successful pregnancies were reported in this series.

Hence, fertility preservation can only be done in the rare cases of early stage unilateral ovarian cancers occurring in strongly motivated young women, where a thorough staging laparotomy confirms no extra-ovarian spread (Table 24.1). The indications are young age, fully informed consent, Stage

Table 24.1: Indications for fertility preservation in invasive epithelial ovarian cancer.

Young, low parity, strong motivation
Fully informed consent
Stage IA/C
Mucinous, serous, endometrioid type, low grade preferable
Negative endometrial biopsy
No other cause for infertility
Preferably no ascites, dense adhesions, capsular involvement or rupture (high-risk)
Close oncological follow-up probable

IA/C, mucinous, serous or endometrioid histology, preferably low grade, tumors with negative endometrial biopsy. Preferably there should be no ascites, no dense adhesions or surface excrescences and the tumor should be unruptured. The pelvis should be otherwise normal with no other impediment to conception. If there are high-risk factors such as Stage IC, grade 3 or rupture, adjuvant chemotherapy is required.

Completion of surgery after childbearing is often recommended to reduce the rate of recurrence. The risk of recurrence is low in IA, grade 1 tumors. Zanetta et al.[8] reported 3.5% recurrence in the opposite ovary after a median follow-up of 7 years. However, in Morice et al's.[7] study, 7 out of 25 conservatively treated patients recurred; 5 out of 7 in the contralateral preserved ovary. Though it may be prudent to advise surgical completion after childbearing, more evidence should accrue before strong recommendations can be made for it. Until then each case should be individually discussed with the patient and family.

Diagnosis of epithelial ovarian cancer at a young age should raise the suspicion of a hereditary cancer syndrome. Careful history-taking and genetic testing may help to identify such cases in which surgery is strongly advocated after childbearing.

Fertility Preservation in Borderline Epithelial Ovarian Cancer (Flowchart 24.1)

Fertility preservation can be considered in many cases of borderline epithelial ovarian cancer because:
- Most (75%) borderline tumors present in early stages.
- Only one-fourth of Stage I borderline tumors are bilateral. (Overall, 10% of mucinous borderline tumors are bilateral as compared to 30–60% of serous borderline tumors.)
- The average age of occurrence is in the forties.

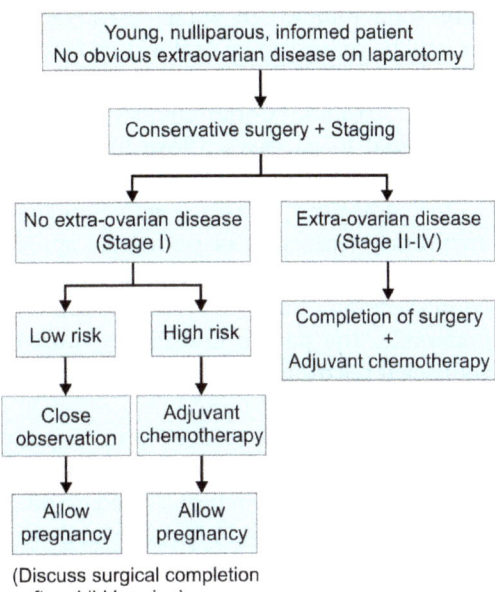

Flowchart 24.1: Algorithm for postoperative management after conservative surgery in apparent Stage I invasive epithelial ovarian cancer.

- If recurrences do occur, most can be cured with another surgery.
- The 5 years survival rate is excellent: approximately 95% in Stage I and up to 90% even in advanced stages.

Frozen section diagnosis of borderline tumors is difficult and best left to an expert pathologist. The reports of frozen section correspond with the final histopathology reports in about 60% of cases. About 6–27% are upgraded to invasive cancer on permanent section.[9] This is an additional reason to perform staging procedures in all cases. These issues should be carefully discussed with patient and relatives.

The conservative surgical options are unilateral adnexectomy/cystectomy for unilateral tumors and bilateral cystectomy for bilateral tumors. If one ovary is involved, unilateral adnexectomy is preferable to cystectomy as patients undergoing cystectomy had a significantly higher recurrence rate than those undergoing unilateral salpingo-oophorectomy. Cystectomy should be limited to cases where both ovaries are involved with borderline tumor.[10] In such cases, fertility can still be preserved by performing bilateral cystectomy with preservation of normal ovarian stroma. Comprehensive staging is essential in all cases. Close follow-up is mandatory to detect recurrences.

In advanced cases with bilateral involvement, capsular or peritoneal spread, total hysterectomy with bilateral salpingo-oophorectomy and cytoreduction is preferable. The patient and family must be counseled regarding the best chance of cure in such cases.

There is ample evidence to support conservative surgery in borderline tumors. Julian and Woodruff[11] demonstrated no difference in 5 years survival rates after unilateral adnexectomy (100%) versus total hysterectomy with bilateral salpingo-oophorectomy (90%). Though recurrence rates are seen to be higher with conservative surgery, survival rates are not affected as the recurrences are amenable to secondary excision. Zanetta et al.[12] showed that in Stage I, recurrence rates were higher (15.2%) with conservative surgery compared to radical surgery (2.5%). In Stages II and III, the respective recurrence rates were 40% versus 12.9%. With cystectomy, the recurrence rates are even higher (36%). However, these recurrences are usually in the form of borderline malignancy and can be salvaged with a second surgery. Hence, all series show excellent survival rates after repeat surgery for recurrence. In Lim Tan's[13] series of 35 cases with uni- or bilateral cystectomy in serous LMP tumors, ipsilateral recurrence was seen only when margins of removed cyst were positive or with multicystic lesions. In spite of recurrences, all patients were alive and well with a mean follow-up of 7.5 years.

Pregnancy rates of 13–44% have been documented in most series after conservative surgery, even in Stage III. Gotleib et al.[14] reported a total of 22 successful pregnancies in 15/39 patients, up to Stage III. In those 15, 5 had undergone cystectomy and 10/15 unilateral salpingo-oophorectomy. There is no consensus on the use of ovulation inducing drugs for conception in these cases. Assisted reproduction (ART) has been used for infertility after conservative management, without any increase in recurrence rates. However, informed consent should be taken before ART regarding the potential risk of recurrence.

The role of "surgical completion" after childbearing is not established. It may be considered in order to decrease the risk of recurrence. However, there is no strong evidence to support this as yet.

Unfortunately, the term "borderline" produces a false sense of security among some physicians and patients. It can, in some cases, be progressive and fatal. Hence, all cases warrant very close follow-up, just as in any ovarian cancer. After conservative surgery, the recommendation for follow-up is with six monthly ultrasound/trans-vaginal sonography, clinical examination and serum Ca 125 estimation. Follow-up should be long-term as the average time to recurrence is 5.5 years.

Pregnancy and Epithelial Ovarian Cancer

Though the incidence of ovarian malignancy in pregnancy is low, a suspicious ovarian mass should be removed surgically in order not to miss a malignancy. Surgical outcomes in a well-controlled setting are excellent during pregnancy.[15]

Most epithelial ovarian tumors diagnosed during pregnancy will be of the borderline type. Invasive epithelial ovarian cancer is not commonly seen in pregnancy. It may be incidentally diagnosed during a clinical examination or ultrasound, and is usually in the early stage.

Surgical management is best accomplished in mid-trimester. The tumor must be excised and staging performed. Usually this can be achieved without any harm to the pregnancy. In advanced cases, cytoreduction is required. The advisability of aggressive surgical debulking during pregnancy will be dictated by the extent of disease, the gestational age of the fetus and maternal wishes. If the patient desires to continue pregnancy, conservative cytoreduction (with the goal of avoiding a prolonged and traumatic procedure that could result in harm to the fetus) followed by adjuvant chemotherapy is appropriate. Hysterectomy during pregnancy is rarely indicated, unless it contributes significantly to debulking.[16] Hysterectomy and more extensive cytoreduction can be performed at the time of cesarean section, or in the immediate postpartum stage if the patient desires vaginal delivery.[17]

There are not many reports of chemotherapy for epithelial ovarian cancer during pregnancy. Most of these are of the use of cisplatin/cyclophosphamide with no deleterious effects on the pregnancy or fetus. Reports on the use of Paclitaxel are rare. Taxanes are teratogenic when administered in early pregnancy. However, they can probably be used in later stages of pregnancy with no deleterious effects on the pregnancy or fetus.

Fertility Preservation in Germ Cell Ovarian Tumors

These are rare tumors, constituting 5–15% of all ovarian cancers. However, they are the commonest malignant tumors occurring in young girls and women. They are very virulent, highly malignant, and rapidly growing. Fortunately, most produce sensitive tumor markers, present in early stages and are unilateral (except 10–15% of dysgerminomas). Also, they are exquisitely chemosensitive. Hence, a higher cure rate can be achieved, with fertility preservation in most cases.

Unlike their epithelial counterparts, fertility preservation is possible in most cases of germ cell ovarian tumor. There are certain inherent differences between germ cell and epithelial ovarian tumors, due to which cure rates are better and conservative surgery is possible (Table 24.2).

Tumor markers play an extremely important role in these tumors. Identification of sensitive tumor markers, especially serum alpha fetoprotein, lactate dehydrogenase and human chorionic gonadotropin have played a large role in improving results. They are very helpful in preoperative diagnosis, monitoring of treatment and detection of subclinical recurrence.

Table 24.2: Characteristics of epithelial and germ cell ovarian tumors.

	Epithelial ovarian cancer	Germ cell ovarian tumors
Age	Peri/Menopausal	< 40 years
Stage	¾ in late stage	¾ in early stage
Growth rate	Slower	Rapid
Early symptoms	Vague, nonspecific	Pain/distension
Laterality	Often bilateral	Almost always unilateral (except 10–15% dysgerminomas)
Recurrence in contralateral normal ovary	Common	Rare
Chemosensitivity	Variable	Exquisite
Fertility sparing surgery	Very few, selected cases	Almost all cases, even advanced

During surgery, the tumor should be removed intact, and sent for frozen section if necessary. The opposite ovary should be closely inspected (Fig. 24.1). Wedge biopsy of an opposite normal-looking ovary is not indicated. Bilaterality is almost unknown in germ cell tumors, except in dysgerminomas. Hence a biopsy is unnecessary and may produce hemorrhage or mechanical infertility. Hence, in non-dysgerminomatous tumors, if there is a mass on the opposite ovary, it is almost always a dermoid cyst, which can be shelled out, leaving behind normal ovarian tissue. Dysgerminomas may be bilateral in about 15% of cases. In such cases, even if both ovaries are removed, the uterus can be left *in situ* for future assisted reproduction. If with bilateral dysgerminoma, one of the tumors is small, it can be excised, leaving behind normal ovarian tissue.[18] This can be done because dysgerminomas are highly chemosensitive. All staging procedures must be carried out to search for microscopic spread, just as in epithelial ovarian cancer. These include peritoneal cytology, omentectomy, peritoneal biopsies and lymphadenectomy (Fig. 24.2).

If the disease is advanced, cytoreduction of gross disease should be done. *However, in these highly chemosensitive tumors, the normal opposite ovary and uterus should*

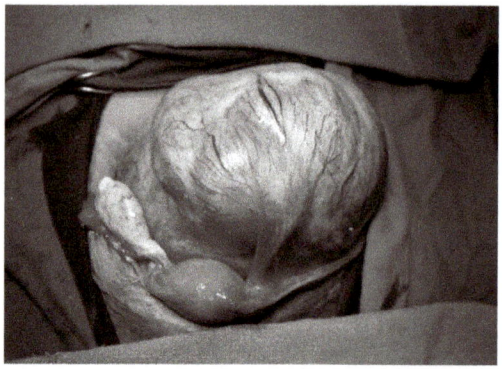

Fig. 24.1: Dysgerminoma of right ovary: Normal uterus and contralateral ovary.

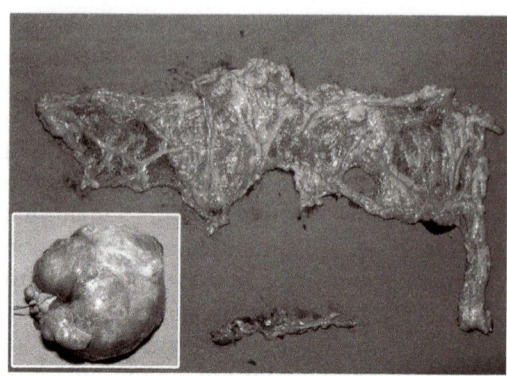

Fig. 24.2: Mixed germ cell tumor: Staging biopsies and omentectomy must be done along with even fertility sparing surgery.

be preserved in spite of advanced disease. The exquisite chemosensitivity results in good cure rates even with bulky residual or recurrence.

Germ cell tumors have a propensity to arise in dysgenetic gonads. *Hence, in premenarchal girls, a karyotype should be obtained before surgery.* If the karyotype contains a Y chromosome, *both ovaries should be removed, regardless of stage.* The uterus can be left behind for future assisted reproduction.

Most patients will require adjuvant chemotherapy. Surgery alone with no further treatment is possible only in Stage I dysgerminoma (pure and properly staged) and Stage IA/grade 1 immature teratoma with no ascites. *All others, even if Stage I, require chemotherapy, which should be initiated as early as possible after surgery.* Before the advent of modern chemotherapy, the survival rates for even Stage I endodermal sinus tumors were dismal. Nowadays an excellent cure rate is possible in all stages. The regime of choice and the current standard of care is BEP chemotherapy (Bleomycin, Etoposide, Cisplatin).

The GOG 93 is the largest study of adjuvant BEP in optimally cytoreduced Stages I–III, now updated. In those 93, 91 patients who took three courses of adjuvant BEP are free of disease.[19] Modern chemotherapy has produced a dramatic reversal in survival. The cure rates are 95–100% in Stage I. Even in advanced stages, the cure rate is 95% for dysgerminomas and 75% for non-dysgerminomas.[20] At present, the standard of care is to give adjuvant chemotherapy to all, except those mentioned above, i.e. Stage I dysgerminoma (pure and properly staged) and Stage IA/grade 1 immature teratoma with no ascites. In order to reduce toxicity, studies are ongoing at centers such as Mount Vernon Hospital/Charing Cross Hospital, to omit chemotherapy in Stage I of other histological types.[21] Some authors now suggest surveillance alone in 50% of early stage I germ cell tumors.[22] Cases of early Stage I yolk sac tumor treated with only sugery, did show higher recurrence rates, but no difference in overall survival as relapses were chemosensitive. With this approach, about 77% could be saved from chemotherapy.[23] However, this approach requires very close, strict follow-up and must be used judiciously.

Most patients have normal menstrual function after chemotherapy, though some may develop treatment-induced menopause. Factors such as older age, cumulative dose and duration of therapy influence the rate of treatment induced menopause. The pre-pubertal ovary is less at risk of drug-induced gonadal dysfunction.

Pregnancy should be avoided for 1–2 years to allow proper follow-up. Many healthy live births have been reported, and the miscarriage rate is no more than in the general population. Gershenson[24] reported that of 16 patients who attempted conception, only one had true, persistent infertility. Eleven patients delivered 22 healthy infants, none with major birth defects.

Hence, appropriate surgery and chemotherapy, the availability of sensitive tumor markers and a better understanding of these tumors have markedly increased the survival rates of these previously fatal tumors, along with preservation of fertility in most cases.

Pregnancy and Germ Cell Tumors

Germ cell tumors occur in the childbearing age. Hence, they may be encountered during pregnancy. The commonest malignant germ cell tumor seen in pregnancy is dysgerminoma. Management will depend on the stage of the disease and the duration of pregnancy. Usually the pregnancy can be continued after excision of the tumor and staging. If the disease is advanced, then continuation of pregnancy must be individually decided, taking gestational age into consideration. Chemotherapy can be given in and after the second trimester without harming the fetus.

Fertility Preservation in Granulosa Cell Tumors

Granulosa cell tumors are bilateral in only 2% of cases. Hence, in young girls and women who desire fertility, conservative surgery along with staging procedures is appropriate. If fertility sparing surgery is planned, an endometrial biopsy must be previously taken to rule out endometrial hyperplasia, which co-exists in 25–50% cases or adenocarcinoma which co-exists in at least 5% cases.

Stage is the most important prognostic factor. Meticulous long-term follow-up is essential, even in Stage I. In later stages, appropriate references should be made for adjuvant treatment.

FERTILITY AND CERVICAL CANCER

Fertility sparing options are nowadays applicable in selected cases of microinvasive and early, small volume, invasive cervical cancer.

Cone Biopsy in Stage IA1 Microinvasive Disease

According to the FIGO 1995 definition, Stage IA1 cervical cancer is preclinical, with

measured stromal invasion of ≤3.0 mm in depth and ≤7.0 mm horizontal spread. In such cases:
- The rate of lymph node metastases is negligible (<1%). Elliot et al.[25] reported a 0.8 child incidence of positive nodes (1 of 121 cases). After cone biopsy, dysplasia of the internal cone margin or in the endocervical curettage (ECC) specimen is a significant factor for residual disease. Roman et al.[26] reported 87 cases of Stage IA (microinvasive) disease. Residual disease was present in 22% of women with dysplasia at the internal margin as against only 3% with a negative margin. This increased to 33% if the ECC was also positive.
- Lymph vascular space involvement (LVSI) is not included in the staging. However, it should be considered during treatment planning, as the risk of recurrence is higher.

The standard treatment for Stage IA1 cervical cancer is extrafascial hysterectomy. However, if the patient is young and keen for fertility preservation, she can be treated with a cone biopsy, preferably a knife cone or by large loop excision of the transformation zone (LLETZ). The factors mentioned above must be kept in mind. Therefore, the treatment is considered adequate only if the surgical margins and post-cone ECC are clear. If the margins or ECC reveal dysplasia, a repeat cone should be performed to rule out invasion, and then further surgical treatment planned accordingly. Lymph node dissection is not necessary in stage IA1. (However, if extensive LVSI is present, she may be a candidate for pelvic node dissection, or should be managed similarly to Stage IA2.) If adequate and complete resection is performed, with negative margins and no lympvascular space invasion, the oncological outcome is not impaired with this fertility sparing approach.[27] Fertility is not impaired though premature rupture of membranes or preterm delivery may occur.[28]

Stage IA2 Microinvasive Disease

According to the FIGO 1995 definition, Stage IA2 cervical cancer is preclinical, with measured stromal invasion of >3.0 mm and ≤5 mm in depth and ≤7.0 mm horizontal spread. In such cases, the rate of lymph node metastases is quite significant, i.e. 7.1% (0–13.8% in different series). Elliot et al.[25] reported a 3.4% incidence of positive nodes (2 of 59 cases). Hence, in cervical cancer Stage IA2, the regional lymph nodes also need to be addressed. The incidence of invasive recurrence and death are 3.6% and 2.9% in several series.[37]

The standard treatment for Stage IA2 cervical cancer is type 1 or 2 hysterectomy with pelvic node dissection. However, if the patient is young and keen for fertility preservation, the options are cervical conization with pelvic node dissection, or, more commonly, radical trachelectomy with pelvic node dissection. This technique, pioneered by Dargent, is dealt with below.

Radical Trachelectomy with Node Dissection in Stage IA2/IB1 Cervical Cancer

The standard treatment for invasive cervical cancer stage IB1 is radical (Type III) hysterectomy along with bilateral pelvic nodded dissection. Cervical cancer is known to spread laterally from the cervix and via lymphatics. Hence, the essential component of the surgery is the extensive central dissection, which aims at resecting the parametrial, paracervical and paravaginal tissue, along with lymphadenectomy. The other option is curative radiation which gives similar results, but has certain disadvantages, one of the main being radiation castration.

In certain selected cases of stage IB1 small volume disease, if the patient is young and very keen for fertility sparing, radical trachelectomy with pelvic node dissection is a feasible alternative to radical hysterectomy.

The indications, according to Dargent,[29] are: age < 40 years, desire for fertility, IA2 or IB1/IIA lesions of small volume, protruding from the endocervix. Patients must be compliant for close follow-up to detect recurrence.

Laparoscopic vaginal radical trachelectomy (LVRT) was pioneered by Daniel Dargent et al.[29] in the 1980s. Laparoscopic lymphadenectomy was first performed, followed by vaginal radical trachelectomy (VRT). The decision to proceed with the VRT was made in one of two ways. In the first method, the nodes were sent for frozen section, and VRT was carried out if they were negative. In the second method, results of the final paraffin section are awaited before deciding to proceed for VRT. VRT entails removal of the cervix along with the surrounding parametrial tissue and a vaginal cuff. The vaginal cuff was re-anastomosed to the isthmus and a cerclage was inserted. The VRT specimen was also subjected for frozen section. The patients were counseled that if the upper margin was positive on frozen or final section, or if nodes were positive, radical hysterectomy and/or radiation would be necessary.

Since then several centers have reported data on radical trachelectomy by vaginal, abdominal, laparoscopic or robotic assisted techniques. Most selection criteria include tumor size less than 2 cm, and absence of lymph node involvement or LVSI. Patients were counseled that if margins or nodes are found to be positive either at frozen section or later on final section, fertility preservation was not an option and they should be treated with radical hysterectomy. Lymphadenectomy (laparoscopic, extraperitoneal or open) is performed first to assess nodes, followed by radical abdominal or vaginal trachelectomy. If nodes are positive, fertility sparing is to be abandoned.

Data from several centers shows survival comparable with traditional surgery and good pregnancy rates. The recurrence rates are comparable to those with standard radical hysterectomy. Dargent[29] reported a 4.3% recurrence rate, i.e. 2 of 47 patients. Both had LVSI, and one had tumor diameter > 2 cm. Burnett et al.[30] reviewed data from five centers. The overall recurrence rate was 2.6% (4/154 cases). Three-fourth recurrences occurred in patients with tumor size > 2 cm and presence of LVSI. The significance of LVSI in choosing candidates for conservative surgery is yet to be established.

Fertility is not impaired after radical trachelectomy. Pregnancy outcome is quite good, though there is a higher risk of cervical insufficiency, spontaneous abortions and preterm labor. In Dargent's[29] series, 13 of 16 women who attempted pregnancy conceived. Twenty pregnancies were achieved, resulting in 10 normal children. They also operated on 5 women with early pregnancy, of which 3 had live healthy births. Of the total 25 pregnancies, there were 13 deliveries, 3 abortions, 3 first trimester and 3 second trimester miscarriages. Shepherd[31] reported 14 pregnancies among 8 women. Nine were delivered by cesarean section. There were 5 early miscarriages. Hence, cerclage is an important component of this surgery, though there is some debate as cerclage related complications may occur. Pregnancy rates of 60% have been reported, though the rate of pregnancy loss may be higher than normal.[32]

In summary, evidence reveals that the oncological outcome of this surgery is similar to the traditional radical approach if patients are carefully selected and if the surgeon is well trained. Fertility is not impaired. The procedure provides a reasonable chance for healthy live births, in spite of an increased incidence of miscarriage and preterm delivery.

An alternative to radical trachelectomy in carefully selected cases with small volume (<20 mm) disease is large knife conization with laparoscopic lymphadenectomy. Some studies report 5 year disease free survival of 7% and conception rates of 47%.[33,34] However, data is still to accrue regarding this technique.

If the disease is more than 2 cm and the patient is still keen for fertility preservation, neoadjuvant chemotherapy followed by radical trachelectomy has been proposed.[35] However, data is scarce and long-term oncolgical outcomes are unknown.

Ovarian Transposition

The rationale for ovarian preservation in young women undergoing radical hysterectomy for cervical cancer is that ovarian metastases are very rare in squamous cell cervical cancer. The incidence is higher (about 2%) in adenocarcinoma and hence ovarian preservation should be probably avoided in these cases.

The preserved ovaries may be transposed outside the radiation field in anticipation of postoperative radiotherapy. The ovary must be transposed as high as possible, at the lower pole of each kidney, so that even scatter radiation can be avoided. Care must be taken to avoid torsion of the pedicle. Even so, it is estimated that function is maintained in only about half of the transposed ovaries.

These patients will have the benefit of natural hormone secretion. They can also avail of assisted reproduction, such as ovum retrieval and surrogate IVF pregnancy. The transposed ovaries are often difficult to access for ovum pickup. Patients must also be warned that the ovaries may need to be removed at a later date if ovarian remnant syndrome occurs.

Pregnancy and Cervical Cancer

It is not rare to encounter cervical cancer during pregnancy. Hacker et al.[36] reported an incidence of 1 in 2,205 pregnancies. One in 34 cases of cervical cancer was diagnosed during or within 12 months of pregnancy.

Management decisions must be made after fully informed consent of the patient and her partner. If a cone reveals Stage IA1 with clear margins, the pregnancy may be continued with close observation. With invasive disease, decisions will depend on the stage of the disease and the stage of the pregnancy.

If the disease is diagnosed before 20 weeks, there is no scope for delay. Treatment must be begun as soon as possible: radiotherapy or surgery depending on disease stage. Radiation can be begun, and spontaneous abortion will usually occur, or evacuation can be done at the time of brachytherapy. Some centers prefer to perform hysterotomy before radiation is started. If the patient is a candidate for curative surgery, then radical hysterectomy with bilateral pelvic node dissection can be performed with the fetus *in situ* or with hysterotomy.

If the disease is diagnosed after 28 weeks, then treatment may be delayed a few weeks, till the fetus is viable.[37] After fetal viability, treatment will depend on the stage of the disease. Delivery should ideally be by classical cesarean section. Vaginal delivery is not unknown, but may lead to cervical trauma/hemorrhage. There is also the theoretical concern for embolization and disease dissemination during cervical dilatation and delivery.[16] This can be followed by curative radiation. If she is a candidate for curative surgery, then radical hysterectomy with bilateral pelvic node dissection can be performed along with classical cesarean section.

For those cases diagnosed in mid-trimester, individualization is important. If the patient refuses to sacrifice the pregnancy, all risks must be explained to her. In such a case, she can be treated with neoadjuvant chemotherapy after 20 weeks, in an attempt to prevent disease progression till the fetus reaches viability.[38]

FERTILITY AND ENDOMETRIAL CANCER

Most cases of endometrial cancer occur in the perimenopausal and postmenopausal group, where fertility preservation is not an issue. However, about 5% occur in women younger than 40 years. In many of these women, the disease is low grade, with no myometrial invasion and very good prognosis with standard treatment. These younger women are usually under treatment for infertility, polycystic disease or are obese and anovulatory. Many of them are still to complete their families and may be interested in a fertility preserving approach.

Progesterone has been known to cure 70% of atypical endometrial hyperplasias. It has also been used for relapses of endometrial cancer, with regression of metastatic lesions. These results are extrapolated to primary management of early endometrial cancers, in an attempt to spare fertility.

Standard treatment of endometrial cancer includes total hysterectomy with bilateral salpingo-oophorectomy and staging procedures. The cure rates in early cases are excellent, but fertility is sacrificed. In an attempt to avoid hysterectomy and preserve fertility, hormonal treatment, usually with progesterone, has been used.

Counseling and fully informed consent of the risks involved is very important before attempting fertility preservation. Advanced disease may be missed. The disease may progress during treatment with progesterone. There may be microscopic metastases in the ovaries or lymph nodes. A synchronous ovarian tumor may be present. The patient and family must be counseled regarding these risks, and the need for surgery if there is no regression. They must be explained regarding strict follow-up and the fact that some form of treatment will have to continue until surgery is performed. The patients must be therefore strongly motivated before proceeding with this conservative approach. Conservative treatment in endometrial cancer, without surgery, is still controversial. There are no guidelines and many series show different results.

Selection criteria are not yet established. The patient should be young, strongly motivated, and compliant for follow-up. The lesion should be well differentiated, endometrioid type and confined to the endometrium. There should be no myometrial invasion, ovarian involvement or lymphadenopathy. MRI is the best method and should be used to assess myometrial invasion, though it is not fool-proof. Radiological methods also cannot detect subclinical ovarian or lymph node involvement, and this must be carefully discussed. In patients who failed hormonal treatment and proceeded to hysterectomy, a high incidence of myometrial invasion has been reported. Mitsushita et al.[39] reviewed the literature and found that of 10 patients operated after progesterone failed to induce response, 3 had myometrial invasion and one had extrauterine spread. With this, one can also expect an increased risk of lymph node metastases.

In Hacker et al's.[40,41] series, the rate of synchronous ovarian cancer was as high as 29.4%, and secondary involvement 17.7% in women less than 45 years. One fourth of Sardi's[42] cases had unsuspected ovarian metastases. He suggested laparoscopic exploration, peritoneal cytology and bilateral ovarian biopsy before proceeding for fertility sparing.

The type of progesterone, dose and duration of treatment, and follow-up are not yet established. In a review of the literature, 60% regression rates have been achieved with progesterone therapy. Medroxyprogesterone acetate 300–600 mg/day, or megestrol acetate orally, 160–320 mg/day are usually administered in carefully selected cases. After two months of continuous treatment, the case is reassessed with hysteroscopy and biopsy. At that point if there is no regression, hormonal treatment must be discontinued and standard surgery performed. If the lesion has completely regressed, then the treatment is continued for at least 6 to 9 months. The patient is then encouraged to conceive. Ovulation induction is often required and pregnancies have been achieved.

Kim et al.[43] proposed combining oral progesterone with a levonorgestrel-intrauterine device (LNG-IUD). Recent studies highlight the fact that LNG-IUD has the advantage of less weight gain in these already obese women. For this reason, some centers prefer to initiate therapy with the LNG-IUD and add oral progesterone if the response is inadequate after 3 months.[44] However, there are no randomized controlled trials, and any therapy must be used with extreme caution. The first goal must always be adequate management of the cancer.

In Wang et al's.[45] series, 8 out of 9 patients achieved complete remission with hormonal therapy. They used a combination of megestrol acetate and tamoxifen for 6 months. Four patients conceived, with 3 full-term pregnancies, one abortion, one ovarian pregnancy and one ectopic pregnancy. Four of the 8 responders subsequently developed recurrences which were treated with definitive surgery/further hormonal therapy. All 9 patients were free of disease at follow-up. Kim et al.[46] reviewed the data of several series. Initial response was 62%. Three initial responders later developed recurrence, one extra-uterine. Three patients delivered 6 viable infants. Nineteen of 21 patients were alive and well at follow-up.

There is no guideline as to continued treatment after tumor regression. Hysterectomy after childbirth is advisable. Recurrence is common, up to 50%, in these inherently high-risk patients. Some therapy must be continued, along with close surveillance, frequent imaging, hysteroscopy, endometrial sampling, etc. Also, hormonal therapy may not completely eradicate the lesion. Mitsushita et al.[39] reported a case in which the patient conceived after response to progesterone. Post-delivery endometrial biopsy revealed residual disease. The hysterectomy specimen revealed a small focus of adenocarcinoma abutting the myometrium. "Consolidation" hysterectomy after childbirth is therefore advisable, even in responders.

In summary, fertility preservation with hormonal treatment in endometrial carcinoma can be attempted in carefully selected cases, with fully informed consent. There is yet no consensus on selection criteria, type and dose of progesterone, duration of treatment, maintenance therapy and consolidation therapy after childbirth. The risks of conservative management must be well understood by both treating physician and patient. It should be explained that the goal is only to delay surgery till childbirth is achieved. A recent meta-analysis showed a pooled complete response rate of 76.2% and a recurrence rate among complete responders of 40.6%.[47]

Ovarian Preservation in Endometrial Cancer

Unlike cervical cancer, ovarian preservation is not recommended in endometrial cancer. The current recommendation is bilateral oophorectomy regardless of age. The reasons are several: ovarian micro-metastases are seen in 3–11% cases, an occult synchronous epithelial or granulosa cell tumor may co-exist, these patients are epidemiologically at risk for future ovarian cancer, endometrial tissue is estrogen-dependent. In Hacker et al's.[40,41] series, the rate of synchronous ovarian cancer was as high as 29.4%, and secondary involvement 17.7% in women less than 45 years. Hence, the standard of care is to remove the ovaries even in younger patients.

However, recent reports have questioned the need to remove normal-appearing ovaries in early stage endometrial cancer in younger women. Lee et al.[48] described independent risk factors for co-existing malignancy such as non-endometrioid histology, intraoperative extrauterine disease, lymph node metastases, and age. In absence of these factors, the risk of ovarian disease was low (0.97%) and the ovaries could be preserved. However, more large-scale studies are required before the current recommendation for bilateral oophorectomy can be changed.

FERTILITY AND GESTATIONAL TROPHOBLASTIC DISEASE

After vesicular mole, the patient requires strict post-molar surveillance with serial beta hCG estimation to detect malignant sequelae. Contraception is advised throughout this surveillance period. Pregnancy can be allowed after the follow-up period of about one year. Conception is not affected. In the following pregnancy, an ultrasound at 10 weeks should be done to rule out a second molar pregnancy. hCG should be estimated 6 weeks postpartum to exclude occult disease. Berkowitz[49] reported 68.6% live births from 1,239 conceptions following complete mole.

For gestational trophoblastic disease, the cornerstone of management is chemotherapy, with surgery playing only a secondary role. Hence, in most cases, fertility can be spared. With the identification of prognostic factors, sensitive tumor marker, individualization and appropriate chemotherapy, excellent results are achieved. Secondary hysterectomy is indicated only in drug resistant disease, which is uterine-confined. There is no indication for removing normal ovaries, either during primary or secondary hysterectomy. Theca lutein cysts will resolve spontaneously.

The results in low-risk disease are almost 100%, and even in high-risk cases, 60–80% success rates are achieved with correct management. After treatment and the recommended follow-up period, fertility goals can usually be achieved. The course of pregnancy is normal and there is no evidence of malformation in the resultant progeny.

PRESERVATION OF OVARIAN FUNCTION IN CANCER PATIENTS

Situations where the ovaries can be preserved either in position or after transposition have been described through this chapter. However, often the ovaries must be removed, or they may be subjected to the deleterious effects of radiation or chemotherapy. Options are now available to preserve ovarian function in such cases.

Ovarian transposition has already been discussed under the section on fertility preservation in cervical cancer.

Many chemotherapeutic agents are known to be gonadotoxic, and may produce premature ovarian failure. Hence, in many clinical situations, the drug or number of cycles of chemotherapy are reduced to prevent the gonadotoxic effects. A good example is combination chemotherapy with bleomycin, etoposide and cisplatin used in young girls with germ cell ovarian tumors. The number of cycles have now been reduced from six to only two or three in order to reduce gonadotoxicity.

Attempts have been made to suppress ovarian function during chemotherapy. Formerly oral contraceptive pills were used throughout the course of chemotherapy, but their efficacy in protecting the ovaries is questionable. Later on Blumenfeld et al.[50] proposed the use of GnRH agonists for this purpose. They demonstrated a much higher rate of resumption of spontaneous ovulation and menses than in the control group. Further studies are required before firm recommendations can be made.

Cryopreservation of Embryos/Oocytes or Ovarian Tissue

If the ovaries are to be removed, or radiated, they can first be stimulated and mature oocytes retrieved before treatment is started. The embryos (or even mature oocytes in case there is no partner), can be cryopreserved. However, this would entail a delay of definitive treatment by at least a month or two for stimulation, maturation and retrieval of oocytes. If delay is not advisable, strips of ovarian tissue can be removed and cryopreserved. After treatment is over, they can be transplanted to their natural location or to other sites.[51] The results so far are ambiguous and concern has also been expressed regarding recurrence of malignancy in the transplanted ovary. However, several livebirths have now been reported after ovarian transplantation.

The first successful livebirth after uterine transplant with a uterus donated by a post-menopausal woman was reported recently by Brannstorm et al.[52]

Many of these methods must at present be considered experimental. However, with advances in medical technology, they will in future help to preserve fertility in cancer subjects where ovarian function would otherwise be sacrificed as part of the treatment.

REFERENCES

1. Munnel. Is conservative surgery ever justified in stage IA cancer of the ovary? Am J Obst Gynecol. 1969;103:641.
2. Ditto A, Martinelli F, Bogani G, et al. Long term safety of fertility sparing surgery in early stage ovarian cancer: Comparison to standard radical surgical procedures. Gynecol Oncol. 2015;138:78-82
3. Kottmeier HL. Surgical management—conservative surgery. In: Gentil F, Junqueria AC (Eds). Ovarian Cancer. Vol 2. New York: Springer Verlag; 1968.
4. Brown CL, Dharmendra B, Barakat R. Preserving fertility in patients with epithelial ovarian cancer: the role of conservative surgery in treatment of early stage disease. Gynecol Oncol. 2000;76:40.
5. Schilder JM, Thompson AM, Depriest PD, et al. Outcome of reproductive age women with Stage IA or IC invasive epithelial ovarian cancer treated with fertility-sparing surgery. Gynecol Oncol. 2002;87:1-7.r
6. Fruscio R, Ceppi L, Corso S, et al. Long term results of fertility-sparing treatment compared with standard radical surgery for early-stage epithelial ovarian cancer. Br J Cancer. 2016;115(6):641-8.
7. Morice P, Wicart-Poque F, Rey A, et al. Results of conservative treatment in epithelial ovarian carcinoma. Cancer. 2001;92(9):2412-18.
8. Zanetta G. Chiari S, Rota S, et al. Conservative surgery for Stage I ovarian carcinoma in women of childbearing age. Br J Obstet Gynecol. 1997;104:1030-5.
9. Houck K, Nikrui N, Duska L, et al. Borderline tumors of the ovary: Correlation of frozen and permanent histopathologic diagnosis. Obstet Gynecol. 2000;95:839-43.
10. Ines Vasconcelos, Miguel de Sousa Mendes. Conservative surgery in borderline tumours: a meta-analysis with emphasis on recurrence risk. European Journal of Cancer. 2015:51:620-31.
11. Julian CG, Woodruff JD. The biologic behavior of the low grade papillary serous carcinoma of the ovary. Obstet Gynecol. 1973;40:60.
12. Zanetta G, Rota S, Chiari S, et al. Behavior of borderline tumors with particular interest to persistence, recurrence and progression to invasive carcinoma: a prospective study. J Clin Oncol. 2001;19:2658-64.
13. Lim-Tan S, Cjigas H, Scully R. Ovarian cystectomy for serous borderline tumors: a follow-up of 35 cases. Obstet Gynecol. 1988;72:775-80.
14. Gotleib WH, Flikker S, Davidson B, et al. Borderline tumors of the ovary: fertility treatment, conservative management and pregnancy outcome. Cancer. 1998;82:141-6.
15. Leiserowitz GS, Xing G, Cress R, et al. Adnexal masses in pregnancy; how often are they malignant? Gynecol Oncol. 2006;101:315-21.
16. Zanotti KM, Belinson JL, Kennedy AW. Treatment of gynecologic cancers in pregnancy. Semin Oncol. 2000;27(6):686-98.
17. Bahador A, Lowe PM, Cheng J, et al. Gynecologic cancer in pregnancy. In: Gershenson DM, McGuire WP, Gore M, Quinn MA, Thomas G (Eds). Gynecologic Cancer: Controversies in Management. Philadelphia: Elsevier Ltd; 2004. pp. 921-30.
18. Berek JS, Hacker NF. Nonepithelial ovarian and fallopian tube cancers. In: Berek JS, Hacker NF (Eds). Practical Gynecologic Oncology, 4th edition. Philadelphia: Lippincott Williams and Wilkins; 2005. pp. 511-41.
19. Williams S, Blessing JA, Liao S, et al. Adjuvant therapy of ovarian germ cell tumors with cisplatin, etoposide and bleomycin: a trial

of the Gynecologic Oncology Group. J Clin Oncol. 1994;12:701-06.
20. Gershenson DM. Management of ovarian germ cell tumors. J Clin Oncol. 2007; 25:2938-43.
21. Dark GG, Bower M, Newlands ES, et al. Surveillance policy for Stage I ovarian germ cell tumors. J Clin Oncol. 1997;2:620-4.
22. Bilmire DF, Cullen JW, Rescoria FJ, et al. Surveillance after initial surgery in for pediatric and adolescent girls with stage I ovarian germ cell tumors: report from the Chilgren's Oncology Group. J Clin Oncol. 2014;32:465-70
23. Park JY, Kim DY, Suh DS, et al. Outcomes of surgery alone and surveillance strategy in young women with stage I malignant ovarian germ cell tumors. Int J Gynecol Cancer. 2016;26:858-64
24. Gershenson DM. Menstrual and reproductive function after treatment with combination chemotherapy for malignant ovarian germ cell tumors. J Clin Oncol. 1988;(2):270-5.
25. Elliot P, Coppleson M, Russel P, et al. Early invasive (FIGO stage IA) carcinoma of the cervix: a clinicopathologic study of 476 cases. Int J Gynecol Cancer. 2000;10:42-52.
26. Roman LD, Felix JC, Muderspach LI, et al. Risk of residual invasive disease in women with microinvasive squamous cancer in a conisation specimen. Obstet Gynecol. 1997;90:759-64.
27. Wright JD, NathavithArana R, Lewin SN, et al. Fertility-conserving surgery for young women with stage IA1 cervical cancer: safety and access. Obstet Gynecol. 2010;115: 585-90.
28. Kyrgiou M, Koliopoulos G,, Martin-Hirsch P, et al. Obstetric outcomes after conservative treatment for intraepithelial or early invasive cervical lesions: systematic review and meta-analysis. Lancet. 2006;367:489-98
29. Dargent D, Martin X, Sacchetoni A, et al. Laparoscopic vaginal radical trachelectomy. A treatment to preserve the fertility of cervical carcinoma patients. Cancer. 2000;88(8):1877-82.
30. Burnett AF, Roman LD, O'Meara AT, et al. Radical vaginal trachelectomy and pelvic lymphadenectomy for preservation of fertility in early cervical carcinoma. Gynecol Oncol. 2003; 88:419-23.
31. Shepherd JH, Mould T, Oram H. Radical trachelectomy in early stage carcinoma of the cervix: outcome as judged by recurrence and fertility rates. Br J Obstet Gynecol. 2001;108:882-5.
32. Pareja R, Rendon GJ, Sanz-Lomana CM, et al. Surgical, oncological and obstetrical outcomes after abdominal radical trachelectomy – a systematic literature review. Gynecol Oncol. 2013;131:77-82.
33. Xu L, Sun FQ, Wang ZH. Radical trachelectomy versus radial hysterectomy for the treatment of early cervical cancer: A systematic review. Acta Obstet Gynecol Scand. 2011;90:1200-9.
34. Zapardiel I, Cruz M, Diestro MD, et al. Assisted reproductive techniques after fertility sparing treatments in gynaecological cancers. Hum Reprod Update. 2016; 22(3):281-305.
35. Robova H, Halaska MJ, Pluta M, et al. Oncological and pregnancy outcomes after high dose-intensity neoadjuvant chemotherapy and fertility-sparing surgery in cervical cancer. Gynecol Oncol. 2014;135:213-6.
36. Hacker NF, Berek JS, Lagasse LD, et al. Carcinoma of the cervix associated with pregnancy. Obstet Gynecol. 1982;59:735-46.
37. Hacker NF. Cervical cancer. In: Berek JS, Hacker NF (Eds). Practical Gynecologic Oncology, 4th edition. Philadelphia: Lippincott Williams & Wilkins; 2005. pp. 337-95.
38. Tewari K, Capuccini F, Gambino A, et al. Neoadjuvant chemotherapy in the treatment of locally advanced cervical carcinoma in pregnancy. Cancer. 1998;82:1529-34.
39. Mitsushita, Toshiko Toki, Kiyoshi Kato, et al. Endometrial carcinoma remaining after term pregnancy following conservative treatment with medroxyprogesterone acetate. Gynecol Oncol. 2000;79:129-32.
40. Hacker NF. Uterine cancer. In: Berek JS, Hacker NF (Eds). Practical Gynecologic Oncology, 4th edition. Philadelphia: Lippincott Williams & Wilkins; 2005. pp. 397-42.
41. Gitsch G, Hanzal E, Jensen D, Hacker NF. Endometrial cancer in premenopausal

women 45 years and younger. Obstet Gynecol. 1995;85:504-08.
42. Sardi J, Anchezar Henry JP, et al. Primary hormonal treatment for early endometrial carcinoma. Eur J Gynecol Oncol. 1998;19:565-68.
43. Kim MK, Seong SJ, Kim YS, et al. Combined medroxyprogesterone acetate/levonorgestrel-intrauterine system treatment in young women with early-stage endometrial cancer. Am J Obstet Gynecol. 2013;209:358.
44. Chlakian D, Hacker K, Fader AN,. Effect of oral versus intrauterine progestins on weight in women undergoing fertility preserving therapy for complex atypical hyperplasia or endometrial cancer. Gynecol Oncol. 2016;140:234-8.
45. Wang CB, Wang CJ, Huang HJ, et al. Fertility-preserving treatment in young patients with endometrial adenocarcinoma. Cancer. 2002;94/8:2192-8.
46. Kim YB, Holschneider CH, Ghosh K. Progestin alone as primary treatment of endometrial carcinoma in premenopausal women. Cancer. 1997;79:320-7.
47. Gallos ID, Yap J, Rajkhowa M, et al. Regression, relapse and live birth rates with fertility sparing therapy for endometrial cancer and atypical complex endometrial hyperplasia: a systematic review and metaanalysis. Am J Obstet Gynecol. 2012;207:266e1-266.12.
48. Lee TS, Jung JY, Park NH, et al. Feasibility of ovarian preservation in patients with early stage endometrial carcinoma. Gynecol Oncol. 2007;104:52-7.
49. Berkowitz RS, Tuncer S, Bernstein MR, et al. Management of gestational trophoblastic diseases: subsequent pregnancy experience. Semin Oncol. 2000;27(6):678-85.
50. Blumenfeld Z, Dann E, Avivi I, et al. Fertility after treatment of Hodgkin's disease. Ann Oncol. 2002;13(Suppl 1):138-47.
51. Radford JA, Lieberman BA, BrisonDr, et al. Orthotopic reimplantation of cryopreserved ovarian cortical strips after high dose chemotherapy for Hodgkin's lymphoma. Lancet. 2001;357:1172-5.
52. Brannstrom M, Johannesson L, Bokstrom H, et al. Livebirth fter uterus transplantation. Lancet. 2015;385:607-16.

CHAPTER 25

Ectopic Pregnancy: Current Management

Majumdar Abha, Singh Tejshree A

Chapter outline

- Incidence
- Risk Factors
  - Cilia Damage and Tubal Occlusion
  - Altered Tubal Motility
  - Idiopathic
  - Previous History of Ectopic Pregnancy
  - Infertility Treatment
  - Other Risk Factors
- Clinical Presentation
- Diagnosis
  - Tubal Ectopic Pregnancy
  - Ovarian Ectopic Pregnancy
  - Cervical Ectopic Pregnancy
  - Abdominal Pregnancy
  - Cesarean Scar Ectopic
  - Heterotopic Pregnancy
- Treatment
  - Expectant Management
  - Nonsurgical Management
  - Surgical Management
- Current Evidence on Surgery, Systemic Methotrexate and Expectant Management in the Treatment of Tubal Ectopic Pregnancy
- Ectopic Pregnancies in Unusual Locations
  - Interstitial (Cornual) Pregnancy
  - Cervical Ectopic Pregnancy
  - Ovarian Pregnancy
  - Abdominal Pregnancy
  - Cesarean Scar Ectopic
  - Heterotopic Pregnancy
- Chance of Future Pregnancy

INTRODUCTION

Ectopic pregnancy (EP) is a complication of pregnancy in which the fertilized ovum implants in any tissue other than the endometrium of the uterus. About 1–3% of all pregnancies are ectopic in location and of these 98% occur in the fallopian tubes. Of tubal pregnancies, the ampulla is the most common site of implantation (80%), followed by the isthmus (11%), interstitia or cornua (5%) and fimbria (4%).[1] Apart from the fallopian tube, implantation can also occur in the cervix, ovaries and abdomen. An embryo implanted in places other than the uterus can cause great tissue damage in its effort to reach a sufficient supply of blood for its growth.

INCIDENCE

Over the last 40 years, the incidence has been increasing steadily and is at present estimated to be 1 in 40 pregnancies or approximately 25 cases per 1000 pregnancies.[1]

RISK FACTORS

There are a number of risk factors for ectopic pregnancies. However, in as many as one-third to one half, no risk factor can be identified.[2]

Cilia Damage and Tubal Occlusion

Hair-like cilia located on the internal surface of the fallopian tubes are responsible for carrying the fertilized egg to the uterus:
- Women with pelvic inflammatory disease (PID) or tuberculous salpingitis[3] resulting from build-up of scar tissue in the fallopian tubes.
- Tubal surgery for damaged tubes.
- Failure of tubal ligation especially when done by destructive methods such as by cautery carries a higher risk of ectopic pregnancy (70%) when compared to tubal clips (30%).
- Reversal of tubal sterilization also predisposes to ectopic pregnancy, the risk being lowest if the sterilization was done by less traumatic methods such as laparoscopic clipping.
- Smoking.[3]

Altered Tubal Motility

- *Hormonal contraception*: Both progesterone only contraceptive pills and progesterone intrauterine contraceptive devices (IUCDs).[3]
- Copper IUCDs.[3]

Idiopathic

In certain women fallopian cilia are genetically less in number, thus predisposing them to recurrent ectopic pregnancies.[4]

Previous History of Ectopic Pregnancy

Previous ectopic increases the risk of future ectopic pregnancy in the same tube to about 10% due to damage to the tubal mucosa and muscularis.

Infertility Treatment

Assisted reproductive techniques involving ovarian stimulation or surgical resurrection of pelvis.[3]

Other Risk Factors

- Advancing age[3]
- Vaginal douching
- Women exposed to diethylstilbestrol (DES) *in utero*
- Prior medical induction of abortion is associated with higher risk of ectopic pregnancy compared to surgical abortion.[3]

CLINICAL PRESENTATION

Clinical presentation of ectopic pregnancy occurs within 4 to 8 weeks of the last menstruation and historically presents with a triad of symptoms.[5]

The subtle symptoms and signs are:[5]
- Amenorrhea of varying duration
- Pain in lower abdomen
- Vaginal bleeding

The subtle presentation can be confusing, since symptoms overlap with early normal pregnancy or spontaneous abortion. Nine percent women have no symptoms and almost 35% have no clinical signs at the first prenatal visit.[1]

The severe symptoms and signs are:[5]
- Severe lower back, abdominal, or pelvic pain because of internal bleeding
- Shoulder pain caused by free blood tracking up and irritating the diaphragm
- Tenderness over lower abdomen without rebound tenderness
- Cervical movement tenderness with pelvic tenderness usually much worse on the affected side. An adnexal mass may or may not be palpated
- Hypotension, collapse and shock (20% cases).

A serum β-hCG level at this point will be able to rule out pelvic inflammatory disease (PID), ovarian torsion, ruptured corpus luteal cyst, appendicitis, other gastrointestinal disorders and urinary calculi. However, the most challenging aspect is to differentiate between an ectopic pregnancy, spontaneous abortion and an early ongoing intrauterine pregnancy (IUP).[1]

DIAGNOSIS

Tubal Ectopic Pregnancy

Transvaginal Ultrasound (TVS)

This has a sensitivity of 90%, specificity of 99.8%, with positive predictive value (PPV) and negative predictive values (NPV) of 93% and 99.8% respectively.[1]

If the location of the gestational sac and viability of the pregnancy at an ectopic location can be confirmed on TVS, it establishes the diagnosis right away. However, the hormonal environment in ectopic pregnancy can produce an intrauterine fluid collection that mimics a gestational sac, known as the pseudogestational sac. The spectrum of sonographic findings can be manifold and include the following:[1]

1. *Tubal ring*: An echogenic ring like structure found outside the uterus.
2. *Extrauterine mass*: A tender adnexal complex mass outside the uterus, with or without a small yolk sac present within it.[6]
3. *Ruptured ectopic pregnancy*: Echogenic free fluid or clotted blood in the cul-de-sac or in the intraperitoneal gutters, such as the Morrison pouch.
4. *Interstitial pregnancy*:
   a. *Timor-Tritsch criteria (1992)*: 88% specific but 40% sensitive[7]
      - Empty uterine cavity
      - Chorionic sac seen separately and >1 cm from the most lateral edge of the uterine cavity
      - Myometrial mantle is the amount of uterine myometrium surrounding the gestational sac and echogenic decidual layer. Myometrial mantle of less than 5 mm clinches the diagnosis of interstitial pregnancy.
   b. *The interstitial line*: It is as an echogenic line extending into the cornual region and abutting the gestational sac. Ackerman reports it to be 98% specific and 80% sensitive.[1]

Beta-Human Chorionic Gonadotropin (β-hCG)

If the ultrasound proves inconclusive, a β-hCG level is ascertained. It is difficult to distinguish between an ectopic pregnancy, spontaneous abortion and early ongoing intrauterine pregnancy using a single β-hCG measurement. However, the value of β-hCG measurement in ectopic pregnancy is based on two crucial concepts.[8-11]

1. The first relates β-hCG concentrations to ultrasound findings using the concept of a 'discriminatory zone'.[8] The 'discriminatory zone' was classified as the minimum β-hCG concentration at which an intrauterine gestational sac could be reliably identified on ultrasound and was labeled around 1500 mIU/mL, which equates to just over 5 weeks gestation. However, more recently the 'discriminatory zone' has been redefined to 1,500–2,500 IU/L, and it is now accepted widely that with hCG levels above this zone an intrauterine pregnancy, should be visible by transvaginal ultrasound. A more conservative discriminatory zone, that is, a higher hCG level, may be used to minimize the risk of terminating a viable pregnancy[10]
2. The second concept is the use of serial β-hCG measurements 2 days apart.[9] In 48 hours the normal increase in β-hCG should be at least 66%, whereas this would not be the case in ectopic pregnancy. However, 15% of normal intrauterine pregnancies show a suboptimal increase and a strict cut-off for the diagnosis of ectopic pregnancy would lead to unnecessary laparoscopies. Recently it has been suggested that the minimum rise, over 48 hours, to predict normal viable intrauterine pregnancy was 53%[10] or even as low as 35%.[11]

Transvaginal Ultrasound and β-hCG Levels Together

1. A high resolution, vaginal ultrasound scan showing no intrauterine pregnancy,

at a β-hCG level of around 1500 mIU/mL, is a presumptive evidence of an ectopic pregnancy.
2. If the diagnosis is still uncertain, it may be necessary to repeat β-hCG levels and an ultrasound 48 hours later. If the β-hCG falls on repeat examination, this suggests a biochemical pregnancy or tubal abortion. If β-hCG levels remain static or rise but do not double, then the diagnosis of ectopic pregnancy should be kept in mind. In such a situation, a three-dimensional ultrasound with Doppler may be able to confirm the diagnosis.

Serum Progesterone Levels

1. Using a cut-off of 20 ng/mL, women with an ectopic pregnancy, could be predicted with a sensitivity of 92%, a specificity of 84%, a PPV of 90% and NPV of 87% when compared with ongoing intrauterine pregnancy.[12]
2. However, there is no significant difference in serum progesterone concentrations in women with an ectopic pregnancy when compared with those who have a spontaneous abortion, as the levels are low in both these situations, reducing its predictive value.

Uterine Curettage: Uterine curettage and evaluation of uterine contents may be helpful in differentiating an abnormal intrauterine pregnancy from an ectopic pregnancy. Alternatively, if hCG levels continue to rise after curettage, the diagnosis of ectopic pregnancy is established.[12-37]

Other Biochemical Markers under Evaluation

A tubal ectopic pregnancy often evades diagnosis at an early stage. Also, the requirement of serial β-hCG measurements involves multiple clinic attendances, which are time consuming and costly, both psychologically to the patient and financially to health services.

Consequently, a serum biomarker of tubal implantation, which could accurately identify an ectopic pregnancy at first presentation, would be a major clinical advance.[12] A serum biomarker has been defined by the biomarkers definitions working Group as 'a characteristic that is objectively measured and evaluated as an indicator of normal biological processes, pathogenic processes, or pharmacologic responses to a therapeutic intervention'.

Apart from β-hCG and progesterone other markers which have been investigated are:
1. *Markers indicating abnormal trophoblast growth:* Activin A and Cell-free fetal DNA
2. *Peptides from the corpus luteum:* Renin and Inhibin A
3. *Markers of a growing pregnancy in the fallopian:* Creatine kinase (CK) and vascular endothelial growth factor (VEGF)
4. *Uterine markers of normal implantation:* Glycodelin.

Out of all these markers the following appear to be of some clinical significance:
- *Activin A:* It is secreted from the ovary and placenta, but in pregnancy, the main source of secretion is the trophoblast. Activin A levels in women with tubal ectopic pregnancy have been found to be markedly lower than those with ongoing intrauterine pregnancy and spontaneous miscarriage. More importantly, it performed better than a single measurement of β-hCG in diagnosing ectopic pregnancy. Tubal ectopic pregnancy could be identified with a sensitivity of 100% and specificity of 99.6%, if the cut-off was <0.37 ng/mL, however another study showed less encouraging results, with a much lower specificity and sensitivity.[12]
- *Inhibin A*: It is a major peptide product of the corpus luteum whose secretion is regulated by β-hCG. It is also produced by the trophoblast. Serum inhibin A and pro-α-C inhibins are lower in women with tubal ectopic pregnancies, than ongoing intrauterine pregnancies and fall more precipitously than β-hCG after treatment, due to their shorter half-life.

A recent prospective study has suggested that inhibin A may be a better marker to differentiate between a failing pregnancy and tubal ectopic pregnancy, than β-hCG.[12]
- *Vascular endothelial growth factor (VEGF):* Implantation in the unfavorable fallopian tube is associated with increased tissue hypoxia and hence serum VEGF would be increased in tubal pregnancy. Use of an cut-off of 700 pg/mL, VEGF was able to distinguish a normal intrauterine pregnancy from a tubal pregnancy with a PPV of 70% and an abnormal intrauterine pregnancy from a tubal ectopic pregnancy with a PPV of 88%.[12]
- Recent attention has focused on metalloprotease 12 (ADAM 12) and fibronectin as potentially promising candidate markers[38,39]
  - *Triple marker analysis:* The combination of three independent markers in the formula VEGF/(PAPP-A × P) was found to be largely superior to the measure of any single marker. The "triple marker analysis" VEGF/(PAPP-A × P) allows a clear discrimination between normal IUP and EP.[13]

Laparoscopy

Laparoscopy can also be performed to visually confirm an ectopic pregnancy. Often if a tubal abortion has occurred, or a tubal rupture has occurred, it is difficult to find the products of conception. A laparoscopy in very early ectopic pregnancy may show a normal looking fallopian tube.

Ovarian Ectopic Pregnancy

Spiegelberg Criteria[14]

- The gestational sac is located in the region of the ovary
- The ectopic pregnancy is attached to the uterus by the ovarian ligament
- The tube on the involved side is intact.
- Ovarian tissue proven in the wall of the gestational sac histologically.

Criteria, Other than Spiegelberg, when Present Together Confirm Ovarian Pregnancy[15]

- β-hCG level ≥1000 mIU/mL and empty uterine cavity at TVS
- Presence of an atypical cyst on the ovary with normal tubes
- Surgical exploration with bleeding seen around the ovary
- Absence of serum β-hCG after treatment of the ovarian mass.

Doppler ultrasonography offers little additional diagnostic value due to the high vascularity of the ovary. It may be useful to perform intraoperative ultrasound to distinguish an ovarian pregnancy from an ovarian cyst.

Cervical Ectopic Pregnancy

Paalman and McElin Criteria (1959)

- Uterine bleeding without pain
- Hourglass uterus with a soft enlarged cervix on ultrasound
- Products of conception entirely confined within and firmly attached to the cervix
- A closed internal cervical os
- A partially open external cervical os.

The sliding sac sign and Doppler flows are helpful in distinguishing abortions in progress from those with vascular implantation in the cervix.

Abdominal Pregnancy

Abdominal pregnancy presents with abdominal pain, nausea, vomiting, painful fetal movements, and less frequently vaginal bleeding.
- *Studdiford criteria (1942)*: (1) Normal bilateral fallopian tubes and ovaries, (2) absence of uteroperitoneal fistula, and (3) presence of a pregnancy related to the peritoneal surface exclusively.[17]
- The classic ultrasound finding is the absence of myometrial tissue between the bladder and pregnancy.

- Magnetic resonance imaging (MRI) may aid ultrasound findings.

Cesarean Scar Ectopic

- Ultrasound criteria for diagnosis and prediction of rupture by Vial et al. (1) trophoblast between bladder and anterior uterine wall, (2) no fetal parts in the uterine cavity, and (3) discontinuity of the anterior uterine wall in the sagittal plane. Ultrasound appearance of an anterior bulging mass outside the contour of the uterus may be indicative.[17]
- Three-dimensional Doppler ultrasound and MRI.
- Hysteroscopy.

Heterotopic Pregnancy

This is a combined IUP and ectopic pregnancy. It may occur in approximately 1 in 30,000 pregnancies. Often the intrauterine pregnancy is discovered later than the ectopic, mainly because of the painful or emergency nature of ectopic pregnancies. Ultrasound helps in early detection. The survival rate of the uterine fetus of a heterotopic pregnancy is around 70%.

TREATMENT

Expectant Management

Selection of Patients as per RCOG Guidelines[18]

1. Clinically stable women with minimal symptoms and a pregnancy of unknown location.
2. Clinically stable asymptomatic women with an ultrasound diagnosis of ectopic pregnancy.
   - Initial β-hCG levels are below 1000 mIU/mL.
   - β-hCG levels are (continually) falling.
   - Less than 100 mL fluid in the pouch of Douglas.

Favorable Prognostic Indicators for Expectant Management[19]

- No evidence of blood in the pouch of Douglas
- Tubal mass < 4–5 cm
- Absence of recognizable fetal parts and heart-beat.

Women managed expectantly should be followed twice weekly with serial β-hCG measurements and weekly by transvaginal examinations to ensure a rapidly decreasing β-hCG level (ideally less than 50% of its initial level) and a reduction in the size of adnexal mass, respectively by seven days. Thereafter weekly β-hCG levels are advised until they are less than 20 mIU/mL. In addition, women selected for expectant management should be counseled about the importance of compliance with follow-up and should be within easy access to the hospital.[18]

Nonsurgical Management

Local Therapy

Early detection of unruptured ectopic pregnancies allows a more conservative course of management. Sonographically guided minimally invasive treatment protocols for ectopic pregnancy may be a safe and effective alternative to surgical and systemic medical therapy. These protocols in addition to resolving the ectopic pregnancy also help in preserving the tube for subsequent pregnancies.

Selection criteria include intact tubal pregnancy not exceeding 4 cm in diameter, rising or plateauing β-hCG levels but less than 3000 mIU/mL, and no evidence of intra-abdominal bleeding.[20]

Although a multitude of agents (sodium chloride, actinomycin D, etoposide, mifepristone and danazol) have been proposed, the most widely used ones are as follows:

- *Methotrexate:* A single dose of 10–25 mg of methotrexate can be injected into the gestational sac under sonographic control. Few patients may require a second administration 4 days after the first one. β-hCG levels of less than 10 mIU/mL reach within 42 days after treatment, with complete resolution.[21] Apart from methotrexate, the following agents have been tried in varying doses with variable results.
- *Prostaglandin F2α* (10 mg).[22]
- *Potassium chloride (KCL)* (2 mL of 2 mEq).[23]
- *Hyperosmolar glucose* (3 mL of 50% solution).[20]

The latter two agents are mostly used intracardiac in cases of ectopic pregnancies with fetal cardiac activity.

The main potential advantages are greater anti-trophoblastic effect, shorter treatment period, and reduced dosage, absence of side effects and preservation of tubal patency.[21] The overall success rate is 66.3–82.1%. The disadvantages are immediate severe hemorrhage requiring surgery, repeat doses, persistent trophoblast and infection.[24]

Therefore, local delivery of chemotherapeutic agents may be used for pregnancies in which a laparoscopic approach is not ideal and systemic therapy either has failed or is not desired. These therapies remain experimental at present since their efficacy and advantages over standard systemic methotrexate protocols have not been established.[1]

Systemic Therapy

Methotrexate, a folic acid antagonist, has remained the most effective and popular drug used in medical therapy for an ectopic pregnancy since the late 1980s and has now become widely accepted as primary treatment for ectopic pregnancy. Folic acid normally is reduced to tetrahydrofolate by the enzyme dihydrofolate reductase (DHFR), a step in the synthesis of DNA and RNA precursors. Methotrexate inhibits DHFR, causing depletion of cofactors required for DNA and RNA synthesis and hence cell multiplication. Folinic acid (leucovorin) is an antagonist to methotrexate (MTX) that can help reduce otherwise prohibitive side effects, particularly when higher doses of MTX are used.[40–49]

Methotrexate has also been used orally in a total dose of 60 mg/m² (in 2 doses 2 hours apart). But treatment success rates are lower with oral use than with injections.[25] If medical therapy is offered, women should be given clear information (preferably written) about the possible need for further treatment and adverse effects during and following treatment.[18]

Principles[26]

1. Selection of patients.
2. Choosing protocol for methotrexate and surveillance:
   - Multi-dose regimen
   - Single-dose regimen
   - Two-dose regimen
3. Patient counseling and education concerning side effects of methotrexate.

Selection of Patients

Recent criteria for methotrexate therapy for ectopic pregnancy as per RCOG guidelines:[18]
1. Hemodynamically stable
2. Reliable, compliant patient who will return for follow-up
3. β-hCG levels below 3000 mIU/mL
4. Minimal symptoms.
5. Tubal mass less than 4–5 cm.

The presence of cardiac activity is associated with reduced chance of success following medical therapy and should be considered a contraindication to medical therapy.[18]

Mechanism of action: Methotrexate, a folic acid antagonist, inhibits DNA synthesis in actively dividing cells, including trophoblasts.[1]

Laboratory investigations prior to starting methotrexate therapy:
1. Pretreatment β-hCG levels and transvaginal ultrasound.
2. Complete blood counts, kidney and liver function tests.
3. Blood grouping and cross-matching (all Rh-negative patients to be given 50 micrograms of Rh immunoglobulin, intramuscularly).

Protocols and Surveillance

Certain key points to be kept in mind by the clinician while using systemic methotrexate therapy (Table 25.1):
- The day 4 β-hCG may be higher than the pretreatment level. This is due to continued β-hCG production by syncytiotrophoblast despite cessation of production by cytotrophoblast. Therefore, the day 4 β-hCG level is the baseline level against which subsequent levels are measured.
- Differentiating the so-called 'separation pain' which occurs within 24–48 hours after the injection (due to tubal abortion), from pain due to tubal rupture can be difficult and a proportion of women will need to be admitted for observation and assessment by transvaginal ultrasound following methotrexate therapy.[18]
- The patients should be advised not to take folic acid, refrain from alcohol consumption and intercourse, until complete resolution of the ectopic pregnancy occurs.
- They should also be advised to use reliable contraception for three months after methotrexate has been given because of a possible teratogenic risk.

Patient Counseling and Education Concerning Side Effects of Methotrexate

Adverse effects associated with methotrexate treatment:

- Methotrexate affects all rapidly dividing tissues within the body including bone marrow, gastrointestinal mucosa and the respiratory epithelium, therefore it should not be given to women with blood dyscrasias, active gastrointestinal and respiratory disease. Methotrexate is directly toxic to the hepatocytes and is cleared from the body by renal excretion; therefore, it should not be used in women with liver or kidney disease.[26]
- Methotrexate morbidity usually is dose and treatment duration dependent. Gastrointestinal side effects, such as nausea, vomiting, and stomatitis, are the most common. Alopecia is a rare side effect.[26]

Contraindications

Absolute contraindications to methotrexate therapy:[26]
- Breastfeeding
- Overt or laboratory evidence of immunodeficiency
- Alcoholism, alcoholic liver disease, or other chronic liver disease
- Pre-existing blood dyscrasias, such as bone marrow hypoplasia, leukopenia, thrombocytopenia, or significant anemia
- Known sensitivity to methotrexate
- Active pulmonary disease
- Peptic ulcer disease
- Hepatic, renal, or hematologic dysfunction.

Relative contraindications to methotrexate therapy:[26]
- Gestational sac larger than 3.5 cm
- Embryonic cardiac motion.

Recent Recommendations and Conclusions by ACOG

The following conclusion is based on good and consistent evidence (Level A):

Comparing systemic methotrexate with tube-sparing laparoscopic surgery,

Table 25.1: Protocols of systemic methotrexate therapy and surveillance.

Protocols	Surveillance
Multiple-dose methotrexate therapy[27] **Goldstein 1976** Methotrexate, 1 mg/kg intramuscularly, days 1, 3, 5, 7 Leucovorin, 0.1 mg/kg intramuscularly, days 2, 4, 6, 8 (24 hours later) **Bagshawe 1989** Methotrexate, 50 mg intramuscularly, days 1, 3, 5, 7 Leucovorin, 6 mg intramuscularly, days 2, 4, 6, 8 (30 hours later)	Continue alternate-day injections until β-hCG levels decline by 15% in 48 hours or four doses of methotrexate given.[28,29] Then weekly β-hCG measurements until undetectable If the weekly levels plateau or increase, surgical therapy is indicated
Single-dose methotrexate therapy Methotrexate (50 mg/m²) intramuscularly The Mosteller formula:[30] Body surface area (BSA) in m² = square root [(height in cm × weight in kg)/3600]	Measure β-hCG levels on day 4 and 7 If difference is more than or equal to 15%, repeat weekly until undetectable If difference is less than 15%, repeat methotrexate dose and begin new day 1 If fetal cardiac activity present on day 7, repeat methotrexate, begin new day 1 Surgical treatment if β-hCG levels not decreasing or fetal cardiac activity persists after three doses of methotrexate
"Two dose" methotrexate regimen Methotrexate (50 mg/m²) intramuscularly, days 0 and 4	Measure β-hCG levels on day 7 If β-hCG levels decline by more than 15%, repeat weekly until undetectable If β-hCG levels do not decline by 15% on day 7, additional doses of methotrexate are given on day 7 and/or day 11 If the weekly levels plateau or increase, surgical therapy is indicated
Systemic methotrexate in combination with mifepristone Methotrexate (50 mg/m²) intramuscularly and 600 mg mifepristone (antiprogesterone)[31]	Same as single-dose methotrexate therapy

randomized trials have shown no difference in overall tube preservation, tubal patency, incidence of repeat ectopic pregnancy, or in occurrence of future pregnancies.

The following recommendations and conclusions are based on limited or inconsistent evidence (Level B):

- An increase in β-hCG level of less than 53% in 48 hours confirms an abnormal pregnancy
- Failure of the β-hCG level to decrease by at least 15% from day 4 to day 7 after methotrexate administration is considered treatment failure requiring therapy with either

additional methotrexate administration or surgical intervention
- Post-treatment β-hCG levels should be monitored until a nonpregnancy level is reached.

The following conclusion is based primarily on consensus and expert opinion (Level C):
- If the initial β-hCG level is less than 200 mIU/mL, 88% of patients experience spontaneous resolution.

Predictors of Success of Methotrexate Therapy (Table 25.2)

- Initial β-hCG level is the best predictor for success of medical therapy. Medical therapy using methotrexate is cost-effective only if β-hCG levels are less than 3000 mIU/mL[18]
- Fetal cardiac activity is associated most often with treatment failure
- Tubal diameter and measure of fetal size is unrelated to outcome
- Yolk sac present in the gestational sac may be associated with treatment failure.[11]

Surgical Management

Surgical management should be reserved for:
- Patients who refuse or have contraindications to medical treatment
- Medical treatment failure
- Hemodynamically unstable patients.[1]

Surgical therapy may be either open laparotomy or laparoscopy. Compared with laparotomy, laparoscopic treatment of ectopic pregnancy is associated with lower cost, shorter hospital stay, less operative time, less blood loss, less analgesic requirement and faster recovery. Patients randomly assigned to laparoscopy also have fewer adhesions than patients treated with laparotomy (19% vs 64%). Risk factors for converting laparoscopy to laparotomy should be considered and include multiple prior surgeries, pelvic adhesions, skill

Table 25.2: Benefits and success rates of various methotrexate protocols.

Protocols	Selection criteria	Advantages and disadvantages	Success rates
Multiple-dose methotrexate therapy	β-hCG < 3000 mIU/mL	Better efficacy Forty percent of women may have side effects Women who have side effects are more likely to have successful treatment[29]	93%[29]
Single-dose methotrexate therapy	β-hCG < 1500 mIU/mL	As effective as multidose methotrexate therapy[32] The incidence of complications similar to multidose therapy[33] Less toxicity Leucovorin rescue not required Approximately 15–20% of women will require a second dose. Less than 1% of patients will need more than two doses[28]	94–96%[1]
"Two dose" methotrexate regimen	β-hCG < 3000 mIU/mL	This protocol may optimize the balance between convenience and efficacy	87%[34]

of the surgeon, surgical staff, availability of the equipment and condition of the patient.[1]

Preoperative Details and Decision-making

Obtain large-bore venous access and start fluid resuscitation; make sure blood is available. Do not delay the operation. The patient may have an active bleeding site, which must be taken care of immediately. Placement of a Foley's catheter prior to starting the operation is optional.[1]

Regardless of the route of approach, indications for salpingectomy are:
- Ruptured ectopic pregnancy or hemorrhage continues after salpingostomy
- Future fertility is not desired or ectopic has resulted from sterilization failure or sterilization is requested
- Ectopic in a previously reconstructed tube or in a blind tube with previous partial salpingectomy
- Chronic tubal pregnancy.

In the absence of any of the above indications for salpingectomy, salpingotomy may be performed. If the ectopic pregnancy is at the fimbria, then fimbrial evacuation is feasible. Partial salpingectomy of the ectopic segment only, preserving the distal end, may be indicated if the pregnancy is in the mid portion of the tube, none of the indications for salpingectomy are present, and the patient may be a candidate for later tubal reanastomosis.[1]

Surgical Technique

Salpingostomy

Infiltrate the mesosalpinx with vasopressin (20 IU in 50 mL of isotonic sodium chloride solution). Avoid intravascular injection because it causes hypertension and is contraindicated in patients with ischemic heart disease. With the knife or needle electrode, make a 1-2 cm incision on the antimesenteric side of the tube. Fluid from the aqua-dissector, under pressure helps to dissect and dislodge the ectopic pregnancy. If any trophoblastic tissue remains, the use of vasopressin may lead to anoxia of the trophoblasts, preventing postoperative growth. Applying pressure with grasping forceps for 5 minutes may control bleeding. Arterial bleeding may require pinpoint bipolar desiccation. Diffuse venous bleeding is best controlled with monopolar current. Uncontrollable bleeding may require suturing of the mesosalpingeal vessels.[1]

Salpingotomy

Seldom performed today, salpingotomy is essentially the same procedure as salpingostomy except that the incision on the tube is closed with 7-0 Vicryl or similar suture. There is no difference in prognosis with or without suturing. Both the terminologies of salpingostomy and salpingotomy are often used interchangeably in literature.[1]

Salpingectomy

Desiccate the tube between the uterus and the ectopic pregnancy using bipolar cautery. Compress and desiccate the tubo-ovarian artery, while preserving the utero-ovarian artery and ligament. Cut along the desiccated path, closer to the ectopic, leaving a pedicle for hemostasis. Repeat until the tube is free and can be removed.[1]

Segmental Resection with or without Reanastomosis

Perform bipolar desiccation across the tube on both sides of the isthmic unruptured ectopic pregnancy. Divide the tube at the sites of desiccation. The mesosalpinx under the ectopic pregnancy can then be either desiccated or ligated with an endo loop. Reanastomosis can be done at the same sitting or later on.[1]

Fimbrial Evacuation Technique

Grasp the fimbria and rotate it to allow insertion of the aquadissector. Fluid under pressure dissects and dislodges the ectopic pregnancy.[1]

Efficacy of Surgery

Tube-sparing salpingostomy is preferred to salpingectomy, as the former is less invasive and conserves the tube but has comparable rates of subsequent fertility and ectopic pregnancy. However, 8% of patients have persistent ectopic pregnancy after salpingostomy. Follow-up is required until β-hCG is undetectable. Regardless of the type of surgery, contralateral tubal abnormalities predispose the patient to recurrent ectopic pregnancy. In a retrospective study of 276 women with ectopic pregnancy, the cumulative rates of spontaneous intrauterine pregnancy over 7 years were 89% after conservative surgery and 66% after radical surgery. There was no significant difference in the risk of repeat ectopic pregnancy (17% after conservative surgery and 16% after radical surgery). Salpingectomy may be necessary for women with uncontrolled bleeding, recurrent ectopic pregnancy in the same tube, a severely damaged tube or a tubal gestational sac greater than 5 cm in diameter.[35]

Postoperative Care

Most patients are able to leave the hospital as soon as they have left the recovery room. In patients who were in shock or had to receive blood transfusions, the postoperative observation should be longer and should include observation that the kidneys are functioning normally and the patient has regained normal hemodynamics.[1]

Follow-up

All patients who have not had the entire ectopic pregnancy removed by salpingectomy need to have their weekly β-hCG levels observed until these levels return to nonpregnant values. If, during this period the β-hCG levels plateaus or rises, methotrexate treatment may be required. Patients should all be on some form of non-hormonal effective contraception till their β-hCG levels reach nonpregnant levels.[1]

Complications

1. *Persistent trophoblast*: Following salpingostomy β-hCG levels decline quickly and are at about 10% of preoperative values by day 12. Persistent ectopic pregnancy is the result of incomplete removal of trophoblast during salpingostomy. It occurs in 5–20% cases. A prophylactic single shot methotrexate, given intramuscularly 24 hours postoperatively, significantly reduces **persistent trophoblast** after laparoscopic **salpingostomy**. If the postoperative day 1 β-hCG value is less than 50% of the preoperative value then the risk of persistent ectopic is low. According to Seifer (1997), factors that increase the risk of persistent ectopic are as follows:[36]
   - Small pregnancies less than 2 cm
   - Early therapy before 42 menstrual days
   - β-hCG levels exceeding 3000 mIU/mL
   - Implantation medial to the salpingostomy site.
2. Hemorrhage and hypovolemic shock
3. Infection
4. Loss of reproductive organs/function following surgery
5. Infertility
6. Urinary and/or intestinal fistulas following complicated surgery
7. Disseminated intravascular coagulation.

CURRENT EVIDENCE ON SURGERY, SYSTEMIC METHOTREXATE AND EXPECTANT MANAGEMENT IN THE TREATMENT OF TUBAL ECTOPIC PREGNANCY

Laparoscopic **salpingostomy** is less successful due to a higher rate of **persistent trophoblast**. A prophylactic single shot methotrexate, given intramuscularly immediately postoperatively, significantly reduced **persistent trophoblast** after laparoscopic **salpingotomy**. With systemic multiple dose methotrexate the likelihood of treatment success was higher than with laparoscopic **salpingostomy**, but the difference was not significant. Systemic multiple dose methotrexate was only cost-effective if initial β-hCG concentrations were <3000 mIU/mL. If β-hCG concentrations were <1500 mIU/mL, then the single-dose methotrexate regimen, if necessary with additional injections, was also cost-effective.[31]

ECTOPIC PREGNANCIES IN UNUSUAL LOCATIONS

Interstitial (Cornual) Pregnancy

The interstitial segment of the fallopian tube is the segment that lies within the muscular wall of the uterus. Interstitial pregnancy accounts for up to 1-3% of all ectopic pregnancies. The term cornual pregnancy is used interchangeably in the United States as a synonym for interstitial pregnancies. As the pregnancy grows in the area of the fallopian tube that enters the uterus, surrounding myometrial tissue allows for further development of the pregnancy into the second trimester. Rupture of such an advanced gestation may result in catastrophic hemorrhage, with a mortality rate of up to 2%.[17]

Treatment: Ruptured interstitial pregnancy may present with hypovolemic shock necessitating immediate laparotomy. In the stable patient with early detection, conservative measures may be attempted, including laparoscopy or medical management. Close monitoring (and even hospital admission) should be considered because rupture is possible even after treatment has begun. The overall success rate is 83% for all protocols.[17]

1. *Surgical*:
   - Cornual resection or hysterectomy by laparotomy or laparoscopy
   - Resection may be assisted by direct injection of vasopressin
   - Hysteroscopic resection of interstitial pregnancies under laparoscopic visualization and/or ultrasound guidance.
2. *Systemic methotrexate*: For interstitial pregnancies with β-hCG levels <1000 mIU/mL
   - There is no consensus on the dose or number of methotrexate injections
   - Interstitial pregnancies are less susceptible to methotrexate because of their increased blood supply, although size of the gestation may also be a factor.
3. Local intra-amniotic methotrexate or etoposide
4. Selective uterine artery embolization.

Future fertility is possible for interstitial pregnancy treated conservatively, although there is a concern for uterine rupture secondary to the weakened myometrial wall. This concern is both for interstitial pregnancies treated surgically and with chemotherapeutic measures.[17]

Cervical Ectopic Pregnancy

Cervical ectopic pregnancy is an ectopic pregnancy that has implanted in the cervix. It has an estimated incidence of one in 2500 to one in 18,000. Cervical pregnancy can cause severe hemorrhage, if it starts to separate from the cervix. This is because of the very few muscle fibers in the cervix leading to inadequate constriction of the hypertrophied blood vessels of the pregnancy.

Predisposing factors are previous instrumentation of the endocervical canal, anatomic anomalies (myomas, synechiae), intrauterine device use and IVF.[17]

Treatment

Cervical pregnancies before 12 weeks, without fetal cardiac activity and with β-hCG levels less than 10,000 mIU/mL seem more amenable to conservative treatment.[17]

- Systemic methotrexate in combination with cervical evacuation and the use of hemostatic techniques (vasopressin, balloon tamponade, uterine artery ligation or embolization, cerclage, cervical stay sutures)
- Hysteroscopy may be used in the visualization of cervical pregnancy prior to resection
- Local injections of various chemotherapeutic agents including methotrexate, etoposide, actinomycin D, and cyclophosphamide
- Local prostaglandins are believed to increase uterine contractions, promote vasoconstriction, and therefore, reduce hemorrhage
- Intra-amniotic injections of methotrexate, hyperosmolar glucose, and KCL have been used as adjunctive treatments when the pregnancy has fetal cardiac activity. Nevertheless, there is no clear recommendation about the optimal dosage or route of administration
- Hysterectomy for those who do not desire fertility.

Because patients who receive methotrexate occasionally develop severe hemorrhage, observe these patients closely for 1–2 weeks after therapy. Although the potential complications of cervical pregnancy primarily involve hemorrhage, the impact on future fertility is largely unknown due to its rare occurrence.[17]

Ovarian Pregnancy

Ovarian pregnancy occurs from one in 2100 to one in 60,000 pregnancies. It is a result of secondary implantation of the embryo or failure of follicular extrusion.

Ovarian pregnancies can be classified as extrafollicular and the less common intrafollicular type. Extrafollicular pregnancies can be classified as interstitial, cortical, superficial, and juxtafollicular.[17]

Treatment

- Laparoscopic oophorectomy or wedge resection of the ovary
- Systemic methotrexate may be an option if there is persistent trophoblastic tissue after laparoscopy
- If future fertility is desired, wedge resection may be considered. Oophorectomy should be reserved for cases of advanced gestation.

Abdominal Pregnancy

Abdominal pregnancy may account for up to 1.4% of ectopic pregnancies. The site of implantation and availability of vascular supply are believed to be factors that may influence the possibility of fetal survival. Abdominal pregnancies are believed to be a result of intra-abdominal fertilization of sperm and ovum or secondary implantation from an aborted tubal pregnancy.[17]

Sites of implantations: Omentum, liver, spleen, large vessels, pelvic cul-de-sac, broad ligament, bowel, and pelvic sidewall.[17]

Treatment

- The optimal treatment of abdominal pregnancy is unknown.
- When possible, ligation of placental blood supply and removal should be attempted to reduce maternal complications.
- Alternatively, the umbilical cord may be ligated and expectant management, arterial embolization, or methotrexate used to facilitate involution.
- However, leaving the placenta *in situ* may lead to further complications such as infection, secondary hemorrhage, or intestinal obstruction.
- Laparoscopy may be used in the treatment of some early abdominal pregnancies.

Risks: These pregnancies can go undetected until an advanced gestational age and often result in severe hemorrhage. Rates of maternal mortality have been reported as high as 20%. Advanced abdominal pregnancy carries a risk of hemorrhage, disseminated intravascular coagulation, bowel obstruction, and fistulae. Frequently, these pregnancies are encountered with a viable fetus, which complicates their management.[17]

Cesarean Scar Ectopic

Intramural pregnancies with implantation in a previous cesarean scar or other uterine scars are probably the rarest of ectopic pregnancies.[17]

Risk factors:
- Previous cesarean section
- Myomectomy
- Adenomyosis
- Previous dilation and curettage
- Manual removal of the placenta.

Theories by Vial et al.[17]
- Partially implantation in the uterine cavity proceeding to term
- Deep implantation in the scar predisposing to early rupture in the first trimester
- These pregnancies enter the cesarean scar via microscopic fistulae.

The optimal treatment of cesarean section scar ectopic pregnancies is unknown.
- Presentation of the patient often dictates the mode of treatment, given that many patients present with hemoperitoneum and require hysterectomy
- Dilation and curettage followed by tamponade with a Foley balloon
- Local injections with KCl or methotrexate have been reported
- Systemic methotrexate followed by dilation and evacuation with success
- Uterine artery embolization to reduce hemorrhage has also been described as adjunctive therapy.

There are also reports of successful term pregnancy after cesarean section scar pregnancy. Nevertheless, these patients should be counseled about the weakened nature of their cesarean section scar and should undergo a repeat cesarean section.

Heterotopic Pregnancy

In heterotopic pregnancies with cardiac activity at the ectopic site, intracardiac injection of agents such as, KCl or hyperosmolar glucose are desirable which have no adverse effect on an ongoing intrauterine pregnancy. In pregnancies with no fetal cardiac activity at the ectopic site, expectant management can be undertaken in carefully selected cases, with rigid surveillance which involves frequent ultrasounds and monitoring of clinical symptoms. In the rest surgical intervention is mandatory. Beta hCG evaluation is of no use in these cases as viable intrauterine pregnancy continues to secrete adequate amounts of this hormone.

Pregnancy of Unknown Origin[38-51]

It is a term used to classify a pregnancy until the final clinical location and outcome is known. Such woman needs to be followed-up to determine the final clinical outcome, which may be an ongoing viable IUP, a failed pregnancy, an organ specific EP or rarely a persisting PUL.

New categorization system for initial ultrasound findings for diagnosing PUL was suggested by Barnhart et al. in their consensus paper published in 2011:
  (i) *Definite ectopic pregnancy (EP)*: Extrauterine gestational sac with yolk sac and/or embryo (with or without cardiac activity.
 (ii) *Pregnanncy of unknown location (PUL)- probable EP*: Inhomogeneous adnexal mass or extrauterine sac-like structure.
(iii) *'True' PUL*: No signs of either an intrauterine or extrauterine pregnancy on TVS.

(iv) *PUL-probable IUP*: Intrauterine gestational sac-like structure.
(v) *Definite IUP*: Intrauterine gestational sac with yolk sac and/or embryo (with or without cardiac activity).

A treated persistent PUL is defined as one managed medically with methotrexate without confirmation of the location of the pregnancy by ultrasound, laparoscopy or uterine evacuation. However, treatment should only be considered in cases when a potentially viable IUP has been definitively excluded.[50,51]

CHANCE OF FUTURE PREGNANCY

The chances of future pregnancy depend on the site of ectopic gestation and the status of the adnexa left behind. Recurrent ectopic pregnancy may occur in about 10% of the cases and does not depend on whether the affected tube was conserved or removed. Successful methotrexate therapy is associated with the highest reported future pregnancy rates. Patients, who have had their adnexa removed during surgery, may often have to resort to *in vitro* fertilization (IVF) in order to achieve a successful pregnancy. In cases where hysterectomy has been performed, surrogacy may be the only option available. The use of IVF however does not preclude further ectopic pregnancies, but the likelihood is significantly reduced (1 in 1000 pregnancies).[1]

REFERENCES

1. Allahyar Jazayeri MD, Herbert S Coussons. Surgical Management of Ectopic Pregnancy; online article; Updated: Feb 17, 2010.
2. Farquhar CM. Ectopic pregnancy. Lancet. 2005;366:583.
3. Bouyer J, Coste J, Shojaei T, et al. Risk factors for ectopic pregnancy: a comprehensive analysis based on a large case-control, population-based study in France. Am J Epidemiol. 2003;157(3):185-94.
4. Lyons RA, Saridogan E, Djahanbakhch O. The reproductive significance of human Fallopian tube cilia. Hum Reprod Update. 2006;12(4):363-72.
5. Weckstein LN, Boucher AR, Tucker H, et al. Accurate diagnosis of early ectopic pregnancy. Obstet Gynecol. 1985;65:393-97.
6. Bixby S, Tello R, Kuligowska E. Presence of a yolk sac on transvaginal sonography is the most reliable predictor of single-dose methotrexate treatment failure in ectopic pregnancy. J Ultrasound Med. 2005;24(5):591-8.
7. Susie Lau, Togas Tulandi. Conservative medical and surgical management of interstitial ectopic pregnancy. Fertil Steril. 1999;72(2):207-15.
8. Kadar N, DeVore G, Romero R. Discriminatory hCG zone: its use in the sonographic evaluation of ectopic pregnancy. Obstet Gynecol. 1981a;58:156-61.
9. Kadar N, Caldwell BV, Romero R. A method of screening for ectopic pregnancy and its indications. Obstet Gynecol. 1981b;58:162-66.
10. Barnhart KT, Sammel MD, Rinaudo PF, et al. Symptomatic patients with an early viable intrauterine pregnancy: hCG curves redefined. Obstet Gynecol. 2004;104:50-5.
11. Seeber BE, Sammel MD, Guo W, et al. Application of redefined human chorionic gonadotropin curves for the diagnosis of women at risk for ectopic pregnancy. Fertil Steril. 2006;86: 454-9.
12. Cartwright J, Duncan WC, Critchley H, et al. Serum biomarkers of tubal ectopic pregnancy: current candidates and future possibilities. Horne Reprod. 2009;138:9-22.
13. Mueller MD, Raio L, Spoerri S, et al. Novel placental and nonplacental serum markers in ectopic versus normal intrauterine pregnancy. Fertil Steril. 2004;81(4):1106-11.
14. Spiegelberg's criteria; Who Named It? Online article.
15. Sergent F, Mauger-Tinlot F, Gravier A. Ovarian pregnancies: revaluation of diagnostic criteria. J Gynecol Obstet Biol Reprod (Paris). 2002;31(8):741-6.

16. Gosakan R, Arutchelvam S, Gergis HH, et al. Medical management of a cervical ectopic pregnancy. J Obstet Gynacol. 2005;25(1):82-83.
17. Molinaro A, Barnhart KT. Ectopic pregnancies in unusual locations. Semin Reprod Med. 2007;25(2):123-30.
18. Royal College of Obstetricians and Gynaecologists (RCOG). The management of tubal pregnancy. London (UK): 2004, p. 10 (Guideline; no. 21).
19. Schreiner A, Singh U, MacDermott R, et al. Guidelines for the Management of Ectopic Pregnancy 2007. Ref: MA052 (v2).
20. Sadan O, Ginath S, Debby A, et al. Methotrexate versus hyperosmolar glucose in the treatment of extrauterine pregnancy. Arch Gynecol Obstet. 2001;265:82-84.
21. Mesogitis SA, Daskalakis GJ, Antsaklis AJ, et al. Local application of methotrexate for ectopic pregnancy with a percutaneous puncturing technique. Gynecol Obstet Invest. 1998;45:154-58.
22. Spitzer D, Steiner H, Graf A, et al. Conservative treatment of cervical pregnancy by curettage and local prostaglandin injection. Hum Reprod. 1997;12:860-6.
23. Salomon LJ, Fernandez1 H, Chauveaud A, et al. Successful management of a heterotopic caesarean scar pregnancy: potassium chloride injection with preservation of the intrauterine gestation: Case report. Hum Reprod. 2003;18(1):189-91.
24. Lauren Ferrara, Victoria Belogolovkin, Manisha Gandhi, et al. Successful management of a consecutive cervical pregnancy by sonographically guided transvaginal local injection. J Ultrasound Med. 2007;26:959-65.
25. Lipscomb GH, Meyer NL, Flynn DE, et al. Oral methotrexate for treatment at ectopic pregnancy. Am J Obstet Gynecol. 2002;186(6):1192-5.
26. American College of Obstetricians and Gynecologists (ACOG). Medical management of ectopic pregnancy. Washington (DC); 2008. 7 (ACOG practice bulletin; no. 94).
27. Hajenius PJ, Mol F, Mol BWJ, et al. Interventions for tubal ectopic pregnancy (Revision). The Cochrane Library, 2007; Issue 4.
28. Tulandi T. Methotrexate treatment of tubal and interstitial ectopic pregnancy. Last Literature Review Version. 2010;1:18.
29. Barnhart KT, Gosman G, Ashby R, et al. The medical management of ectopic pregnancy: a meta-analysis comparing "single-dose" and "multidose" regimens. Obstet Gynecol. 2003;101(4):778-84.
30. Mosteller RD. Simplified calculation of body surface area. N Engl J Med. 1987;22; 317(17):1098 (letter).
31. Mol F, Mol BW, Ankum WM, et al. Current evidence on surgery, systemic methotrexate and expectant management in the treatment of tubal ectopic pregnancy: a systematic review and meta-analysis. Hum Reprod. 2008;14(4):309-19.
32. Lipscomb GH, Givens VM, Meyer NL, et al. Comparison of multidose and single-dose methotrexate protocols for the treatment of ectopic pregnancy. Am J Obstet Gynecol. 2005;192(6):1844-7.
33. Alleyassin A, Khademi A, Aghahosseini M, et al. Comparison of success rates in the medical management of ectopic pregnancy with single-dose and multiple-dose administration of methotrexate: a prospective, randomized clinical trial. Fertil Steril. 2006;85(6):1661-6. Epub 2006 May 2.
34. Barnhart K, Hummel AC, Sammel MD, et al. Use of "2-dose" regimen of methotrexate to treat ectopic pregnancy. Fertil Steril. 2007; 87(2):250-6. Epub 2006 Nov 13.
35. Bangsgaard N, Lund CO, Ottesen B, et al. Improved fertility following conservative surgical treatment of ectopic pregnancy. BJOG. 2003;110:765-70.
36. David B Seifer. Persistent ectopic pregnancy: an argument for heightened vigilance and patient compliance. Fertil Steril. 1997;68(3):402-4.
37. Barnhart KT, Katz I, Hummel A, et al. Presumed diagnosis of ectopic pregnancy. Obstet Gynecol. 2002;100:505-10.
38. Brown JK, Lauer KB, Ironmonger EL, et al. Shotgun proteomics identifies serum

fibronectin as a candidate diagnostic biomarker for inclusion in future multiplex tests for ectopic pregnancy. PLoS One. 2013; 8:e66974.
39. Rausch ME, Sammel MD, Takacs P, et al. Development of a multiple marker test for ectopic pregnancy. Obstet Gynecol. 2011;117:573-82.
40. Calabresi P, Chabner BA. Antineoplastic agents. In: Gilman A, Goodman LS, Goodman A (Eds). The Pharmacologic Basis of Therapeutics. New York: Macmillan. 1990:1275-6.
41. Rodi IA, Sauer MV, Gorrill MJ, et al. The medical treatment of unruptured ectopic pregnancy with methotrexate and citrovorum rescue: preliminary experience. Fertil Steril. 1986;46:811-3.
42. Ory SJ, Villanueva AL, Sand PK, et al. Conservative treatment of ectopic pregnancy with methotrexate. Am J Obstet Gynecol. 1986;1546:1299-306.
43. Stovall TG, Ling FW, Buster JE. Outpatient chemotherapy of unruptured ectopic pregnancy. Fertil Steril. 1989;51:435-8.
44. Pisarska MD, Carson SA, Buster JE. Ectopic pregnancy. Lancet. 1998;351:1115-20.
45. Lipscomb GH, Stovall TG, Ling FW. Nonsurgical treatment of ectopic pregnancy. N Engl J Med. 2000;343:1325-9.
46. Barnhart K, Coutifaris C, Esposito M. The pharmacology of methotrexate. Expert Opin Pharmacother. 2001;2:409-17.
47. Stovall TG, Ling FW, Gray LA. Single-dose methotrexate for treatment of ectopic pregnancy. Obstet Gynecol. 1991;77:754-7.
48. Lipscomb GH, Bran D, McCord ML, et al. Analysis of three hundred fifteen ectopic pregnancies treated with single-dose methotrexate. Am J Obstet Gynecol. 1998;178:1354-8.
49. Alleyassin A, Khademi A, Aghahosseini M, et al. Comparison of success rates in the medical management of ectopic pregnancy with single-dose and multiple-dose administration of methotrexate: a prospective, randomized clinical trial. Fertil Steril. 2006;85:1661-6.
50. Barnhart K, van Mello NM, Bourne T, et al. Pregnancy of unknown location: a consensus statement of nomenclature, definitions, and outcome. Fertil Steril. 2011;95:857-66.
51. Agency for Healthcare Research and Quality. Medical management of ectopic pregnancy, 2008. Available on: http://www.guidelines.gov/content.aspx?Id=12625#Section 427 (last assessed on 6 August 2013).

CHAPTER 26

Gonadotropins: The Future

Madhuri Patil

Chapter outline

- Structure of Corifollitropin Alfa (Org 36286)
- Method of Administration
- Pharmacokinetics
- Efficacy
- Follicular Growth
- Hormone Levels
- Results with Corifollitropin Alfa
  - Disadvantages of Corifollitropin Alfa
  - Safety
- Cost Effectiveness of Corifollitropin Alfa
- Conclusion on Corifollitropin Alfa
- Recombinant LH-Lutropin Alfa for Injection (Luveris)
- Follitropin Alfa and Lutropin Alfa (2:1 Ratio) (Pergoveris) (r-hFSH 150 IU and r-hLH 75 IU)
- Follitropin Delta
  - Dosing and Administration of Follitropin Delta
  - For Subsequent Treatment Cycles
  - In Research
  - In Humans

INTRODUCTION

The role of the *in vitro* firtilization (IVF) clinician is to make the assisted reproductive technology (ART) treatment safe, patient friendly, cost effective and at the same time offer good and high quality treatment. IVF protocols are a burden for women and are one of the potential reasons why women do not return for subsequent cycles. Frequent injections may increase stress and also result in high error rates. Moreover the ovulation induction protocols can be associated with side effects of gonadotropins and gonadotropin-releasing hormone (GnRH)-analogs, which include a higher risk of ovarian hyperstimulation syndrome (OHSS) and multiple pregnancies. Fertility experts are concerned about the patient compliance.

About 50% of them are also worried if patients were injecting correctly.

Simple short treatment regimen with optimal recovery of good quality oocytes results in development of good quality embryos followed by single embryo transfer (SET) in treatment and cryopreservation cycles are a less burden and result in related lesser discontinuation, side effects, treatment cycles in time and are more cost-effective.

Development of follicle-stimulating hormone (FSH) analogues with longer terminal $t_{1/2}$ and slower absorption to peak serum levels will increase the efficiency, decrease the side effects and also is easy to administer. This makes it convenient for the patients increasing the compliance. Development of corifollitropin alfa is the first step towards a new generation of recombinant gonadotropins.

STRUCTURE OF CORIFOLLITROPIN ALFA (ORG 36286)

Corifollitropin alfa is a hybrid molecule with sustained follicle stimulating activity. It is a recombinant fusion molecule of FSH and the carboxyl terminal peptide (CTP) of hCGb subunit.[1] It is a gonadotropin with different pharmacokinetic properties but similar pharmacologic features as the available FSH in the market today. Presence of CTP component, which contains four O-linked oligosaccharides gives it a prolonged half-life compared with rFSH (Table 26.1).[2] It has a similar *in vitro* receptor binding and steroidogenic activity compared with wild-type FSH but, had significantly enhanced *in vivo* activity and plasma half-life with $t_{1/2}$–65 hours, t_{max} – 25–45 hours.[3] It interacts only with the FSH receptor and lacks LH activity.

FSH-CTP is produced by Chinese Hamster Ovary cells. Using site-directed mutagenesis and gene transfer techniques the CTP extension of hCG-beta was coupled to the FSH-beta unit. It was found that the presence of the CTP sequence did not significantly affect assembly or secretion of the intact dimmer by stable cell lines.[1]

Development of long acting molecules can be done by
1. Linkage of CTP to recombinant hormones[1]
2. Introducing additional sequences containing potential glycosylation sites at the N-terminus of the FSH a-subunit[4]
3. Fusion with the constant region fragment (Fc) domain of immunoglobulin G1—Two forms of FSH were created[5]
4. By creating a contiguous, single-chain, covalently-bound fusion protein containing the common a- and FSH b-subunits separated by the hCG b-CTP.[2,6,7]

METHOD OF ADMINISTRATION

Before the start of ovarian stimulation, pregnancy should be excluded by means of an hCG test, a blood sample taken for hormone assessments, and ultrasound performed to measure and count visible follicles and to rule out the presence of an ovarian cyst.

The treatment cycle was started on menstrual cycle day 2 or 3 as depicted in Figure 26.1. Stimulation starts with a single SC injection of 150 mg (0.5 mL) corifollitropin alfa (NV Organon, The Netherlands). To prevent premature LH surges the GnRH antagonist ganirelix (0.25 mg, Orgalutranw/ganirelix acetate injection, NV Organon, The Netherlands) was administered once daily SC starting on stimulation day 5 up to and including the day of hCG. From stimulation day 8 onwards, treatment is continued with a

Table 26.1: Comparison of corifollitropin alfa with r-hFSH.

Corifollitropin alfa	r-hFSH
• High and sustained levels	• Gradual increasing levels
• Simultaneous recruitment	• Sequential recruitment
• Homogenous/Fixed cohort development	• Heterogenous/dynamic cohort
• No dose adjustments	• Dose adjustment impact response
• All/none response	• Variable manageable response
• Ongoing PR/cycle 38.9%	• Ongoing PR/cycle 38.1%
• 7% patients developed OHSS	• 6.3% patients developed OHSS
• Antagonist cycles	• Agonist/Antagonist cycles
• No control for 7 days after injection	• Controlled ovarian stimulation
• Documented use only for selected patients	• Documented use in variety of patients

(r-hFSH: recombinant human follicle stimulating hormone; OHSS: ovarian hyperstimulation syndrome).

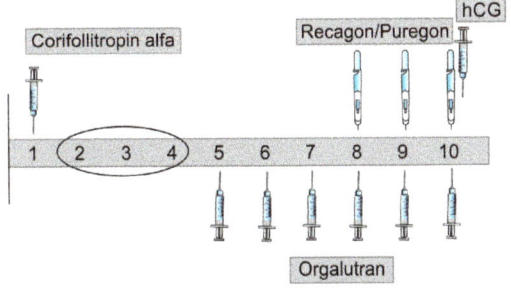

Fig. 26.1: Protocol for corifollitropin.

daily SC dose of (active) 150–200 IU rFSH up to the day of hCG. Urinary hCG (10 000 IU) or Rec hCG 250 mcg should be administered to induce final oocyte maturation as soon as at least three follicles of 17–18 mm are observed by transvaginal USG.[3]

Organon, the human healthcare business unit of Akzo Nobel, announced recently that two out of three Phase III clinical trials with corifollitropin alfa (Org 36286), a new long-acting fertility hormone, have reached their randomization target.

Corifollitropin alfa is a new recombinant fertility hormone. It is the first of a new class of gonadotropins (a sustained follicular stimulant or SFS) of which, due to its long half-life, one single injection may replace the first 7 injections with conventional gonadotropins during a fertility treatment cycle. The objective of the ENGAGE trial, the largest double-blind fertility trial ever performed, is to demonstrate clinical efficacy and safety of corifollitropin alfa 150 μg in a double-blind comparison with Organon's Puregon, one of the most commonly used preparations to treat infertile patients. The recruitment goal of the ENGAGE trial was to include a total of 1400 patients from 34 fertility clinics in Europe, USA and Canada and was started in July, 2006. The study reached its randomization target on June 10, 2007.

A second trial, the ENSURE trial, is an efficacy and safety trial with corifollitropin alfa 100 μg designed specifically for women who weigh less than 60 kg (133 lbs). This double-blind study comparing corifollitropin alfa with Puregon was started in January 2007 in 19 clinical trial centers in Europe and Asia with a recruitment goal of 330 patients by June 30, 2007. All 330 subjects have now been randomized.

A third Phase III trial in the Life program (the Trust trial) focuses on safety of repeated treatments with corifollitropin alfa, and is expected to complete recruitment on target by mid-August 2007.

On the basis of phase I, II, III and Engage and Ensure trial following information was obtained about corifollitropin alfa.

Can Corifollitropin alfa be used with GnRh agonist?

A single-dose of 100 μg or 150 μg corifollitropin alfa in a long GnRH agonist protocol is able to support multifollicular development during the first week of ovarian stimulation.[8] This study observed that number of follicles, serum E2 and number of oocytes retrieved indicate a relatively high ovarian response. However, further controlled studies are needed to support efficacy and safety of corifollitropin alfa in a long GnRH agonist protocol.

PHARMACOKINETICS

The results of Phase I and Phase II trials in pituitary-suppressed volunteers and patients, respectively, show that the mean $t_{1/2}$ of corifollitropin alfa is approximately 65 h for all doses tested between 60 and 240 mg (Fig. 26.2), compared with approximately 35 h for rFSH.[9-12] Peak levels reached within 36–42 hours as compared to 10–12 hours for rFSH. Dose normalized (dn) area under the curve (AUC) and dn C_{max} are similar across all doses, indicating that the PK parameters of corifollitropin alfa are dose-proportional over this range. Median C_{max} of corifollitropin alfa is reached between 25 and 45 h after injection. No differences were observed between the PK in volunteer's pituitary suppressed by oral contraceptives[9]

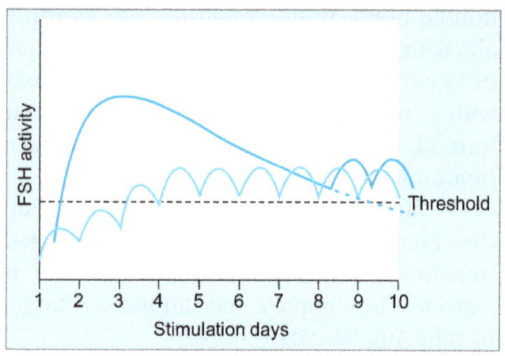

Fig. 26.2: Follicular-stimulating hormone (FSH) activity increased on first seven days of stimulation.

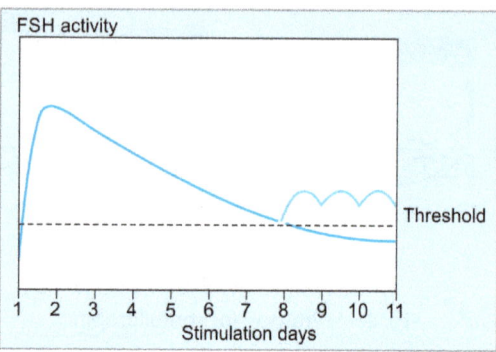

Fig. 26.3: Threshold of FSH declines after 8th day of administration of corifollitropin.

and nonsuppressed patients undergoing ovarian stimulation in a GnRH antagonist protocol. Elimination of corifollitropin alfa is not largely affected by body weight, but exposure is inversely correlated to body weight, exhibiting a linear relationship to both serum clearance and volume of distribution (The Corifollitropin Alfa Dose-finding Study Group, 2008). In summary, the single-dose PK of corifollitropin alfa is characterized by a slow absorption resulting in peak levels within 2 days after injection. Thereafter, serum corifollitropin alfa levels decrease steadily, though the FSH activity may be retained above the FSH threshold for an entire week if the administered dose of corifollitropin alfa is sufficiently high.

EFFICACY

The PK profile of corifollitropin alfa after a single injection implies the highest FSH activity (Fig. 26.3) during the first 2 days of stimulation, followed by decreasing FSH activity until treatment with daily FSH is started. Single injection induces and sustains multifollicular development during the first week of stimulation and is effective in stimulation of multi-follicular growth for IVF but less suitable for induction of monofollicular growth and therefore IUI.[10]

The maximal serum concentration of Org 36286 increased with the doses injected. Maximum serum FSH-CTP concentrations were 0.42, 0.66, 1.49 and 3.27 ng/mL after administration of 15, 30, 60 or 120 µg Org 36286 respectively. When statistical analysis was performed, no statistically significant differences between doses were found for any of the (dose normalized) pharmacokinetic parameters. Thus absorption of FSH-CTP was much slower and the elimination half life was twice as long as that of rFSH. Initial trials studies a dose range of 15–120 µg and the elimination half-life (ranging from 60–75 h) was dose independent.

Dose-finding Trial of Corifollitropin Alfa was initiated in 2008 where 60, 120 and 180 mgs were studied. Single dose of corifollitropin alfa sustains follicular growth for an entire week in all the 3 groups but the number of follicles that are recruited vary with dose. High cancellation rate in the 60 µg dose group (44%) indicated that dose was too low to support the first 7 days of ovarian stimulation.

FOLLICULAR GROWTH

Transvaginal ultrasonography results showed that single FSH-CTP administration induced follicular growth in almost all subjects.

Follicles with a diameter > 8 mm were only observed in the 60 and 120 µg group. The maximum diameter of follicles in the 60 µg group was between 8.0 and 9.9 mm and between 14.0 and 15.9 mm in the 120 µg group. In the higher dose groups, large cohorts of follicles were recruited.

When comparing the ultrasonography results of this study with results from previous work,[13] the effect of a single administration of 120 µg FSH-CTP on follicular growth appears to be slightly reduced compared with 7 days administration of 150 or 225 IU rFSH. This implies that, to obtain an effect similar to that of seven daily rFSH injections, the dose of FSH-CTP should be further increased. Thus, FSH levels would remain above the threshold level for follicular stimulation during a longer time period, and probably weekly administration would be sufficient.[9]

Statistically significant dose-related increase in number of follicles 11 or 15 mm on day 8 of stimulation and hCG administration was noted. There was also a statistically significant increase in number of oocytes retrieved over this dose range.

HORMONE LEVELS

Serum levels of inhibin-B, which is produced by granulosa cells and is an early marker of follicular growth[13] increased dose-dependently after FSH-CTP administration. Serum LH concentrations were lower than observed during GnRH agonist administration and comparable with those of hypogonadotropic hypogonadal women.[3,14-16] Apparently LH levels were too low for adequate E2 production since, even though E2 is a marker of follicular growth, E2 levels were also low. Only in the highest dose groups a small increase in serum E2 levels was seen.

Median serum E2 levels declined from Day 6 onwards in the 60 µg group, reached a plateau in the 120 µg group, and continued to increase in the 180 µg group. For patients who received hCG, serum E2 levels were similar in the 60, 120 µg and rFSH groups, but 1.5-fold higher in the 180 µg group. From Day 6 onwards, inhibin-B levels continued to increase in 180 µg group and daily rFSH group, whereas it reached a plateau from Day 6 to 8 in the 120 µg group and decreased in the 60 µg group.

RESULTS WITH CORIFOLLITROPIN ALFA

Devorey et al. published in human reproduction 2009 an oocyte retrieval rate of 96.8% of the patients in the corifollitropin alfa group and 98.9% in the rFSH group.[17] A higher mean number of cumulus–oocyte complexes were retrieved in the corifollitropin alfa group. There were higher number and percentage of mature oocytes in the corifollitropin alfa group (mean 10.8, 78.9%) compared to rFSH group (mean 9.2, 77.4%).[18] A comparable fertilization rate was observed between corifollitropin alpha and rFSH. A mean of 5.6 embryos were obtained on day 3 of culture in the corifollitropin alfa group and 4.8 embryos in the rFSH group for patients with IVF and/or ICSI. Embryo quality was also reported to be similar in both groups and on average, 1.7 (0.4) embryos were transferred in both treatment groups. For 51.7% and 53.2% of the patients in the corifollitropin alfa and rFSH groups, a mean (SD) of 4.3 (3.6) and 3.9 (2.7) supernumerary embryos have been cryopreserved, respectively. In the dose finding study of 2008 a statistically significant increase in the number of oocytes retrieved with[18] increasing dose was observed. This group also published similar pregnancy rates (confirmed by positive hCG test) of 48.1% and 46.9% for corifollitropin alfa and rFSH groups respectively.[17] Early pregnancy losses during the first 10 weeks were also comparable in the two groups. Percentage of patients who discontinued treatment either for poor or excessive response was also similar in the two groups.

Thus, initial trials concluded that the optimum dose of corifollitropin alfa to sustain follicular development for one week was greater than 60 µg and lower than 180 µg. Later Organon initiated a clinical development program for corifollitropin alfa for the therapeutic indication of COH. This was a Phase III trial and it concluded that 150 µg most appropriate dose for achieving an optimal treatment outcome in terms of the number of oocytes retrieved and fertilized for patients with a body weight >60 kg. However, in women weighing <60 kg lower dose of 100 µg was shown to result in optimal outcome without compromising the follicular support during the first week of stimulation. It was also noted that the dose of rFSH required from day 8 in the patients with a body weight of >60 kg was 200 IU as against 150 IU in patients with body weight <60 kg. On average, two days of rFSH treatment are needed to reach criterion for hCG administration (at least 3 follicles ≥17 mm). The drug and follicular response was similar in both the groups. The number of oocytes retrieved, fertilization rate, number of good quality embryos were also similar. There was also no difference in the total number of embryos and good quality embryos frozen. The ongoing pregnancy rate was also not different in the two groups.

A meta-analysis published in 2015 looks at clinical parameters like live birth rate, ongoing pregnancy rate, clinical pregnancy rate and risk of spontaneous abortion between corifollitropin alfa and rFSH and found no significant differences. When the ovarian response to COS was considered, corifollitropin alfa yielded a higher number of oocytes and embryos than rFSH. Careful selection of patients that are eligible for corifollitropin alfa in order to prevent OHSS and cycle cancellation is required.[19]

Polyzos looked at treatment of poor ovarian responders, as described by the Bologna criteria, with corifollitropin alfa in a GnRH antagonist protocol and concluded a low pregnancy rates, similarly to conventional stimulation with a short agonist protocol.[20]

Later Kolibianakis et al. in 2015 published no significant differences with respect of length of stimulation between corifollitropin alfa with rFSH in poor responder patients but showed a definite reduction in the treatment burden.[21] There was another study which looked at using a single injection of 150 mg of corifollitropin alfa in older women and found it to be as effective as 300 IU of recombinant FSH for the development of multiple follicles during COS, and in also in respect to the number of oocytes reterieved, and clinical pregnancy rate with an adequate safety profile.[22]

Individual responses variation in 3 subsequent cycle with the same protocol of corifollitropin alfa was demonstrated in 25% of women and was not explained by baseline FSH and AFC. It was also seen in this study that the number of follicles on the day of hCG administration correlated well with the number of oocytes retrieved. It was also observed in this study that the inter cycle variability in ovarian response to controlled ovarian stimulation was not strongly linked to individual patient demographics, infertility characteristics, or baseline predictors.[23]

There was a study by Pérez-Calvo A et al., which looked at the pill free interval in an antagonist protocol using corifollitropin alfa in oocyte donors. The results of this study showed that extending the pill-free interval from 5 to 7 days significantly reduces the total dose of gonadotropins, duration of stimulation, total cost of medication and total number of injections (P = 0.015).[24]

Disadvantages of Corifollitropin Alfa

- Dose cannot be reduced to obtain milder stimulation
- Serum FSH levels decline after stimulation day 3 (C_{max}) onwards

- Dose reduction during first week of stimulation cannot be made in case of hyper-response
- Less suitable in cases with known risk of hyper-response—PCOS, previous OHSS
- PR and LBR not yet confirmed to be comparable with daily Rec FSH
- Ovarian response induced may decrease with the patient's age and ovarian reserve.

Safety

No antibodies against FSH-CTP or CHO-derived proteins were detected. The FSH-CTP preparation was well tolerated. No serious adverse events (SAE) were observed and none of the subjects discontinued due to adverse events (AE). There were no clinically relevant adverse events and no relevant changes in laboratory parameters.[25]

The TRUST Trial initiated by Organon's clinical development program focuses on safety of repeated treatments with corifollitropin alfa. All tested doses were safe and well-tolerated, no anti-corifollitropin alfa antibodies were detected and OHSS with hospital admission occurred in 2–3%.

A single dose of corifollitropin alfa for the first 7 days of ovarian stimulation has a similar efficacy and safety profile compared with seven daily injections of rFSH when risk of ovarian hyperstimulation syndrome, pregnancy rate and live birth rate were compared.[26] The same author also looked at pre-treatment AMH values as a single predictor to predict either hypo or hyper response to corifollitropin alfa 150 µg to achieve optimal treatment outcome. AMH at a threshold of 0.91 ng/mL showed a sensitivity of 82.4%, specificity of 82.4%, positive predictive value 52.9% and negative predictive value 95.1% for predicting low response (P-value: 0.853, 0.769–0.936; <0.0001). The optimal threshold for AMH was 2.58 ng/mL for predicting hyper-response, with a sensitivity of 80.0%, specificity 82.1%, positive predictive value 42.5% and negative predictive value 96.1% (P-value: 0.871, 0.787–0.955; <0.0001). Thus patients with serum AMH concentrations between approximately 0.9 and 2.6 ng/mL were unlikely to show extremes of response (<6 or >18 oocytes, for poor and hyper response respectively) to 150 µg corifollitropin alfa stimulation.[27]

COST EFFECTIVENESS OF CORIFOLLITROPIN ALFA

When cost per unit of gonadotropin was calculated and compared according to the manufacturer's sale price, together with the cost of nursing, infrastructure, patient care time and consumables used in each group of the study, it was found that corifollitropin alfa as compared to recombinant FSH and highly purified human menopausal gonadotropin increased the overall cost of the treatment as well as the cost per retrieved and effective oocyte.[28]

CONCLUSION ON CORIFOLLITROPIN ALFA

Corifollitropin alfa is the first long-acting hybrid molecule with sustained follicle-stimulating activity developed for the induction of multi-follicular growth along with GnRH antagonist co-treatment for IVF. The development of corifollitropin alfa is the first step towards a new generation of recombinant gonadotropins.

Using corifollitropin alfa in combination with a fixed daily GnRH antagonist will further simplify treatment and may reduce the treatment burden of IVF for patients. Future trials concerning corifollitropin alfa will need to compare clinical outcomes using GnRH antagonist co-treatment with those achieved using long GnRH agonist protocols.

Pharmacokinetic results for corifollitropin alpha showed that absorption was much slower and the elimination half-life was twice as long as that of rFSH. It is the first long-acting hybrid molecule with sustained follicle-stimulating activity developed for induction of multifollicular growth with GnRH antagonist co-treatment for IVF. It is simpler and more convenient for patients compared with conventional long protocols with GT.

Several meta-analysis have shown that corifollitropin alfa is effective as rFSH in terms of live birth rate, ongoing pregnancy rate and clinical pregnancy rate. Corifollitropin alfa regimen are associated with increased cohort of developing follicles and corresponding increased number of eggs retrieved. This can increase the risk of OHSS in high responder women, which may contraindicate its use in this group of women.[19] High basal anti-Müllerian hormone and/or AFC can identify women with enhanced functional ovarian reserve are at risk of hyper stimulation, and the risk is even higher if maximally stimulated with corifollitropin alpha or high dose of daily recombinant FSH.[29] Using AMH and AFC to select suitable candidates for treatment with corifollitropin alfa may result in a safe and convenient stimulation.[30]

RECOMBINANT LH - LUTROPIN ALFA FOR INJECTION (LUVERIS)

Luveris is pure LH manufactured using genetic recombinant mammalian technology. It is indicated for use in women with profound LH deficiency and to improve outcome in ovarian stimulation protocols using recombinant FSH.

There was no significant difference observed in the probability of live birth with or without rLH addition to FSH with odds ratio, OR – 0.92, 95% CI = 0.65 – 1.31 and P value of 0.65.[31] No significant difference was observed in the gonadotropin consumption, duration of stimulation, estradiol and progesterone levels on the day of hCG, number of cumulus complexes retrieved and fertilization rate.

Cochrane review in 2017 published that there is very low quality evidence for any difference between rLH combined with rFSH and rFSH alone for live birth rates or occurrence of OHSS. This Cochrane review also complained that there is moderate quality evidence that the use of rLH combined with rFSH may lead to more ongoing pregnancies than rFSH alone. There was also moderate-quality evidence suggesting little or no difference between the groups in rates of miscarriage. There was no clear evidence of a difference between the groups in rates of cancellation due to low response or imminent OHSS, but the evidence for these outcomes was of low or very low quality. Thus available evidence does not support or discourage the addition of recombinant LH increases the live birth rate in patients treated with Recombinant FSH alone with GnRH analogues in IVF/ICSI cycles.[32]

Lutropin alfa for injection is contraindicated in:
- Women who exhibit prior hypersensitivity to human LH preparations
- Primary ovarian failure
- Uncontrolled thyroid or adrenal dysfunction
- Uncontrolled organic intracranial lesion such as a pituitary tumor
- Abnormal uterine bleeding of undetermined origin
- Ovarian cyst or enlargement of undetermined origin
- Sex hormone dependent tumors of the reproductive tract
- Pregnancy.

FOLLITROPIN ALFA AND LUTROPIN ALFA (2:1 RATIO) (PERGOVERIS) (r-hFSH 150 IU AND r-hLH 75 IU)

This combination may be used in women with low basal LH, suboptimal responders, young poor responders and older women (>35 yrs). The number of oocytes reterived and the percentage of mature oocytes were significantly more in the combination Pergoveris group. The total dose and days of stimulation were significantly less in the Pergoveris group. There was no difference in the implantation and pregnancy rate between the two groups. The number of cycles cancelled for the risk of ovarian hyperstimulation syndrome was much higher in the pergoveris group (11.1% vs 1.7%).[33]

FOLLITROPIN DELTA

It is well known that FSH is composed of two glycosylated protein subunits and recombinant FSH is derived by introduction of genes encoding for human FSH into mammalian cell line from which FSH is derived and further purified.

Follitropin delta is the first recombinant FSH protein expressed in human cell line (human retinal cell line) with an individualized dosing regimen based on Anti-Mullerian hormone (AMH) levels and body weight. Follitropin delta differs from that of follitropin alfa in their glycosylation although they have similar amino acid sequence. Follitropin delta has a higher proportion of tri- and tetra-sialylated glycans, with both alpha 2,3- and alpha 2,6-linked sialic acid, while follitropin alfa has only alpha 2,3-linked sialic acid. More acidic isoforms of FSH with greater sialic acid modification are less potent *in vitro* at the human FSH receptor compared to more basic FSH isoforms and also display lower serum clearance and longer circulating half-life.[34]

In a pharmacokinetic comparative study wherein 50 women were randomized to receive either 450 IU of subcutaneous follitropin delta or alfa, following findings were recorded for Follitropin delta as compared to follitropin alfa.[35]
- 1.5-fold greater exposure (AUC)
- 1.3-fold higher Cmax
- 1.2 times longer half-life
- 1.3-fold longer tmax, respectively

Dosing and Administration of Follitropin Delta[36,37]

Dosing is individualized for each patient and aims to obtain an ovarian response which is associated with a favorable safety/efficacy profile, i.e. aims to achieve an adequate number of oocytes retrieved and reduce the interventions to prevent ovarian hyperstimulation syndrome (OHSS). REKOVELLE is dosed in micrograms.

The dosing regimen is specific for REKOVELLE and the microgram dose cannot be applied to other gonadotropins. For the first treatment cycle, the individual daily dose will be determined on the basis of the woman's serum anti-Müllerian hormone (AMH) concentration and her body weight. The dose should be based on a recent determination of AMH (i.e. within the last 12 months) measured by Roche ELECSYS AMH Plus immunoassay. The individual daily dose is to be maintained throughout the stimulation period. For women with AMH <15 pmol/L the daily dose is 12 μg, irrespective of body weight. For women with AMH ≥15 pmol/L the daily dose decreases from 0.19 to 0.10 μg/kg by increasing AMH concentration.

For Subsequent Treatment Cycles

The daily dose of REKOVELLE should be maintained or modified according to the patient's ovarian response in the previous cycle.
- If the patient had adequate ovarian response in the previous cycle without developing OHSS, the same daily dose should be used
- In case of ovarian hypo-response in the previous cycle, the daily dose in the subsequent cycle should be increased by 25% or 50%, according to the extent of response observed
- In case of ovarian hyper-response in the previous cycle, the daily dose in the

subsequent cycle should be decreased by 20% or 33%, according to the extent of response observe
- In patients who developed OHSS or were at risk of OHSS in a previous cycle, the daily dose for the subsequent cycle is 33% lower than the dose used in the cycle where OHSS or risk of OHSS occurred. The maximum daily dose is 24 µg.

Clinical Efficacy of Follitropin Delta has been tested through ESTHER 1 trial (Evidence-based Stimulation Trial with Human rFSH in Europe and Rest of World).[38]

This was a randomized, multicenter, assessor-blinded, non-inferiority trial conducted at 37 investigational sites in 11 countries. In this study 1329 women were randomized to receive either follitropin delta individualized on the basis of AMH and body weight or follitropin alfa with a starting dose of 150 IU/day for 5 days. Ongoing pregnancy rate, ongoing implantation rate and live birth rate were similar for individualized follitropin delta and conventional follitropin alfa.

In this landmark trial, individualized follitropin delta resulted in following as compared to follitropin alfa:
- More women with target response (8-14 oocytes) (43.3% vs. 38.4%)
- Fewer poor responses i.e. fewer than four oocytes in patients with AMH <15 pmol/L (11.8% vs. 17.9%)
- Fewer excessive responses i.e. ≥15 or ≥20 oocytes in patients with ≥AMH 15 pmol/L (27.9% vs. 35.1% and 10.1% vs. 15.6%, respectively)
- A fewer measures taken to prevent ovarian hyperstimulation syndrome (2.3% vs. 4.5%).

Currently in practice, clinicians use subjective preferences for predictive parameters as there is no standard position about the weightage that needs to be allocated to each factor. Additionally the heterogeneity of response to ovarian stimulation make it all the more challenging to predict ovarian response in advance. In this scenario, the novel gonadotropin preparation follitropin delta offers a new rFSH derived from human retinal cell line with personalized dosing based on the robust parameter AMH alongwith body weight of patient to pool higher number of patients in the range of target number of oocytes.

Optimizing ovarian response in IVF by individualized dosing with follitropin delta according to pretreatment patient characteristics results in similar efficacy and improved safety compared with conventional ovarian stimulation.

In Research

Oral and pulmonary delivery of FSH-Fc fusion proteins via neonatal Fc receptor-mediated transcytosis.[39]

Heterodimer FSH-Fc is also significantly more active than single chain FSH-Fc. FSH-Fc fusion proteins have increased stability in blood and improved bioactivity *in vivo*, and that heterodimer FSH-Fc is more active in rats and monkeys than single chain FSH-Fc. Data on its use in rats and monkeys suggest that Fc fusion proteins offer the potential for oral and pulmonary delivery of FSH. The half-life of heterodimer FSH-Fc in cynomolgus monkeys is 182-219 h. This is significantly longer than the half-life of rFSH of, 24 h in humans[40] and in non-human primates.[41,42] Thus, an obvious advantage of using heterodimer FSH-Fc in infertility treatments is the potential for a greatly reduced dosing frequency. In addition, pulmonary or oral delivery of FSH-Fc fusion proteins using endogenous FcRn expressed in epithelial cells of the lung and intestine could significantly improve tolerability of current infertility treatments.

In Humans

Low Molecular Weight Gonadotropins

Consistent with other therapeutic areas, novel drug development in the infertility field is likely to concentrate on less invasive delivery methods, such as the use of long-acting compounds or different routes of administration that may include transdermal, inhaled or oral agents. On the horizon is the development of orally active, low molecular weight gonadotropins, for which a first proof-of-concept study has been reported in female volunteers.[43]

Induction of Ovulation by a Potent, Orally Active, Low Molecular Weight Agonist (Org 43553) of the Luteinizing Hormone Receptor

Org 43553 is the first LMW LH-R mimetic with demonstrated *in vivo* efficacy upon oral administration and could therefore replace subcutaneously administered hCG. It is a thienopyrimidine compound class. It is a pure synthetic molecule lacking the variability between batches as observed for proteins of urinary or recombinant origin. It is completely protein free, thus totally excluding the minimal current risk for diseases like Creutzfeld Jacob's, originating from recombinant gonadotropin production in the presence of bovine serum in the culture media.

On the basis of the pharmacokinetic profile of Org 43553 in rat, the anticipated human half-life of Org 43553 was calculated with a method described by Bachman et al. (1996). Using this method, the anticipated human half-life of Org 43553 was found to be between 15 and 30 h after a single-dose oral treatment. In a first human exposure study, the human elimination half-life of Org 43553 after oral administration was proven to vary between 30 and 47 h,[22] which is substantially and remarkably shorter than the elimination half-life of hCG (48–96 h in humans). The shorter half-life of Org 43553 in humans compared with hCG may have a reduced risk for OHSS.

Thus, it can be developed as a safe oral alternative to the current injectable LH/hCG preparations for clinical use to induce ovulation or oocyte maturation for both *in vivo* and IVF therapy. In addition, the compound can also be developed for male indications such as hypogonadism.

Small Molecule Agonists and Antagonists for the LH and FSH Receptors

Luteinizing hormone (LH) and follicle-stimulating hormone (FSH) play a critical role in human reproduction. LH and FSH are secreted from the pituitary and act on their respective G-protein-coupled receptors (GPCRs), LHR and FSHR, in the gonads to either promote follicular growth and differentiation in women or to stimulate the proper progression of spermatogenesis in men. LH and FSH are currently used in the clinic for the treatment of infertility. Small molecule agonists of LHR and FSHR have the potential to become oral therapeutics for infertility treatment, whereas small molecule antagonists of LHR and FSHR may find utility in oral contraception. Advances in molecular biology, high-throughput screening (HTS) and combinatorial chemistry have made significant contributions to the recent discovery of a variety of small molecule LHR and FSHR agonists and antagonists, some of which have shown highly promising efficacy in animal models of fertility control.

CONCLUSION

Although current treatments are increasingly successful, treatment-related burden may be reduced by less intervention. The GnRH antagonist protocol should be considered for each patient as compared to the long GnRH agonist protocol which is time-consuming and stressful for the patient.

Corifollitropin alfa and Follitropin delta are two new gonadotropins with equivalent efficacy, success and safety as compared to conventional gonadotropins.

Addition of Recombinant LH (Luveris) or use of combination of Recombinant FSH and LH in the ratio of 2:1 (Pergoveris) can replace hMG.

New parenteral, transdermal, inhaled and oral fertility drugs and regimens are currently under research and development with the objective to further simplify treatment for ART.

REFERENCES

1. Fares FA, Suganuma N, Nishimori K, et al. Design of a long-acting follitropin agonist by fusing the C-terminal sequence of the chorionic gonadotropin beta subunit to the follitropin beta subunit. Proc Natl Acad Sci USA. 1992;89:4304-8.
2. Boime I, Ben-Menahem D. Glycoprotein hormone structure–function and analog design. Recent Prog. Horm. 1999;54:271-88.
3. Devroey P, Mannaerts B, Smitz J, et al. Clinical outcome of a pilot efficacy study on recombinant human follicle-stimulating hormone (Org 32489) combined with various gonadotrophin-releasing hormone agonist regimens. Hum Reprod. 1994;9:1064-9.
4. Perlman S, van den Hazel B, Christiansen J, et al. Glycosylation of an N-terminal extension prolongs the half-life and increases the in vivo activity of follicle stimulating hormone. J Clin Endocrinol Metab. 2003;88:3227-35.
5. Low SC, Nunes SL, Bitonti AJ, et al. Oral and pulmonary delivery of FSH-Fc fusion proteins via neonatal Fc receptor-mediated transcytosis. Hum Reprod. 2005;20:1805-13.
6. Sugahara T, Sato A, Kudo M, et al. Expression of biologically active fusion genes encoding the common a subunit and the follicle-stimulating hormone b subunit—role of a linker sequence. J Biol Chem. 1996;271:10445-8.
7. Klein J, Lobel L, Pollak S, et al. Pharmacokinetics and pharmacodynamics of single-chain recombinant human follicle-stimulating hormone containing the human chorionic gonadotropin carboxy terminal peptide in the rhesus monkey. Fertil Steril. 2002;77:1248-55.
8. Mousavi Fatemi H, Oberye J, Popovic-Todorovic, et al. First results with corifollitropin alfa in long GnRH agonist protocol. Abstracts of the 25th Annual Meeting of ESHRE, Amsterdam, the Netherlands 2009.
9. Duijkers IJM, Klipping C, Boerrigter PJ, et al. Single dose pharmacokinetics and effects on follicular growth and serum hormones of a long-acting recombinant FSH preparation (FSH-CTP) in healthy pituitary-suppressed females. Hum Reprod. 2002;17:1987-93.
10. Balen AH, Mulders AG, Fauser BCJM, et al. Pharmacodynamics of a single low dose of long-acting recombinant follicle-stimulating hormone (FSH-carboxy terminal peptide, corifollitropin alfa) in women with World Health Organization group II anovulatory infertility. J Clin Endocrinol Metab. 2004;89:6297-304.
11. Devroey P, Fauser BC, Platteau P, et al. Induction of multiple follicular development by a single dose of long-acting recombinant follicle-stimulating hormone (FSH-CTP, corifollitropin alfa) for controlled ovarian stimulation before in vitro fertilisation. J Clin Endocrinol Metab. 2004;89:2062-70.
12. The Corifollitropin Alfa Dose-finding Study Group. A randomized dose-response trial of a single injection of corifollitropin alfa to sustain multifollicular growth during controlled ovarian stimulation. Hum Reprod. 2008;23:2484-92.
13. Voortman G, Mannaerts BMJL, Huisman JAM. A dose proportionality study of SC and intramuscularly administered recombinant human FSH (Follistim/Puregon) in healthy female volunteers. Fertil Steril. 2000;73:1187-93.
14. Groome NP, Illingworth PJ, O'Brien M, et al. Measurement of dimeric inhibin B throughout the human menstrual cycle. J Clin Endocrinol Metab. 1992;81:1401-05.
15. Schoot DC, Coelingh Bennink HJT, Mannaerts, BMJL, et al. Human recombinant follicle stimulating hormone induces growth of preovulatory follicles without concomitant increase in androgen and estrogen biosynthesis in a woman with isolated gonadotropin deficiency. J Clin Endocrinol Metab. 1992;74:1471-3.

16. Mannaerts B, Shoham Z, Schoot D, et al. Single-dose pharmacokinetics and pharmacodynamics of recombinant human follicle-stimulating hormone (Org 34289) in gonadotropin-deficient volunteers. Fertil Steril. 1993;59:108-14.
17. Devroey P, Boostanfar R, Koper NP, et al. A double-blind, non-inferiority RCT comparing corifollitropin alfa and recombinant FSH during the first seven days of ovarian stimulation using a GnRH antagonist protocol. Hum Reprod. 2009;24(12):3063-72.
18. Fauser BCJM, Mannaerts BMJL, Devroey P, et al. Advances in recombinant DNA technology: corifollitropin alfa, a hybrid molecule with sustained follicle-stimulating activity and reduced injection frequency. Hum Reprod. 2009;15(3):309-21.
19. Stefania Fensore, Marco Di Marzio, Gian Mario Tiboni. Corifollitropin alfa compared to daily FSH in controlled ovarian stimulation for in vitro fertilization: a meta-analysis. Journal of Ovarian Research. 2015; 8:33.
20. Nikolaos P. Polyzos, Michel DeVos, Peter Humaidan, et al. Corifollitropin alfa followed by rFSH in a GnRH antagonist protocol for poor ovarian responder patients: an observational pilot study. Fertil Steril. 2013;99:422-6.
21. Kolibianakis EM, Venetis CA, Bosdou JK, et al. Corifollitropin alfa compared with follitropin beta in poor responders undergoing ICSI: a randomized controlled trial. Hum Reprod. 2015;30:432-40.
22. Robert Boostanfar, Bruce Shapiro, Michael Levy, et al. Large, comparative, randomized double-blind trial confirming non-inferiority of pregnancy rates for corifollitropin alfa compared with recombinant follicle-stimulating hormone in a gonadotropin-releasing hormone antagonist controlled ovarian stimulation protocol in older patients undergoing in vitro fertilization. Fertil Steril. 2015;104:94-103.
23. Luk Rombauts, Cornelis B, Lambalk, Askan Schultze-Mosgau, et al. Intercycle variability of the ovarian response in patients undergoing repeated stimulation with corifollitropin alfa in a gonadotropin-releasing hormone antagonist protocol. Fertil Steril. 2015;104:884-90.
24. Alicia Pérez-Calvo, Francisca Martínez, Christophe Blockeel, et al. Importance of a 5-versus 7-day pill-free interval in a GnRH antagonist protocol using corifollitropin alfa: a prospective cohort study in oocyte donors. Reprod Biomed. Online 2017.
25. Bouloux PM, Handelsman DJ, Jockenhövel F, et al. First human exposure to FSH-CTP in hypogonadotrophic hypogonadal males. Hum Reprod. 2001;16:1592-7.
26. Georg Griesinger, Robert Boostanfar, Keith Gordon, et al. Corifollitropin alfa versus recombinant follicle-stimulating hormone: an individual patient data meta-analysis. Reprod Biomed (Online). 2016;33:56-60.
27. Tamara Lerman, Marion Depenbusch, Askan Schultze-Mosgau, et al. Ovarian response to 150 μg corifollitropin alfa in a GnRH-antagonist multiple-dose protocol: a prospective cohort study. Reprod Biomed (Online). 2017;34:534-40.
28. María Cruz, Pilar Alamá, Manuel Muñoz, et al. Economic impact of ovarian stimulation with corifollitropin alfa versus conventional daily gonadotropins in oocyte donors: a randomized study. Reprod Biomed (Online). 2017;34:605-10.
29. Antonio La Marca, Giovanni D'Ippolito. Ovarian response markers lead to appropriate and effective use of corifollitropin alpha in assisted reproduction. Reprod Biomed (Online). 2014;28:183-90.
30. Nikolaos P Polyzos, Herman Tournaye, Luis Guzman, et al. Predictors of ovarian response in women treated with corifollitropin alfa for in vitro fertilization/ intracytoplasmic sperm injection. Fertil Steril. 2013;100: 430-7.
31. Kolibianakis EM, Kalogeropoulou L, Griesinger G, et al. Among patients treated with FSH and GnRH analogues for in vitro fertilization, is the addition of recombinant LH associated with the probability of live birth? A systematic review and meta-analysis. Hum Reprod (Update). 2007;13(5):445-52.
32. Mochtar MH, Danhof NA, Ayeleke R, et al. Recombinant luteinizing hormone (rLH) and recombinant follicle-stimulating hormone (rFSH) for ovarian stimulation in IVF/ICSI cycles. Cochrane Database of Systematic Reviews 2017, Issue 5. Art. No. CD005070.

33. Pacchiarotti A, Sbracia M, Frega A, et al. Urinary hMG (Meropur) versus recombinant FSH plus recombinant LH (Pergoveris) in IVF: a multicenter, prospective, randomized controlled trial. Fertil Steril. 2010;94(6):2467-9.
34. Koechling W, Plaksin D, Croston GE et al. Comparative pharmacology of a new recombinant FSH expressed by a human cell line. Endocr Connect. 2017;6(5):297-305.
35. Olsson H, Sandström R, Grundemar L. Different pharmacokinetic and pharmacodynamic properties of recombinant follicle-stimulating hormone (rFSH) derived from a human cell line compared with rFSH from a non-human cell line. J Clin Pharm. 2014;54(11):1299-307.
36. Rekovelle Solution for Injection, 12 µg, 36 µg, 72 µg. 4.2 Posology and method of administration. Retrieved on 28 August, 2017. Available from: https://www.medicines.org.uk/emc/medicine/33324
37. Nyboe Andersen A, Nelson SM, Fauser BC, et al. Individualized versus conventional ovarian stimulation for in vitro fertilization: a multicenter, randomized, controlled, assessor-blinded, phase 3 noninferiority trial. Fertil Steril. 2017;107(2):387-96.
38. Low SC, Nunes SL, Bitonti AJ, et al. Oral and pulmonary delivery of FSH-Fc fusion proteins via neonatal Fc receptor-mediated transcytosis. Hum Reprod. 2005;20(7):1805-13.
39. le Cotonnec J-Y, Porchet HC, Beltrami V, et al. Clinical pharmacology of recombinant human follicle-stimulating hormone. II. Single doses and steady state pharmacokinetics. Fertil Steril. 1994;61:679–86.
40. Porchet HC, le Cotonnec J-Y, Canali S, et al. Pharmacokinetics of recombinant human follicle stimulating hormone after intravenous, intramuscular, and subcutaneous administration in monkeys, and comparison with intravenous administration of urinary follicle stimulating hormone. Drug Metab Dispos. 1993;21:144-50.
41. Weinbauer GF, Simoni M, Hutchison JS, et al. Pharmacokinetics and pharmacodynamics of recombinant and urinary human FSH in the male monkey (Macaca fasicularis). J Endocrinol. 1994;141:113-21.
42. Mannaerts BMJL, Novel FSH. LH agonists. In: Filicori M (Ed). Proceedings of the fourth world congress on ovulation induction (Bologna, 27–29 May 2004). Rome: Aracne Proceedings. 2005; 159–72.
43. R. van de Lagemaat1, Timmers CM, Kelder J, et al. Induction of ovulation by a potent, orally active, low molecular weight agonist (Org 43553) of the luteinizing hormone receptor. Hum Reprod. 2009;24(3):640-8.

CHAPTER 27

Infertility Treatment: When to give up?

Rohit V Bhatt, Sonia Golani

Chapter outline

- When to Stop Infertility Treatment?
  - Material and Methods
- When should Friends and Relatives Give Up?
- When should Religious Leaders, Soothsayers and Astrologers Give Up?
- When should Quacks Give Up?
- When should Family Physician Give Up?
- When should Obstetric and Gynecologic Specialist and ART Expert Give Up?
- How many Attempts at Induction of Ovulation before Giving Up?
- When to Give Up after Intrauterine Insemination?
- When to Give Up after Donor Insemination?
- When to Give Up after Microtubal Surgery?
- When to Give Up ART Procedures?
- Reactions of Infertile Couple Who Discontinued Further Treatment
- When to Give Up for Medical Reasons?
- Embryo Donation, Surrogacy and Adoption
- Future Hopes for Infertile Couples

WHEN TO STOP INFERTILITY TREATMENT?

Infertility problem is worldwide. Infertility is not only a medical issue. It has ethical, moral, social, psychological, religious and economic aspect. Recent advances in management of infertility have helped many infertile couples to achieve pregnancy. There is a trend to delay pregnancy to achieve their educational and professional goal. Some women delay pregnancy till they are 35+ years. Thus voluntary infertility gets changed to involuntary infertility. There is general consensus on the issue of timing of initiating treatment of infertility. Three years after normal sexual activity in young women and 6 to 12 months in elderly women is generally accepted for initiating treatment of infertility. However, there is no consensus about the time to give up infertility treatment. In India and in many other countries, there are several players involved in infertility treatment. The players are—friends and relatives of infertile couple, religious leaders, soothsayers, astrologers, etc., family physician, Obstetrician and gynecologist and experts in assisted reproductive technology (ART).

Unfortunately, there is no guideline when each player should give up treatment in favor of the next player. Each player continues with the management too long and this causes delay in achieving pregnancy. If each player understands the limitations and refers to another player in time, many more infertile women may achieve pregnancy. There is no consensus about the time to give up infertility treatment. We scanned Indian medical literature and found that there are hardly any studies from India on this issue. There are some studies describing emotional and social aspects due to infertility.[1,2] There are some studies assessing reactions of infertile couple undergoing treatment.[3-6] There is need for more research in order to reach consensus on this issue. Infertility is still considered a social stigma in India and in many other countries. It is more traumatic for most infertile couples to face the fact that they will never have their own child.

A successor is badly needed for social security. The infertile couple, more so the woman continues treatment for infertility because family circle and society do not label her as infertile. Many infertile women go into depression or commit suicide because they cannot withstand the taunts from in-laws and relatives. Infertile couple, more so the woman is under tremendous social and family pressure. Sometimes, infertility is the reason for divorce. Presence of infertile woman in religious ceremonies is considered a bad woman. Partnership is strained by the fact that one partner persistently reproaches the other with his/her unwillingness to help fulfill their wish for a child. Infertile couple does not seek parenthood with the same intensity. Male is more ambivalent and undergoes treatment only to satisfy his wife. The male partner does not suffer as much social pressure as his wife.

In India and in many other cultures, many players are involved in the treatment of infertility. These players are:
- Friends and relatives of infertile couple
- Religious leaders, soothsayers, astrologers
- Quacks
- Family physician
- Obstetrician and gynecologist
- Infertility expert.

The million dollar question is "who decides when each player should give up infertility treatment?" Since, several players are involved, we should put a time limit for giving up treatment in favor of expert person (next in hierarchy). Each player must know when to give up efforts in time so that infertile couple does not suffer. If each player continues the efforts too long, the infertile couple suffers. Sometimes timely reference to other player may help the infertile couple. The players should not consider commercial reasons for continuing the treatment for long. Therefore, by the time infertile couple has failed with standard simple procedure, the woman is already 35+ years. This delay causes problem in conceiving because of the aging ovary and diminishing sperm capacity. Till recently, healthcare providers were satisfied by knowing the sperm count and motility index. Now more information is available about sperm quality. Many morphological and chromosomal changes take place in sperm quality with advancing age, which makes it difficult to penetrate ovum. Many morphological and chromosomal changes take place in sperm and ovum quality with advancing age, which makes it difficult for the sperm, to penetrate the ovum. We used to look to the ova size and time of rupture. Now recent studies have shown that there is more to ova quality other than the size.

Material and Methods

I sent a questionnaire to 200 members of medical fraternity, mostly from India but about 15 from overseas. There were 20 family physicians, 145 obstetrics and gynecology doctors and 35 ART specialists. I received reply from 180 doctors (Table 27.1). I also analyzed my personal series of 94 infertile couples who discontinued treatment for infertility. Some of them came to me before deciding to give up treatment. This study summarizes current views of medical fraternity and infertile couple. The following questions were asked to medical fraternity:
1. When to stop treatment for infertility? Who should decide?—Infertile couple or doctor or both?
2. Indications for primary giving up without initiating treatment

Table 27.1: When to stop infertility treatment: What experts think?

Procedure	Average	Range
Induction of ovulation	4–6 attempts with each regime	12–16 attempts
IUI	4–6 attempts	3–8 attempts
Donor insemination	4 attempts	3–10 attempts
Tubal surgery	6–12 months'	6–24 months
ART	4–6	4 to till patient says No
Adoption	70%	
Surrogacy	30%	

(IUI: intracuterine insemination; ART: assisted reproduction tehnology).

- Absent uterus/ovary, azoospermia, genital tuberculosis
- Age 45+, advance medical disease.

3. When will you give up after initiating treatment in following cases?
    - After how many failed induction of ovulation?
    - After how many unsuccessful IUI?
    - After how many attempts with AID?
    - How long you would wait after tubal microsurgery?
    - How many attempts should be made with ART?
    - Couples inability to bear the cost
    - Development of life-threatening disease.

The general consensus was that it is the prerogative of the infertile couple to decide when to stop infertility treatment. Medical fraternity can suggest about poor chances but the final decision is of the infertile couple. Twenty percent believe that they will give up and advise to seek second opinion if there was no success in two years. Fifteen percent (mainly ART experts) felt that they would never accept defeat and persist with treatment till infertile couples decide to discontinue the efforts. The infertility experts feel that it is impossible to say that the woman will not conceive. They site following reasons.

- Age at menopause is on the increase
- There are documented cases of women conceiving after 50 years of age
- Miracles do occur. Women do conceive when least expected
- Some women do conceive after adoption
- Advising couple to stop trying for conception may cause depression
- If a woman conceives when doctors have given up hope, doctor may cut a sorry figure. Woman may lose faith in the doctor.

I feel that the healthcare provider must give a balanced picture about the success/failure of the procedure. If the healthcare provider is convinced that success is unlikely, he/she should not hesitate in informing the couple.

Sometimes the infertile couple spends a fortune in the treatment and still conception has not taken place. Infertile couple usually the wife, goes into depression and sometimes even ends her life.

WHEN SHOULD FRIENDS AND RELATIVES GIVE UP?

In Indian and many other societies, friends and relatives guide the infertile couple about methods that may help in conception. Couple follows the advice because it is free. This practice is more common in rural settings because healthcare facilities are scarce. Unfortunately even educated couples in urban areas are also guided by the advice of friends and relatives. Most of the time, the advice is based on hearsay or anecdotal experiences. The advice consists of various postures and timing of coitus, consumption of some food articles, use of various herbal preparations, visits to some temples or religious places, etc. (Figs. 27.1A to C). Sometimes the infertile couple continues following the instructions for a long time and then repents for the delay in seeking medical help. It would be proper

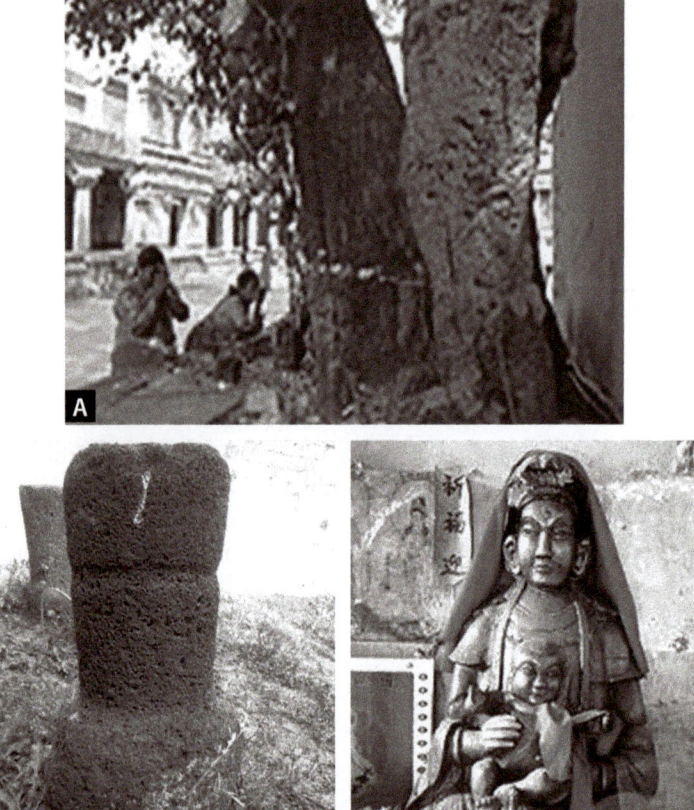

Figs. 27.1A to C: Goddess of infertility (A); Penis temple (B); Mating with Mother Earth (C).

for friends and relatives to advise them to consult healthcare provider if there is no conception in one year after leading normal sex life without contraception. If the woman is already 30 years +, it is better that they straight away refer to healthcare provider.

WHEN SHOULD RELIGIOUS LEADERS, SOOTHSAYERS AND ASTROLOGERS GIVE UP?

There are lots of myths, misconceptions beliefs about fertility in every society. Fertility issue is high jacked by religious leaders, astrologers and soothsayers. The religious leaders advise various rituals, ceremonies and *Gaudan* (donation of a cow). They charge hefty fee for such rituals and ceremonies. If a woman has spontaneous pregnancy during this ritual, they claim the credit. It is a known fact that spontaneous pregnancy does occur when the woman is following any treatment (though pregnancy may not be because of their efforts). Astrology is a science. We do not know how much influence it can have in the process of conception. It is difficult to accept how astrology can help if the fallopian tubes are blocked or the husband has no sperms. They must realize that technology is available to assess factors necessary for conception.

It is likely that in 'unexplained infertility' conception is possible because of release of tension, anxiety or tender loving care (TLC). It is true healthcare providers may cause lot of anxiety and depression in infertile couple because of invasive nature of the modality of treatment and need for frequent visits. Religious leaders and astrologers do not have to do any invasive procedures. They may be able to give more time and confidence. It would be wise for these people to restrict their treatment to cases of 'unexplained' infertility. They should give up treatment if there is no success in 1-2 years in young women and 4-6 months in older women.

WHEN SHOULD QUACKS GIVE UP?

Ideally, the quacks should not be allowed to practice. The quacks flourish because their services are cheap, noninvasive and simple to follow (Fig. 27.2). Quacks flourish all over the world but much more so in India. The business of quacks thrives because most people are ignorant, gullible and god fearing. The quacks succeed in impressing the infertile couple by rituals and religious ceremonies and false claims by advertisements. Some infertile couples, if they conceive, they are told by the quacks to announce the success in local papers and magazines. Unlike the medical person, quacks have plenty of time to gain confidence of their clients. It is difficult to challenge these quacks in the court of law. Women do conceive when they are undergoing treatment from quacks. But this pregnancy is spontaneous and unrelated to their treatment. Ideally, quacks should not be allowed to practice. Education to the community is the only way out. Unfortunately, quacks are rarely challenged in the courts by clients. Quacks flourish in India because government agencies are soft in taking action.

WHEN SHOULD FAMILY PHYSICIAN GIVE UP?

Our survey showed that there are two types of family physicians. One group does not treat cases of infertility but advise where and to whom they should go. The second groups of family physicians, mostly ladies, do offer treatment. They order semen examination, ultrasound to monitor follicular growth and get hysterosalpingography done. They even advise drugs for ovulation. Rarely they do intrauterine insemination (IUI). This is acceptable because it is easy for infertile couple to have access to family physician.

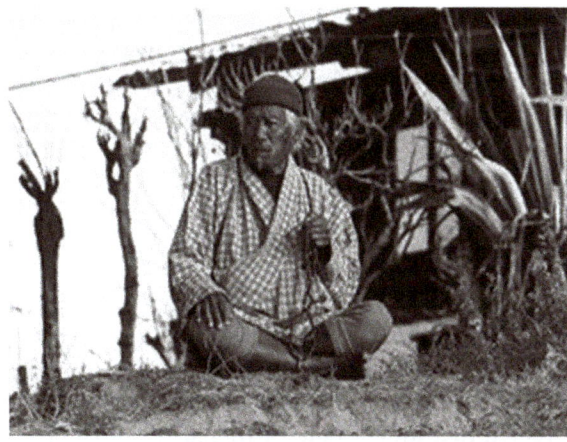

Fig. 27.2: Quacks offering herbs for infertility.

It is cheap. Semen examination, ultrasound and hysterosalpingography are done by experts. The family physician only evaluates. When should family physician give up and refer the infertile couple to gynecologist or infertility expert? It may be difficult to put time limit. However, if the young woman does not conceive after three to four attempts, the family physician should refer the case to specialist. If the woman is 35 years+, it is advisable that the case is referred to specialist straight away

WHEN SHOULD OBSTETRIC AND GYNECOLOGIC SPECIALIST AND ART EXPERT GIVE UP?

We asked questions mentioned earlier to Obstetric and Gynecologic and ART experts from India and a few from overseas. There is consensus to most of the questions. However, there are differences on the range. Fifteen percent of ART experts said they would never give up. Newer technologies are appearing on the horizon and so we must continue to try till the infertile couple wants to call it a day. There was agreement to give up when there is absent uterus. Though most agreed to give up if ovaries are absent. Thirty percent thought that one may consider ovum donation from a volunteer. Ovarian transplant was suggested by 12% in my study. Surrogacy can be another option. There was some agreement among experts about azoospermia. Eighty percent said they would offer donor insemination. Twenty percent of ART experts said they would like to offer sperm retrieval from testes or epidydimis before suggesting donor insemination.

In genital tuberculosis, there was agreement to advise conception if the menstrual cycles and endometrial reaction is normal and she is ovulating. They would give up only if she is amenorrheic or endometrial reaction is poor. In women who are 45 years+ large majority of experts felt that they would advise caution and explain probable chances of conception. If the couple wants to try for conception, they would help the couple. If the woman is suffering from medical condition that would place her life at risk, they would advise to give up. Most ART experts said that if either spouse is suffering from advance medical condition, they would offer cryopreservation of sperms, ovum or embryo. It is useful when chemotherapy or radiotherapy is needed for the medical condition. Embryo donation/adoption is another alternative in such condition.

HOW MANY ATTEMPTS AT INDUCTION OF OVULATION BEFORE GIVING UP?

It is debatable when to call induction of ovulation as failure? There are several protocols for induction of ovulation. Induction of ovulation may not always result in pregnancy. The ovulation rate with clomiphene is 70% but only 30–35% conceive. Pravin Mhatre (personal communication) from Mumbai has achieved some good results with ovarian transplant. The initial method is usually clomiphene or letrazole. If this fails, combination of pituitary hormones (FSH, LH) is advised. Finally Gonadotropin-relusing hormone (GnRH) analogs are advised. Normally 4–6 attempts are made with each method before giving up. Variation of dose of each method is also taken into consideration. Clomiphene dose is increased from 50 mg to 150 mg before changing to another method. Even with pituitary hormones dose variations are common. One of my patients had a successful ovulation after 31 injections of FSH taken on her own without medical guidance. Even with GnRH analogs, various dose schedules are tried with success. Therefore, it is difficult for the clinician to decide when to give up. Pituitary hormones and GnRH analogs being expensive, most patients and clinicians would like to give up after 4 to 6 efforts.

WHEN TO GIVE UP AFTER INTRAUTERINE INSEMINATION?

In our study, 34% clinicians agreed to give up after 3-4 attempts. However, 66% clinicians said they would try 6-8 times. There are several points for consideration. Some clinicians rely on pathologist to prepare the semen sample for IUI. Others prepare the sample themselves. When the sample is prepared by the pathologist, there is a time lag between preparation and introduction in the uterus. It is suggested that IUI should be performed within 30 minutes after preparation. The clinician may feel that semen sample for IUI was not correctly prepared or there was delay in performing IUI after the sample was prepared. This doubt results in more attempts at IUI by the clinician. It is better IUI preparation is done in the gynecologist office so that IUI can be done in time.

WHEN TO GIVE UP AFTER DONOR INSEMINATION?

Donor insemination (AID) has raised several doubts. There is fear of transmission of HIV/hepatitis virus if proper screening is not done. There are several other objections to donor insemination. We are focusing on the issue of number of attempts. In our study the opinion ranged between 3 and 10 attempts with an average of 4 attempts.

WHEN TO GIVE UP AFTER MICROTUBAL SURGERY?

It is assumed that only tubal factor is the cause of infertility. Our study showed that 30% clinicians believed that 2 years is the maximum period before giving up. Whereas 70% felt that 6-12 months are adequate. The study showed that except in cases of tubal reversal procedures after tube ligation, results of IVF are better than tubal surgery. Current trend is to go for IVF when tubes are diseased.

WHEN TO GIVE UP ART PROCEDURES?

Though ART has become an established and increasingly successful form of treatment, it does not guarantee a successful outcome. The Human Fertilization and Embryology Authority (HFEA) in its 9th annual report shows improvement in live birth rate from 14% in 1991-92 to 22% in 2000-2001 for IVF treatment in UK.[8] It is important to identify factors that influence the decision to discontinue ART treatment. The decision not to pursue ART after one or more unsuccessful attempts is an important but difficult decision for the infertile couple. Many couples embarking on ART programs are optimistic with unrealistically high expectations.[9] The first cycle of IVF treatment is statistically the most successful attempt but multiple attempts improve the probability of achieving pregnancy. The estimated cumulative conception rate after four attempts has ranged from 54%[10] to 75%.[3.] Some infertile couples feel that while on treatment, they were frequently given false hopes of success. There are others who give up because of depression resulting from anxiety and tension. The dropout rate in ART is high in all over the world.[11] The reason for high dropout rate are lack of state funding, psychological stress and poor outcome. Olivius[6] from Sweden report dropout rate of 54% with 26% of couples discontinuing treatment for psychological reasons though state funding was available. In Netherlands, where state funding is available for up to three attempts, the dropout rate after three cycles was 62%. Hammerberg[12] reported from Australia, that mean number of cycles in their population was 3 even though funding was available for up to six cycles indicating that lack of funding is not the sole reason for discontinuation of IVF treatment. Rajkhowa[7] states, "Health care providers involved in ART treatment need to be more aware of the psychological stress associated with repeated attempts at

IVF." Boivin et al.[2] has shown that both male and female partners give evidence of stress while undergoing IVF treatment. Laffont[1] has shown that aspiration and waiting to become pregnant can be more stressful than treatment itself. ART has flourished mainly in private sector. In public sector, it is not routinely offered because such facilities are not available in most medical colleges. Assisted reproductive technology (ART) has many subgroups, to name a few, intracytoplasmic sperm injection (ICSI), subzonal insemination (SUZI), partial zona dissection (PZD) and embryo hatching are some of the subgroups. The technology is expanding very fast. The ART experts feel that 4-6 attempts should be tried before calling it a day. This applies to all ART procedures such as ICSI and other similar procedures. There are some ART experts who believe that efforts must be continued till the patient is willing. Sadhana Desai[13] feels that ART is an expensive and high tech procedure with limited success of 15-25% takes home baby rate per cycle. The success rate after IVF is likely to improve with newer technology. Desai has rightly stressed that infertile couple is more concerned with 'take home baby rate' rather than 'pregnancy rate'. There are some infertile couples who switch to another expert who would like to try more attempts at ART. The main reason why couple discontinues is combination of finance and psychosomatic problems. In our study, 85% of experts try for 3-4 cycles whereas 15% feel that they would make more attempts if, the couple is agreeable.

REACTIONS OF INFERTILE COUPLE WHO DISCONTINUED FURTHER TREATMENT

We analyzed 92 infertile couples who decided to call it a day and discontinue further treatment. Some of these couples were under our treatment from the beginning. Others came to us finally before giving up treatment. Table 27.2 gives reasons while the couple decided to discontinue treatment. Large majority (64.8%) discontinued treatment because they could not afford ART. Twelve women gave up after one unsuccessful attempt at IVF. Ten women gave up because husband was uncooperative. Eight had no success after donor insemination. Ovulation could not be induced in 9 women in spite of drugs.

Eleven couples gave up after failed tubal surgery. Thirty women gave up because of emotional stress. Twenty-two couples finally accepted adoption. The male reactions showed insight into male psychology. We give some reactions in couples on words. They were disturbed because they were "asked to masturbate under unaccustomed condition". "The support staff at the clinic was impersonal and at times rude". "The procedures are very stressful". "Repeated clinic visits affect family and professional life". "Gave up because of money problem". "Poor support system when treatment fails" "Doctors have less time to listen to our queries".

Table 27.2: Reaction of unsuccessful infertile couples on infertility treatment (Total 94 couples).

Reaction	Number
Discontinued because could not afford ART	61
Discontinued after 1 attempt at ART	12
Husband uncooperative	10
Failed donor insemination	8
Failed induction of ovulation	7
No success after tubal surgery	12
Accepted adoption	22
Decided for surrogacy	5
Discontinued because of emotional stress	30

Total number. is more than number of patients because some patients have more than one reason for discontinuing treatment.
(ART: assisted reproductive technology)

It appears that infertile couples need lot of emotional support when treatment fails. All infertility clinics must have psychiatric and social support facility.

WHEN TO GIVE UP FOR MEDICAL REASONS?

This is a debatable issue. There may be genuine differences of opinion among clinicians, whether women should be allowed to conceive. This issue is not restricted to infertile woman only. It applies to all women who wish to conceive. There is a general agreement that women with advance heart, liver or kidney disease or advance cancer should not be advised conception. Disease considered untreatable today may be treatable in future. Therefore, the restrictions on conception are relative. In auto-immune disease, it is felt that conception should be permitted when woman is in remission phase. Surrogacy/Adoption are other alternatives.

EMBRYO DONATION, SURROGACY AND ADOPTION

When all attempts at conception fail, surrogacy, embryo donation or Adoption are available at present. Many eggs/embryos are produced during IVF cycles. The extra embryos are cryo-preserved. Such embryos are available for use if the woman permits. In USA where embryo adoption is a decade old, over 1000 babies have been born using embryo donation. Malpani from Mumbai perform three to four embryo adoption every month (personal communication). Adopting an embryo allows infertile woman to experience motherhood, complete with labor pains as against rearing an adopted child, says Indira Hinduja from Mumbai. It must be remembered that though the infertile woman carries through pregnancy and delivers the child, it does not genetically belong to her because the embryo belongs to other couple. Embryo donation is not cheap. In USA it may cost 10,000 US dollars (4.5 lac rupees).

Surrogacy has been in practice since biblical times. Even then it is the cause for great moral, ethical and legal debates. It is defined, "when embryo of infertile couple is placed in the womb of another woman". The woman who bears the pregnancy is called surrogate mother. The surrogate mother is given money for carrying the pregnancy. Surrogacy has remained controversial though it is accepted in UK, parts of USA, Australia and Israel. It is not practiced in most European countries. Islam, Jews and Buddhist forbid surrogacy. It is legal in India but problems arise when the child is to be taken in other countries. Surrogacy could be 'Traditional' or 'Gestational'. Traditional surrogacy is done via artificial insemination with the surrogate using her egg and another man's sperm. Gestational surrogacy is done via IVF, where fertilized eggs from another woman are implanted into the surrogate's uterus. Lot of paper work is necessary for surrogacy. Those interested may refer to review article on surrogacy by Kamini Rao.[14] Simplified details about surrogacy are given by Dr Nayana Patel in her book, 'Last Ray of Hope'.[15] Now In India, parliament is planning to pass a bill to prohibit commercial surrogacy. The bill is very much debated in India. Let us wait and watch whether the bill is passed.

Adoption is another option for infertile couple when all treatment fails. Adoption has an advantage in giving a choice to the infertile couple. The child is tested for health and other diseases. Stress is much reduced in those couple who go for adoption as compared to those who remain childless. The problem is there are not enough children available for adoption and the couple has to wait for long time before child can be adopted. Adoption is permitted only in Hindus. Other communities cannot adopt a child but can be Caretakers. Our survey shows that 70% of obstetricians and gynecologists favor Adoption. Surrogacy is favored by 30%.

FUTURE HOPES FOR INFERTILE COUPLES

Surrogacy, embryo adoption or adoption of fully developed child is available at present.

The way technology is expanding, infertility may be the issue of the past. Procedures for the investigation of female infertility are becoming less invasive and more accurate. The therapies for infertility are becoming more effective. In future, technology may permit every infertile woman to conceive. Some possibilities are summarized below.

Technology is available to retrieve sperms from testes or seminal vesicles and allow them to mature in *in vitro*. These sperms may be capable of fertilizing the ovum.

The role of male may be unnecessary. Stem cell technology may create sperms from the woman herself. Thus male involvement may not be needed.

Egg donation is available for women who have no ovaries or are unable to ovulate. Ovarian transplant may allow a woman with absent ovaries to conceive. Similarly, it may be possible in future to transplant the human uterus. First uterine transplant surgery is done in Sweden. It is planned to do uterine transplant in India also. Japanese scientists have developed technology to have fetus grow outside the body in artificial womb in animal model. In future it may be possible for human fetus to develop outside the body. Reproductive technology will certainly expand and make conception possible for more infertile women. However, there is need to focus attention of psycho-social issues due to ART. It would be nice if all ART centers develop support group in their clinic to address to such problems.

REFERENCES

1. Laffont I, Edelman RJ. Psychological aspects of IVF. J Psychosomobstet Gynecol. 2001;15:85-92.
2. Boivin J, Tafekman JE. Stress level across stages of IVF. Fertil Steril. 1995;64:802-10.
3. Sharma V, Alghar U, Rajkhowa M. Factors affecting cumulative conception rate and discontinuation of IVF treatment. Fertil Steril. 2002;78:40-6.
4. Smeenk JM, Verhaak CM. Reasons for drop out in ART program. Fertil Steril. 2004;81:262-8.
5. Schroder AK, Katalinik A. Cumulative dropout rate in German IVF program. Reprod Biomed on line. 2004;8:600-6.
6. Olivius C, Friden B, Brog G. Why do couples discontinue? Fertil. Steril. 2004;81:258-61.
7. Rajakhowa M, McConnel A, Thomas G. Reasons for discontinuation of IVF treatment. Hum Reprod. 2006;21:358-63.
8. Human Fertilization & Embryology Authority 9th Annual Report 2000 http.//www.hfea.gov.uk
9. Templeton A, Morris JK, Parshi W. Factors affecting outcome of IVF treatment. Lancet 1996;348:1402-6.
10. Tan SL, Rayston P, Campbell S. Cumulative conception rates after IVF. Lancet 1992;339:1390-3.
11. Land JA, Courtar AD. Patient drop out in ART treatment. Fertil Steril. 1997;68:278-81.
12. Hammerberg K, Astbury S. Baker HW Women experience with IVF. Hum Reprod. 2001;16:374-83.
13. Desai Sadhana, Mangoli V. Current concepts in ART Recent Advances in Obst. Gyn. Vol.2. S. Dasgupta Ed. Jaypee Brothers Medical Publishers, New Delhi. 1996;page 99.
14. Rao Kamini. Surrogacy in India. Demystifying Obst Gyn. Mini Sood. Ed. AITBS, Delhi 2006;page 54.
15. Nayana Patel, Karshan Bhandarka. The Last Ray of Hope-surrogate mother Anand surrogate Trust 2009.

CHAPTER 28

The ART Bill: Its Implications

Manish Banker, Pravin Patel, Arati Gupte-Shah

Chapter outline

- Setting Up an ART Clinic
  - Primary (Level 1) Infertility Care Units
  - Secondary (Level 2) Infertility Care Units
  - Tertiary (Level 3) Infertility Care Units
- Requirements of an ART Clinic
  - Space
  - The Nonsterile Area
  - The Sterile Area
  - Staff
- Registration and Accreditation
  - Which Clinics should be Registered?
  - Grant of Registration
- Information and Counseling of Patients
- Confidentiality and Consent
  - Penalties

INTRODUCTION

With the development of new techniques and procedures to treat infertility, the perceptions and concerns of the medical fraternity as well as the public have also evolved. Technology that would have been relegated to science fiction a mere 30 years ago is now used routinely at every assisted reproductive technology (ART) center. In the 21st century we have gained the means to not only regulate growth but actually create life.

But with increase of invasiveness and ethical complexity in these current techniques the scope for mismanagement and unethical actions has also increased. Thus, the need for strict guidelines and an ethical approach to safe practices has rapidly emerged.

At present, there is no official legislation for ART practices in India. The ICMR guidelines are a step in that direction.

SETTING UP AN ART CLINIC

Infertility clinics have been divided into 3 levels depending on their level of expertise (Table 28.1).

Primary (Level 1) Infertility Care Units

These are clinics where preliminary investigations are carried out and the type and cause of infertility diagnosed. They are qualified to carry out all types of infertility treatment that does not require handling of sperm, egg or embryo outside the body. This type of unit can be a doctor's consulting room or a general hospital. The gynecologist in-charge of this type of clinic should have an appropriate postgraduate degree or diploma. Level 1 clinics do not require registration.

Table 28.1: Levels of infertility clinics.

Level 1
- Investigation into the cause of infertility by diligent history taking, physical examination and simple semen analysis
- Treatment of minor anatomical defects
- Confirmation (by diagnostic laparoscopy) and treatment of mild endometriosis
- Induction of ovulation with clomiphene citrate. (Gonadotropins should not be used at primary level)
- Treatment of mild endocrine disorders like thyroid or hyperprolactinemia
- Treatment of oligozoospermia
- Detection and treatment of reproductive tract infections
- Conservative surgery through a laparoscope, hysteroscope or via laparotomy
- Combined medical-surgical therapy by a coordinated team, as in endometriosis
- Assessment of follicular growth and ovulation by serial ultrasonography
- Appropriate referral to higher level clinics

Level 2
- Facilities for investigations:
  - Immunological tests for infertility
  - Sperm function tests
  - Assessment of follicular growth and ovulation by serial TVS
  - Hysteroscopy, laparoscopy and transvaginal sonography
- Facilities for treatment:
  - Facilities for semen preparation and IUI
  - Provision for semen collection in men with functional erectile and ejaculatory problems (use of vibrator or electroejaculator)
  - Provision for extended treatment of infertility except oocyte handling, IVF, ICSI and similar techniques

Level 3

Diagnostic procedures for male infertility:
- Endocrine assays
- Detailed tests for sperm function and integrity
- Assessment of cell contaminants, debris and infection
- Assessment of seminal plasma for viscosity, thinness and blood contamination and biochemical constituents
- Karyotyping

Diagnostic procedures for female infertility:
- Endocrine assays
- Transvaginal sonography
- Karyotyping

Therapeutic procedures:
- Induction of ovulation using gonadotropins, a GnRH agonist and antagonist, and other adjuvants.
- All types of ART including ICSI
- Procedures for IUI using split or pooled ejaculate or using sperm recovered from postcoital specimen of urine in case of retrograde ejaculation
- Cryopreservation of gametes and embryos

Secondary (Level 2) Infertility Care Units

These units have infrastructure for further in-depth investigation and extended treatment of infertility, except where oocytes are handled outside the body. They are to have facilities for artificial insemination and intrauterine insemination using husband's semen as well as donor semen.

Clinics from this level onwards are required to register.

Tertiary (Level 3) Infertility Care Units

These units should perform diagnostic and therapeutic functions at the highest level of specialization with the best of facilities, and research (except on human embryos).

REQUIREMENTS OF AN ART CLINIC

Space

A well-designed ART clinic of Level 2 or Level 3 should have a nonsterile and a strictly sterile area. Some of the spaces could be combined as long as such a step does not compromise the quality of service. For Level 1 clinics, a strictly sterile area in not required. The Guidelines do not specify the minimum areas required for each purpose, but specially designed spaces are mandatory, as follows.

The Nonsterile Area

- A reception and waiting room for patients.
- *A room with privacy*: A room with privacy for interviewing and examining male and female partners independently is essential. The room must be equipped with an examination table and gynecological instruments, an appropriate ultrasonographic machine with a probe for transvaginal examination of the female and examination of the male reproductive tract.
- A general-purpose clinical laboratory.
- *Store room*: Facilities must be available for storing sterile (media, needles, catheters, Petri dishes and such items) and nonsterile material under refrigerated and nonrefrigerated conditions as appropriate.
- *Record room*: Recordkeeping must be computerized as far as possible so that data is easily accessible.
- Autoclave room.
- Steps for vermin proofing.
- Semen collection room should be located in a secluded area close to the laboratory. This room must have a washbasin with availability of soap and clean towels. The room must also have a toilet and must not be used for any other purpose.
- *Semen processing laboratory*: There must be a separate room with a laminar air flow for semen processing, preferably close to the semen collection room. This laboratory must also have facilities for microscopic examination of postcoital test smears. Care must be taken for the safe disposal of biological waste and other materials (syringes, glass slides, etc.).
- *Clean room for IUI*: This should be a separate area/room with an appropriate table for IUI.
- Back-up power supply.

The Sterile Area

Entry to the sterile area must be strictly controlled by an anteroom for changing footwear, area for changing into sterile garments and a scrub-station. The sterile area must be airconditioned where fresh air filtered through an approved and appropriate filter system is circulated at an ambient temperature.

1. *The operation theater:* This must be well-equipped with facilities for carrying out surgical endoscopy and transvaginal

ovum pick-up as well as for emergency resuscitative procedures.
2. *Room for intrauterine transfer of embryo*: This room must be a sterile area having an examination table on which the patient can be placed for carrying out the procedure and rest undisturbed for a period of time.
3. *The embryology laboratory complex*: The embryology laboratory must have facilities for the control of temperature and humidity and regular flow of filtered air. Walls and floors must be composed of materials that can be easily washed and disinfected.

The embryology laboratory must have the following:
- A laminar flow bench with a thermostatically controlled heating plate
- A stereo microscope
- A routine high-powered binocular light microscope
- A 'high resolution' inverted microscope with phase contrast or Hoffman optics, preferably with facilities for video recording
- A micromanipulator (if ICSI is done)
- A CO_2 incubator, preferably with a back up
- A hot air oven
- A laboratory centrifuge
- Equipment for freezing embryos in a programmed manner
- Liquid nitrogen cans
- A refrigerator.

Also,
- Appropriate steps for the correct identification of gametes and embryos
- Correct and rigorous labeling
- Immediate disposal of used pipettes and other disposables
- Maintenance of a daily logbook to record all the day's activities including performance of equipment.

4. *Ancillary laboratory facilities*: ART clinics can send certain investigations to specialty laboratories, as long as they are located in the neighborhood. These can be used for:
   - Hormone and other assays
   - Microbiology and histopathology.
5. *Laboratory maintenance*:
- All sterile areas to be checked periodically for microbial contamination using standard techniques. Records of such checks to be maintained.
- Log books to maintain records of temperature, carbon dioxide content and humidity of incubators and manometer readings of laminar air flow.
- Calibration of all instruments periodically.
- Culture media and disposable plastic wares to be procured from reliable sources, and confirmed to be nontoxic.
- Testing of each batch of culture media for sterility, endotoxins, osmolality and pH.

Staff

The practice of ART requires a well-orchestrated teamwork between the gynecologist, the andrologist and the clinical embryologist supported by a counselor and a program coordinator/director. The following staff requirements would be mandatory for Level 2 and Level 3 clinics.

Gynecologist

Should have a postgraduate diploma or degree in gynecology, having experience in diagnosis and treatment of infertility, with knowledge of the clinical aspects of reproductive endocrinology, and skills in gynecological ultrasonography. He/she must also be well versed in the pharmacology of hormone action. For a Level 3 clinic, the gynecologist must also have the expertise of ovum pick-up and embryo transfer.

Clinical Embryologist

He/she must be knowledgeable in mammalian embryology, reproductive endocrinology, genetics, molecular biology, biochemistry, microbiology and *in vitro* culture techniques. The biologist must also be familiar with ART. He/she must be either a medical graduate or have a postgraduate degree or a doctorate in an appropriate area of life sciences. An embryologist must not be associated with more than two centers.

Andrologist

Must have knowledge of the occupational hazards, infections and fever that cause reversible or irreversible forms of infertility, and knowledge of ultrasonographic or vasographic studies. He/she should be able to interpret the fertility status of the male from the result of semen analysis. He/she should be familiar with the surgical procedures available for correcting an anatomical defect in the reproductive system and with procedures for sperm extraction like testicular/epididymal sperm extraction (TESE), percutaneous epididymal sperm aspiration (PESA) and micro epididymal sperm aspiration (MESA).

Counselor

This should be a person who has at least a degree (preferably a postgraduate degree) in social sciences, psychology, life sciences or medicine, and a good knowledge of the various causes of infertility and its social and gender implications, and the possibilities offered by the various treatment modalities. He/she should have a working knowledge of the psychological stress that would be experienced by potential patients, and should be able to counsel them to assuage their fears and anxiety.

An andrologist or counselor can work for more than one clinic, as long as they are able to handle the workload and their quality of work is not compromised.

Program Coordinator/Director

He/she should be a senior person who has had considerable experience in all aspects of ART. He should have a postgraduate degree in an appropriate medical or biological science and should also have a reasonable experience of ART. He/she should be able to coordinate the activities of the rest of the team and take care of staff administrative matters, stock keeping, finance, maintenance of patient records, statutory requirements, and public relations.

REGISTRATION AND ACCREDITATION

The central government has proposed the establishment of a national advisory board as well as state boards to exercise the jurisdiction and powers and perform the functions and duties laid down in the guidelines.

Which Clinics should be Registered?

Clinics involved in any one of the following activities should be regulated, registered and supervised by the registration authority:

1. Any treatment involving the use of gametes which have been donated or collected or processed *in vitro, except for* AIH, and for IUI by Level 1A clinics who will not process the gametes themselves.
2. Any infertility treatment that involves the use and creation of embryos outside the body.
3. The processing or/and storage of gametes or embryos.
4. Research on human embryos.

Level 1 clinics do not require registration. For Levels 2 and 3 clinics, registration is mandatory.

All ART clinics that are already operative when this Act comes into force, will receive a temporary registration within 6 months and a permanent registration within 18 months. Those clinics that were set-up before the guidelines were implemented will have 18 months to change over to the new guidelines.

Grant of Registration

If the registration authority (RA) is satisfied that all the criteria laid down in the rules have been met, and after inspection of the premises, it can grant a registration for a term of 3 years.

Within one month the RA will report the registration to the state board, which maintains records of all registrations.

Certificate of Registration

This will be issued by the RA, in duplicate. One copy must be displayed in a prominent location in the clinic.

The certificate is considered nontransferable. In case a clinic changes ownership, both copies of the certificate have to be returned to the RA, and the new owner should apply separately for a registration.

Renewal, Suspension or Revocation of Registration

Renewal can be obtained by applying to the RA before the date of expiry of the previous registration.

If the RA feels at any time that the terms and conditions of the rules are not being met, it could suspend the registration. The owner of the clinic may then have to furnish whatever documents the RA demands for inspection. If the evidence presented is not satisfactory, the RA has the right to revoke the registration after having first heard the arguments of the applicant.

INFORMATION AND COUNSELING OF PATIENTS

Patients should be informed about:
- The basis, limitations and possible outcome of the treatment proposed, variations in its effectiveness over time, success rates and recommended treatments. This data should be available as a printed document with references.
- The possible side-effects and risk of treatment to the woman as well as the resulting child, including risks associated with multiple pregnancy.
- The techniques involved, including the possible deterioration of gametes or embryos associated with storage, and possible pain and discomfort.
- The cost (with suitable break-up) of the proposed treatment, as well as any alternative treatment that may be required.
- Transparency should be maintained with regards to costs as well as success rates of all procedures.
- The couple should be made aware of the rights of a child born through embryo donation or surrogacy.
- All registered clinics should have procedures for acknowledging and investigating complaints.

CONFIDENTIALITY AND CONSENT

Any information about clients and donors must be kept confidential. No information about the treatment of couples provided may be disclosed to anyone other than the accreditation authority or persons covered by the registration, except with the consent of the person to whom the information relates, or in a medical emergency, or a court order. It is the person's right to decide what information will be passed on and to whom. The ICMR guidelines also provide an 'Oath of Secrecy', to be signed by every member/staff of an ART clinic which prohibits them from disclosing any information pertaining to the patient, donor or surrogate. Violation of this declaration makes the person liable to prosecution.

Consent forms an important first step for all ART procedures. The ICMR guidelines have formulated specific consent forms for different ART procedures. Consent forms should be signed by both the patient and the spouse before undergoing any treatment.

Penalties

Prenatal sex determination, sale of embryos for research, monetary dealings with donors or surrogates, or any other contraventions of the provisions specified in the guidelines are all considered cognizable and punishable offences, with imprisonment up to 3 to 5 years as well as a fine specified by the court.

There is a special clause for offences committed by companies which states that if an offence has been proved to be committed by a corporate body or firm, every person working in that organization, as well as the organization itself, can be deemed guilty of the offence.

Many prominent members of the infertility community are lobbying to convert these guidelines into an Act of Parliament. Safe and ethical practice is the goal for the future, and compliance will make for better success rates and happier patients.

INDEX

Page numbers followed by *f* refer to figure, *fc* refer to flowchart, and *t* refer to table

A

Abdomen 287
Abdominal pregnancy 291, 300
    treatment 300
Abstinence, short period of 20
Acanthosis nigricans 66
Accessory gland
    infection 20
    inflammation 20
Acne 66
Acquired immunodeficiency
    syndrome 4
Acrosome reaction 21, 182
    assessment of 38
    test 38
Actinomycin D 292
Adamyan classification 126
Adenomas, pituitary 97
Adnexal mass 271
Adnexectomy 273
Agenesis 139
Air purification system 252, 253*f*
Alloimmune factors 30
Amenorrhea 97, 102, 150, 159
American College of Obstetricians
    and Gynecologists 31, 69
American Fertility Society
    Classification 123
American Society for Reproductive
    Medicine 64, 126, 172, 193
Amino acid 9, 93, 241, 242, 262
    metabolism 242
Anastrozole 57, 153
    pharmacodynamics 153
Ancillary laboratory facilities 332
Androgenic alopecia 66
Androgens 10, 110
Anemia 159
Antagonist ganirelix 306
Antibiotic therapy 188
Anti-corifollitropin alfa antibodies
    311

Antifibrotic drugs 155
Antiglobulin reaction, mixed 202
Anti-Mullerian hormone 8, 65, 231,
    313
Antioxidants 241
Antipaternal complement dependent
    antibodies 32
Antiphospholipid antibody 29, 74
    syndrome 29
Antisperm antibody 47, 181
    evaluation hormonal analysis 20
Antral follicle 13, 224*f*
    count 13, 180*f*
Appendicitis 288
Arcuate uterus 141
Aromatase inhibitors 56, 57, 153, 191
    plus gonadotropins 191
    safety of 59
Arterial thromboembolism 148
Arteries, intrinsic 165
Artificial insemination 192
    of donor 209
    techniques 205
Asherman's syndrome 178
Asoprisnil 149, 158, 159
    dosage 149
    long-term benefits 150
    side effects 150
Aspirin 33, 116
Assisted reproductive medical
    technology 220
Assisted reproductive technology 19,
    23, 28, 34, 37, 79, 85, 108,
    127, 193, 196, 204, 235,
    248, 258, 288, 305, 319,
    321, 326
    bill 329
    center 329
    clinic 333
        requirements of 331
        setting up 329
    procedures 325, 334
    treatment 325

Asthenospermia 20
Atmospheric oxygen 239
Atresia 8
Atrigel 154
Autoimmune polyendocrine
    syndrome 31
Ayurveda 2
Azoospermia 20, 24, 47, 209, 227, 324
    causes of 25*t*
    management of 24
    nonobstructive 20
    obstructive 20

B

Balloon
    catheter 134
    tamponade 300
Basal body temperature 174, 175,
    206
Beta-human chorionic gonadotropin
    289
Bicornuate uterus 133, 134, 134*f*,
    140, 143, 179*f*
    complete 140
    computed tomography images of
        137*f*
    hysterosalpingographic image of
        133*f*
    magnetic resonance image of
        137*f*
Bicorporeal uterus 138, 141
Biopsy
    endometrial 175, 178
    peritoneal 271
Blastocoel fluid study 266, 267
Blastocyst
    development 239
    formation 235, 263
    grading system for 262
    scoring system for 264, 265*f*,
        265*t*
    stage 235

Bleomycin 276
Blood
   circulation 231
   dyscrasias 294
Body mass index 9, 52
   abnormal 188
Body temperature 237
Borderline epithelial ovarian cancer 273
Bowel endometriosis 126
Boyle's machine 250
Bromocriptine 100
Bulls-eye pronuclei 263
Cabergoline 100, 154

C

Calcium
   channel blockers 44
   ionophore 182
Cancer
   advance 327
   borderline 270
   endometrial 63, 280-282
   gynecological 270
Carbon dioxide 237, 253
   incubators 253f
Carboxy terminal peptide 83, 306
Cardiac anomalies, congenital 59
Centers for Disease Control and Prevention 193
Central nervous system 10
Cerebral carotid artery 102
Cerebrospinal fluid 100
Cervical
   ectopic pregnancy 291, 299
   factor 186, 204
      infertility 215
   insemination 204
   mucus, depression of 53
   pregnancy 299
   trauma 280
Cervicothoracic somite dysplasia 133
Cervix 138, 287
Cetrorelix 152
Chemical air contaminants 253
Chemotherapy 20, 25, 277
Chlamydia 23
Chromosomal analysis 224
Cirrhosis, biliary 65
Cisplatin 276
Cleavage embryos, scoring system for 264t

Clomiphene 51, 56, 57, 115, 324
   citrate 21, 51, 52, 54, 116, 189, 192, 214
   adverse effects 189
   complication of 54
   cycles of 218
   dosage 52
   flare protocols 114
   induced pregnancies 189
   resistant 53
   treatment
      cycle 53
      results of 53
Clostridium histolyticum 156
Clozapine 95
Collagen producing cells 155
Comet assay 40f, 183, 183f
Conception, probability of 214t
Contraception 283
   hormonal 288
Corifollitropin
   administration of 308f
   alfa 116, 306-309, 311, 312, 315
      cost effectiveness of 311
      disadvantages of 310
      structure of 306
Cornual pregnancy 299
Cornual resection 299
Corpora lutea 85
Corpus hemorrhagicum 14
Corpus luteum 175f
Creatine kinase 290
Critical ovarian hyperstimulation syndrome 72f
Cryomyolysis 160, 161
Cryptorchidism 20
Cumulus
   cells 240, 261
   corona complex 259
   oocytes complex 82
Cushing's syndrome 65
Cycle fecundity rate 194
Cyst 288
Cystectomy 125f, 273, 274
Cytokines 30
Cytomegalovirus 23
Cytoplasm 235
   homogeneous 259
Cytotrophoblast 294

D

Danazol 292
Dehydroepiandrosterone 63, 110
Density gradient technique 207, 207f

Deoxyribonucleic acid 4, 155
Desogestrel 66
Dexamethasone, doses of 53
Diabetes insipidus 102
Diabetes mellitus 172
Didelphys uterus 140
Diminished ovarian function 180
Dizziness 99
Donor insemination 23, 324
Donor semen, use of 209
Dopamine agonist 76, 99
   resistance 101
   treatment 101
   withdrawal 101
Doxycycline, course of 188
Ductal obstruction 20, 25
Dupuytren's contracted joint, treatment of 156
Dutch uterine artery embolization 163
Dysgerminoma 276f
   bilateral 276
Dysmorphic uterus 141

E

Ectopic endometriotic lesions 59
Ectopic pregnancy 287, 288, 290, 291, 293, 297-301
   persistent 298
   previous history of 288
   ruptured 289
Ejaculatory duct
   obstruction 20
   transurethral resection of 22
Ejaculatory failure 204
Elagolix 152
Elective single embryo transfer 230
Electricity control room 250
Embolization 300
Embryo 234, 236, 241, 243, 262, 327, 329
   abnormal 28
   cryopreservation of 116, 283
   culture 221, 237
      system 234, 235, 242
      techniques 243
   donation 327
   freezing 221, 247
   hatching 326
   intrauterine transfer of 332
   investigations 265
   quality, lower 85
   transfer 78, 227, 230

catheters 251f
multiple 236
Embryonic morphology, assessment of 228
Endocervical curettage 278
Endocrine 20
evaluation 215
factors 186
neoplasia, multiple 106
Endometrial cancer, treatment of 281
Endometrial cavity, normal 178f
Endometrioma 125
excision 129
ovary 125f
Endometriosis 58, 123, 215, 271
deep infiltrating 126
diagnosis of 123
etiopathogenesis of 122
fertility index 123, 124f
focusing, laparoscopic treatment of 122
management of 129
mild 215
minimal 215
moderate 125
severe 123f, 125
Endometrium, triradiate appearance of 179f
Endoscopy 138
Enigmatic disease 122
Enzymatic degradation 46
Enzyme 239
dihydrofolate reductase 293
Epididymal sperm extraction 333
Epididymis 18
Epithelial cell, synchronous 282
Epithelial ovarian cancer
diagnosis of 273
fertility preservation in invasive 270
Erectile dysfunction 105
Estradiol 112, 262
serum 58
Estrogen 10, 159
Ethylene-diamine-tetra-acetic-acid 240
Etoposide 276, 292
European Society for Human Reproduction and Embryology 64, 128, 195
Excess body weight 52
Exemestane 153
Extrafollicular pregnancy 300

Extrapituitary prolactin 92
Extrauterine disease, intraoperative 282
Extrauterine mass 289

F

Fadrozole 153
Fallopian tube 45, 133, 176, 287, 288
Fatty acids 258
Female genital anomalies 135, 143
Female genital tract 132, 133
anomalies 141, 141t
congenital abnormalities of 132
embryology of 132
Female reproductive endocrinology 7
Fertile control 183
Fertility 279
and cervical cancer 277
and endometrial cancer 280
and gestational trophoblastic disease 283
and ovarian cancer 270
long-term 128
preservation 271, 273, 280
preserving surgery 272
rates 4
sparing surgery 276f
treatment 143
Fertilization 40, 239, 242
rate 310
Fertilized eggs 327
Fertilized oocyte 262f
Fertilizing ovum, capable of 328
Fetal cardiac activity 296, 299
Fetal development 242
Fibroid 155
medical management of 146
Registry for Outcomes Data 162
symptomatic 161
Fimbria 287
Fimbrial evacuation technique 298
Final oocyte maturation 85
Fixed versus flexible antagonist administration 81
Flexible regimen 82
Folic acid
antagonist 293
metabolism 187
Folinic acid 293
Follicle
aspiration pump 251f
dynamics 259
number of 189

preovulatory 192
production 85
required per ovary 65
stimulating hormone 8, 17, 20, 52, 63, 69, 111-113, 180, 205, 315
development of 305
recombinant 87
Follicular
development 225
monitoring of 205, 223
fluid 261
growth 308
heritage 108
phase 13
stimulating hormone 308f
Follitropin alfa 312f
Follitropin delta 313, 315
administration of 313
dosing of 313
efficacy of 314
Free androgen index 65
Freeze autologous oocytes 87
Fungal contamination 247

G

Galactorrhea 98, 105
pre-existing 99
Galactose-1-phosphate uridyltransferase 133
Gametes 43, 241, 258
donation 35
function 43
intrafallopian transfer 205, 213
Ganirelix acetate injection 306
Gastrinoma 106
Gastrointestinal disorders 288
Genes 187
Genetic disorders 209
Genital ducts, primordial 8
Genitalia, external 132
Germ cell
ovarian tumors 275t, 276
fertility preservation in 275
primordial 7
tumor, mixed 276f
German measles 203
Gestational sac 289
Gestational trophoblastic disease 283
Gestodene 66
Gestrinone 154
Giant oocytes 260
Giant prolactinomas 106

Gland, pituitary 152
Glucagon-like peptide-1 155
Glucocorticoid 61
　steroid 53
Glucose 240, 258
　concentration 240
Glycolysis, stimulation of 235
Glycopeptides 17
Gonadotropin 59, 74, 85, 114, 191, 193, 225, 305, 311
　adverse effects 191
　cycles of 218
　dosage 226
　dose of 223, 310
　long acting 83
　lower doses of 60
　preparations 51
　releasing hormone 9, 17, 51, 54, 63, 111, 122, 148, 149, 158, 225, 305, 324
　　agonist 79-81, 84, 85, 111, 112, 151
　　analog 78, 112, 148
　　antagonist 76, 83-85, 111, 112f, 152, 226, 227
　　types of 81
　secretion 190
　therapy 51, 214
Gonorrhea 23
Good quality embryos
　development of 305
　frozen 310
　number of 310
G-protein-coupled receptors 315
Granular cytoplasm 259f
Granulocyte-macrophage colony-stimulating factor 266
Granulosa
　activity of 261
　cell 13, 282, 309
　　tumors 277

H

Halofuginone 155
Halosperm 183, 184f
Hamster penetration test 38
Headaches 99
Hemizona
　binding assay 182
　surfaces 183
Hemorrhage 276, 280
Heparin 33, 154
Hepatic insulin-like growth factor 258

Hepatitis 23, 203
High oxygen concentrations 236
Hirsutism 66
Hormonal contraception, combined 148
Hormone 9, 262
　adaptive multifaceted 91
　adrenocorticotropic 65
　ancient 91
　growth 92, 116, 258
　levels 309
　pituitary 97
　polypeptide 92
　replacement therapy 148
　secretion 30
Horse-shoe kidney 137f
Human chorionic gonadotropin 14, 23, 29, 54, 74, 80, 84, 85, 112, 113, 204, 226, 275
　dose of 53
Human embryos, pre-implanting 247
Human Fertilization and Embryology Authority 325
Human follicle stimulating hormone, recombinant 306
Human healthcare business 307
Human immunodeficiency virus 23, 203
Human in vitro fertilization 154, 239
Human menopausal gonadotropin 25, 59, 112, 205, 225
Human monoclonal anticardiolipin antibodies 29
Human oocytes 183
　and embryos, selection of 258
Human serum albumin 241
Human sperm 46
　technique of cryopreservation of 209
　thawing, technique of 209
Human zona
　binding assay 21
　pellucida 182
Hyaluronan binding assay 39
Hybrid molecule 306
Hydrophilic acrylic acid 155
Hydroxyethyl starch solution 75
Hyperandrogenism 55, 66
Hyperinsulinemia 52, 66
Hyperosmolar glucose 293
Hyperplasia
　endometrial 159
　parathyroid 106

Hyperprolactinemia 91, 95, 97, 98, 102-104, 176
　etiology of 95t
　frequency of 95
　mild 98
　signs of 98
　symptoms of 98
　treatment of 97
Hypertension, portal 65
Hyperthyroidism 65
Hypogonadism 98, 99
　symptoms of 98
Hypogonadotropic hypogonadism 25, 60, 104
Hypogonadotropism 20
Hypomenorrhea 97
Hypo-osmotic swelling test 21, 182
Hypoplasia 139
Hypotension, postural 99
Hypothalamic-pituitary-ovarian axis 11, 11f
　maturation of 63
Hypovolemia 54
Hysterectomy 159, 275, 282, 299
　radical 279
Hysterosalpingo contrast sonography 137
Hysterosalpingogram 123
Hysterosalpingography 133, 172
　normal 172f, 174f
Hysteroscopy 138, 159

I

Immature sperm cells 20
Immunobead test 172
In vitro embryo culture 239
In vitro fertilization 13, 19, 21, 24, 30, 37, 43, 45, 52, 78, 187, 194, 205, 213, 220, 234, 246, 248, 258, 302, 305
　chamber 253, 254f
　laboratory layout 248f
　treatment 123
In vitro maturation 258
In vitro receptor binding 306
In vitro sperm nuclear chromatin decondensation test 182
Indian Council of Medical Research 255
Infertile couple
　embryo of 327
　reactions of 326
Infertile couples 327

Infertility 2, 4, 5, 28, 91, 95, 105, 213, 220
  care units, secondary 331
  causes of 29t, 214t
  complaints 122
  duration of 188, 216
  Goddess of 322f
  idiopathic 204
  involuntary 319
  male factor 214
  male immunological 215
  mechanical 276
  multiple causes of 213
  services 213
  treatment 288, 319, 320, 326t
    conventional 213
Inflammatory cells 47
Injected progestogen, high-dose 148
Inner cell mass 264
  number of 236
Insemination
  cycles 195
  intracervical 203, 211
  intrafallopian 204
  intraperitoneal 204
  intravaginal 203
  number of 217
  subzonal 326
  techniques 203
  timing of 217
Insulin 53, 258
  sensitivity 56
  stimulates luteinizing hormone 52
Insulinoma 106
Interstitial cell stimulating hormone 9
Intracranial malignancies 102
Intracytoplasmic morphologically selected sperm injection 40
Intracytoplasmic sperm 237
  injection 21, 23, 24f, 37, 45, 194, 215, 220, 248, 254, 259, 326
  workstation 255f
Intrauterine
  adhesions 179f
  contraceptive devices 288
  insemination 19, 22, 37, 47, 53, 187, 188, 196, 202, 203f, 204, 213, 218, 249, 321, 323, 325, 331
  procedure 204
  system, progestogen-releasing 150

Invasive epithelial ovarian cancer 271, 272t
Isthmica nodosa 174

K

Kallmann's syndrome 25
Kidney disease 327
Klinefelter's syndrome 20, 25
Kruger's strict criteria 38
Lactate dehydrogenase 275
Lactotrophs 92
Laminar airflow hood 251f, 252
Lanreotide 153
Laparoscopy 134, 138, 151, 159, 176, 176f, 291
Laparotomy 151, 159
Laser machine 255f
Leiomyomas 158
  submucus 178
Leptin 258
Letrozole 57, 153, 190
  advantages 191
  dose 190
  flare protocols 114
  mechanism of action 190
  side effects 191
Leucovorin 293
Leukemia inhibitory factor 30
Leukocytes, quantitation of 181
Leukocytosis 47
Levonorgestrel intrauterine system 148, 150
Leydig cells 8, 10, 17
Lipoprotein, high density 258
Liquogel 155
Lisuride 100
Live birth rate 110t
Liver disease 327
Long acting molecules, development of 306
Low molecular weight gonadotropins 314
Low viscosity density gradient 207f
Luteal phase defect 175
Luteal phase support 85, 86, 230
Luteinizing hormone 8, 17, 78, 79, 93, 152, 174, 175, 315
  detection of 206
  premature 78
  recombinant 74
Lymph node 278

Lymph vascular space involvement 278
Lymphadenectomy 279
  para-aortic 271, 272

M

Macroadenoma 97
Macromolecules 75
Macroprolactin 94
Macroprolactinemia 94, 96, 104
Makler chamber 252f
Malate-aspartate shuttle 235
Male infertility 17, 173, 223
  mild 215
  severe 224t
Mammalian embryology 332
Mammary gland development and lactation 93
Mature oocyte 259f
Maximal serum concentration 308
Mayor-Rokitansky-Kuster-Hauser syndrome 139
Meiotic spindle 260, 261
Meningitis 102
Menopause 15
Menstrual bleeding, heavy 148
Menstrual cycle 12, 178
  dysfunction 98
  hormonal changes during 11f
Menstrual flow 15
Menstrual irregularity 66
Metabolic syndrome 67
Metformin 51, 54, 55
  dosage 55
Methotrexate 293, 294
  local intra-amniotic 299
  protocols 296t
  side effects of 294
  therapy 293, 294, 296
Microdose bonadotropin releasing hormone agonist protocol 113f
Micro-epididymal sperm aspiration 333
Microinvasive disease 278
Microprolactinoma
  management of 104fc, 105fc
  treatment 103
Microsurgical epididymal sperm aspiration 24, 209
Microtubal surgery 325
Microtubule organization 237
Mid-luteal serum progesterone 172

Mifepristone 32, 149, 292
  dosage 149
  long-term benefits 149
  side effects 149
Milk proteins 93
Mitochondria 235, 241
Molar pregnancy, second 283
Monitor follicular growth 323
Motile sperm
  organelle morphology
    examination 40
  proportion of 46
Motility and sperm survival test,
    assessment of 39
Müllerian abnormalities 131, 133
  genetics of 132
Müllerian agenesis 133
Müllerian anomalies 132, 141
  ASRM classification of 139f
Müllerian aplasia 132, 142
Müllerian assessment 131
Müllerian duct
  aplasia 133
  system 8
Müllerian inhibiting substance 8
Müllerian system 131, 132
Müllerian tubes 132
Multifollicular growth 311
Multiple dose methotrexate therapy
    295, 296
Multiple gestations, delivery of 230
Multiple pregnancy 334
  rate of 59-61
Mumps 25
Myolysis 160
Myoma
  bed after enucleation 160f
  enucleation 151
  intramural 178f
  screw 160f
  submucous 177f, 178f
Myomata, size of 151
Myomectomy 159, 160
  laparoscopic 160

N

Nasal septal perforation 102
National Institute for Health and
    Care Excellence 195
National Institute of Child Health
    and Human Development
    64
Natural killer cells 30
Nausea 54

Neoplasm, pituitary 106
Newer sperm function tests 39
N-isopropylacrylamide 155
Nonsteroidal anti-inflammatory
    drugs 73, 148
Noonan syndrome 25
Norgestimate 66
Normal ovarian stroma, preservation
    of 274
Normal uterus 141, 276f
  helical CT images of 136f
Nucleic acids, biosynthesis of 235
Nucleolar organizing regions 262

O

Obesity, treatment of 52
Olanzapine 95
Oligospermia 20
Oligozoospermia 47
Oliguria 54
Omentectomy 271, 276f
Oocyte 116, 154, 221, 247, 259, 261
  collection 226, 241
  cryopreservation of 283
  cytoplasm, structure of 259
  development 239
  fertilization of 40
  identification 221
  investigations 260
  number of 116, 310
  production 85
  pronuclear 263
  quality 259
  with cytoplasmic granularity 260f
  with vacuoles 260f
Oral contraceptive 99,158
  low dose combined 151
  pill 83, 111, 113, 146
    side effects 146
  side effects of 146
Oral progestogen, high-dose 147
Orchitis 25
Organon's Clinical Development
    Program 311
Osteoporosis 95, 159
Ovarian antral follicles 224f
Ovarian cancer 274, 282
  endometrioid 271
  epithelial 271, 273fc
Ovarian cyst development 79
Ovarian ectopic pregnancy 291
Ovarian endometrioma 127
Ovarian factors 186
Ovarian follicular development 226

Ovarian function 189
  preservation of 283
Ovarian hyperstimulation 51, 225
  complication of 230
  controlled 78, 79, 192, 214, 225
  syndrome 54, 60, 67, 71, 72, 76,
      79, 84, 205, 208, 208f, 225,
      230, 305, 306, 313
    classification of 71, 71t
    early form of 71
    management of 72, 74f
    mechanisms of 74f
    mild 73
    moderate 73
    primary risk of 74
    secondary prevention 75
    severe 72f
Ovarian malposition 140
Ovarian micro-metastases 282
Ovarian pregnancy 291, 300
  treatment 300
Ovarian preservation 282
Ovarian reserve 108
  assessment of 180
Ovarian response, prediction of 109,
    109t
Ovarian stimulation 83, 192, 195,
    205, 288
  controlled 108, 109, 191
  protocols 312
  start of 306
Ovarian suppression 124
  postoperative 124
  preoperative 124
Ovarian tissue 283
Ovarian transplant 324
Ovarian transposition 280, 283
Ovarian tumors, epithelial 275t
Ovarian volume 109, 180f
Oviductal oxygen tension 239
Ovulation 13
  induction 108, 188, 189, 226, 324
  predictor kits 175
  signs of 176f
  spontaneous 78
  trigger agent, modification of 75
Ovulatory disorder 203
Ovum pick-up 113
  embryo transfer room 249f
Oxygen concentration 239

P

Pain, abdominal 54
Partial cell necrosis 99

Pelvic inflammatory disease 4, 288
Pelvic lymphadenectomy 271
Penile deformities, surgical
	correction of 22
Percutaneous epididymal sperm
	aspiration 24, 333
Pergolide 100
Phosphate buffered saline 241
Photo-oxidation 240
Pirfenidone 155
	oral administration of 155
Pituitary gland, anterior 92
Pituitary hormones, combination
	of 324
Plasma half-life 306
Plasminogen activator inhibitor 187
Polycystic ovarian disease 125
Polycystic ovarian syndrome 51,
		63, 64
	diagnosis of 63, 65, 66
	etiology of 63
	management 63, 66
	pathophysiology 63
	recent advances 63
Polyethylene glycol precipitation 94
Polyp 178f
Poor support system 326
Postcoital test 21, 180
Postwash motile sperm count 47
Potassium
	chloride 293
	supplemented simplex
		optimization medium 242
Potent antioxidant 235
Pouch of Douglas 134
Pramipexole 100
Prednisolone 116
Pregnancy 277
	and cervical cancer 280
	and epithelial ovarian cancer 274
	and germ cell tumors 277
	complication of 287
	heterotopic 292, 301
	interstitial 289, 299
	intramural 301
	intrauterine 288, 301
	loss 29t
		rate of 218
		recurrent 28, 29, 34
	normal 202
	rate 116t, 216t
	test, positive 231
Pre-intrauterine insemination
		workup 202
Prenatal sex determination 335

Primary infertility care units 329
Progesterone 230, 262, 281
	receptor agonists and modulators
		149
	supplementation 32
	types of 281
Progestins 158
Prolactin 9, 91, 92
	functions of 93
	gene 92
	levels 97
	radioimmunoassay 94
	receptor, activation of 93
	secreting adenoma 97
	secretion
		and assays 94
		regulation of 93
	variants 92
Prolactinoma 97, 99, 103, 106
	malignant 106
	management of 102, 103
	medical management of 100t
Pronuclear morphology 263f
Prostaglandin 293
Prostatitis 20, 47
Proteins, oxidation of 239

Q

Quetiapine 95
Quinagolide 100

R

Radiation 20
Radiotherapy 25
	role of 102
Raloxifene 154
Randomized controlled trial 55,
		151, 162
Rapid progressive motility 18
Rectovaginal endometriosis,
		diagnosis of 126
Rectovaginal septum, deep
		endometriosis of 126
Recurrent pregnancy loss, causes
		of 28
Renal agenesis 140
Renal aplasia, unilateral 133
Reproductive
	functions 93
	organs 132
	tract 189
Residual disease 278
Retrograde ejaculation 20, 25

Rhinorrhea 100
Ribonucteic acid 155
Ropinirole 100
Roxindole 100

S

Saline infusion sonography 134, 134f
Salpingectomy 297, 298
Salpingostomy, laparoscopic 298
Salpingotomy 299
Scrotal temperature 20
Selective estrogen receptor
		modulator 153
Selective progesterone receptor
		modulator 158
Semen 18
	analysis 18t, 43, 44, 45fc, 171f,
		173t, 248
	basic 173
	computer-aided 19, 181
	diagnostic use of 48
	role of 43
	collection room 248
	cryopreservation 209
	parameters 20t, 172, 217, 227
	processing laboratory 331
	volume 20, 44
Seminal plasma 206, 227
Seminal vesicles 20
	absence of 20
Septate uterus 134, 140, 141, 143,
		179f
Sertoli cells secrete Müllerian
		inhibiting substance 10
Serum alpha fetoprotein 275
Serum progesterone 175
	levels 290
Serum prolactin 101
Sex hormone binding globulin
		55, 65
Sex steroids 149
Sexually transmitted
	disease 4
	infections 4, 172
Simple cyst drainage 111
Single-dose methotrexate therapy
		295, 296
Skeletal abnormalities 131
Society for Assisted Reproductive
		Technology 193
Society of Reproductive Medicine 53
Sodium chloride 292
Somatic cell nuclear transfer 255
Somatostatin analogs 152

Sperm 329
- abnormal 19
- analysis, computer-assisted 39
- and ovum, intra-abdominal fertilization of 300
- antibodies 21
- binding 182
- cells 184
- chromatin
  - dispersion 47
  - structure assay 47, 183
- concentration 20
- count 45
  - biological significance of 45
  - total 45
- DNA
  - fragmentation test 39, 183
  - integrity tests 47
- donor 209
- function
  - biochemical tests of 184
  - tests 19, 21t
- mitochondrial activity index 182
- morphology 207
  - assessment of 46
- motility 46
- nuclei 40f
- number of 45
- penetration assay 38
- preparation 206, 207f
  - techniques 192
- washing 206
  - safety of 211

Spermatogenesis 18
Spermatozoa 18, 37
- head 40f
- incidence of 182
- proportions of 183

Spermatozoon 262
Sperms per inseminate, total number of 23
Stem cell technology 328
Stereozoom microscope 254f
Stress 5
Subfertility 67
Subseptate uterus, hysteroscopic image of 137f
Sulfasalazine 44
Surrogacy 35, 324, 327
Swim-up technique 206, 206f
Syncope 99
Syphilis 23
Systemic methotrexate 298, 299

therapy and surveillance 295t

T

Tamoxifen 65, 154, 282
Teflon coated tubing 247
Telapristone 150
Teratospermia 20
Terguride 100
Tertiary infertility care units 331
Tesarik zygote-grading system, advantages of 263
Testicular sperm 24
- aspiration 24, 209
- extraction 24, 209, 333
Testosterone 262
Therapeutic donor insemination 23
Thiazolidinediones 56
Three dimensional sonography 134, 136f
Thrombophilia 74, 187
Thyroid
- disorders 176
- stimulating hormone, serum 176
Thyrotropin releasing hormone 10, 92
Tissue culture grade 242
Torsion 25
Toxic oxygen 227
Trachelectomy, radical 278, 279
Tranexamic acid 147, 148
- dosage 148
- long-term disadvantages 148
- side effects 148
Transient uterine ischemia 165
Transrectal ultrasound 20, 25
Transvaginal ultrasonography 289, 308
Triptorelin 75
Troglitazone 56
Trophectoderm 236
Trophoblast
- cells 178
- persistent 298, 299
Troublesome leucorrhea 143
Tubal ectopic pregnancy 289, 290
- treatment of 298
Tubal factors 186
Tubal ligation 288
Tubal occlusion 288

Tubal pregnancy, aborted 300
Tubal ring 289
Tube sparing salpingostomy 298
Tuberculosis, genital 324
Tuberoinfundibular cells 93
Tubo-ovarian relationship, restoration of 126f
Tumors
- malignant 275
- necrosis factor alpha 72
- non-dysgerminomatous 276
Tunel assay 183, 184f
Tunel positive nuclei 183
Two-cell two-gonadotropin hypotheses 12, 12f

U

Ulipristal acetate 148, 150
- dosage 150
- long-term usage 150
- side effects 150
Unexplained infertility 58, 170, 171, 184, 187, 195, 214, 215
- diagnosis of 170
Unicornuate uterus 139, 143
Upper respiratory diseases 172
Ureteric agenesis, ipsilateral 140
Urinary bladder 126
Urinary calculi 288
Urinary luteinizing hormone 175
Uterine
- anomalies 142f
- artery 164
  - branches of 165
  - Doppler-guided 164, 165
  - embolization 301
  - intrinsic 165
  - laparoscopic 163
  - ligation 300
  - occlusion 164, 165
- bleeding, abnormal 150
- cavity 134f, 139, 177, 202
- curettage 290
- device 164
- fibroids 146, 156, 158
  - removal of 159
  - tumors, symptomatic 163
- leiomyomas 146
- polyps 178
- synechiae 178

transplant 284
wall thickness 138, 139
Uterosacral disease 126
Uterus
　congenital malformations of 131, 139, 140t
　didelphys 143
　infantile 138
　surrogate 327

V

Vagina 138
　partial duplication of 140
Vaginal delivery 275
Vaginal radical trachelectomy 279
　laparoscopic 279
Vaginal septum
　nonobstructive 143
　obstructive 143
Vaginal sonography 224f
Varicocele 20, 22
Vas deferens
　absence of 20
　congenital bilateral absence of 20
Vascular endothelial growth factor 30, 72, 74, 291
Vasectomy 20
Vasopressin 300
Volatile organic carbons 242
　compounds 247, 253
Vomiting 54

W

Water-insoluble biodegradable polymer 154
Wedge biopsy 272
Wolffian duct 8
World health organization 1, 18
Wunderlich-Herlyn-Werner syndrome 140

Y

Y-chromosome 276
　microdeletions 224
　sex determining region of 8
Young syndrome 20

Z

Zona free hamster
　egg 38
　oocyte test 21, 181
Zona pellucida 240, 259, 260
Zygote 235, 241
　grades 263f

Milton Keynes UK
Ingram Content Group UK Ltd.
UKHW052309070524
442372UK00003B/19